JULIAN LEFF

Psychiatry Around the Globe
A Transcultural View

GASKELL

ISBN 0 902241 24 9

Gaskell is an imprint of the Royal College of Psychiatrists,
17 Belgrave Square, London SW1

Distributed in North America
by American Psychiatric Press, Inc.

First published 1981 by Marcel Dekker, Inc.
Second edition 1988

Typeset by Dobbie Typesetting Limited, Plymouth, Devon
Printed in Britain

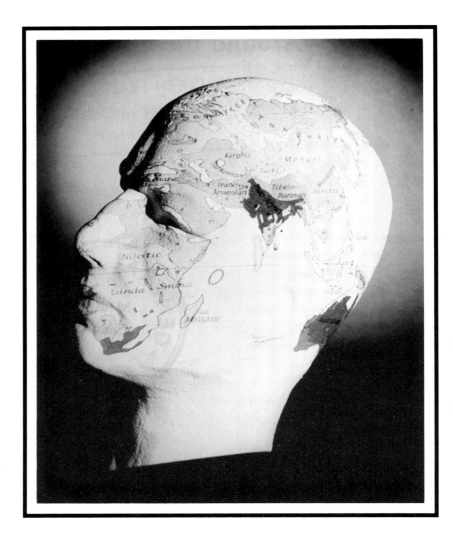

Contents

Foreword

ARTHUR KLEINMAN

Substantial cross-cultural research has been conducted in psychiatry over the past decades, yet the more important results of this increasingly extensive undertaking are not well appreciated by mental health professionals or educated laymen, even though these studies address some of the most fundamental questions about mental illness and hold practical significance for patient care. What is even more surprising, most psychiatrists do not seem to understand what progress has been made and its implications for the profession. The chief reason for this lack of awareness, I believe, is simply a failure to communicate effectively the key concepts and findings in a language that readers, who are not themselves experts, can readily comprehend. Often one hears this notable defect rationalised away as inevitable — after all, it is lamented, so complex, fragmented and obscure a subject just doesn't lend itself to successful synopsis or persuasive popularisation.

Julian Leff's highly readable book demonstrates that this is nothing but a poor excuse. For in it the major conundrums and concerns of cross-cultural psychiatry are presented with such compelling clarity and fluent grace, yet at the same time with fidelity to the scholarly discourse from which they emerge, that readers from all the mental health disciplines, as well as educated laymen, whether or not they possess prior knowledge of the field, will be able to grasp what this subject is about and why it is of considerable significance. Leff clarifies which questions have been answered, which problems remain to be solved, and which have been refined and restated. He not only directs attention to the major issues for future research, but points out the available methodologies that can be applied in their examination. (Researchers will find entire projects set out for them.) This fine volume is popularisation in the best sense. I believe it deserves and will receive a very wide readership, and that it will become a standard source for introducing comparative international and cross-cultural aspects of psychiatry to students, practitioners, and just about anyone who has wondered whether mental illness is universal and how it differs in different cultures.

Leff ducks none of the hard questions, nor hedges on the answers. His chapters are organised to respond to four fundamental questions whose stark simplicity contrasts with the technical obfuscation that often surrounds them in the academic literature and thereby introduce a refreshing clarity by clearing the deck, so to speak, of a great deal of confused and confusing qualifications. Do psychiatric conditions look the same in different cultures? Do they have the same frequency? Are they treated differently? And do they have a different course?

In responding to these questions, Leff reviews a large number of studies that set out the chief findings of psychiatric epidemiology on the major psychoses. He also describes the clinical data that frame our understanding of cultural influences on their symptomatology and that contribute to our knowledge of the culture-bound disorders and historical and cross-cultural changes in hysteria. Each of the studies that he adduces to clarify the debate on these subjects is described concisely and yet with such admirable attention to concrete detail that the reader gets a first-hand view of the quality of the evidence and the uncertainties of its interpretation. Leff is particularly good when discussing difficulties in developing cross-culturally valid and reliable psychiatric assessment methodology.

One of his most provocative contributions is the extended discussion of the language of the emotions and how this both varies for distinctive cultures yet exhibits certain universal features. Leff presents a developmental/ evolutionary model of affective communication that is impressively well-illustrated from a variety of cultures and languages. This model offers a fascinating account of different forms of somatisation, especially in developing societies and historically in the West. Leff views hysteria as the somatisation of anxiety and catatonia as the somatisation of schizophrenia. The model also attempts to explain the emergence of the individual as a psychocultural concept. He rightly argues that in cross-cultural and historical perspective somatisation is normative and psychologisation is deviant.

Throughout, Leff very effectively presents a psychopathological and ethno-psychological orientation to critical issues in cross-cultural psychiatry. The 'natural' follow-up to this volume is one that is as clear and compelling in presenting a social structural and meaning-centred approach to the same questions. Now that the case has been made for a wide audience from epidemiological and clinical-phenomenological perspectives, the ball is in the court of anthropologists to popularise a culture analysis view that complements and completes our necessarily interdisciplinary understanding of this multi-sided subject. Again Leff opens the way for such an analysis by his straightforward critique of ethnocentrism and his balanced defence of a biopsychosocial position that maintains both universalist and cultural relativist features. Not the least of his accomplishments is writing in a direct and simple style about an extraordinarily complex subject whose epistemological bases, methodological difficulties, and practical implications for the planning and delivery of clinical care combine at the end in the mind of the reader in a crescendo of questions that one imagines will stimulate supporters and provoke critics for volumes to come to rethink the discourse that Leff so successfully recreates in these pages.

Arthur Kleinman, MD

Professor of Anthropology and Psychiatry
Harvard University
Cambridge
Massachusetts

Preface to the first edition

People are very curious about each other. There is a fascination in watching people from a far-off land behaving in exotic and often incomprehensible ways. Sometimes, though, their behaviour strikes a chord and causes us to think about aspects of our own behaviour which are so much part of our background that we take them completely for granted. For example, when we see Hindus burning their dead in public places and casting the ashes in the river, the suspicion may arise that our habit of enclosing the dead in wooden boxes, which we keep underground, might appear equally peculiar to the Hindu.

In this book I have attempted to provide a transcultural perspective on psychiatry in order to question the unspoken assumptions that form the background to this branch of medicine. To this end, the nature of psychiatric symptoms and conditions is examined in a variety of cultures (Part I), leading inevitably to the question of what may be considered mentally abnormal and whether an absolute standard of abnormality can be determined. Cultural influences on the form taken by psychiatric disorders are explored, particularly the effect that language has on the expression of emotional distress. In Part II, the issue of variation in the frequency of psychiatric conditions throughout the world is tackled in order to seek out clues to their origins.

Part III is devoted to a description of traditional methods of healing the psychiatric patient, and these are compared with Western scientific medicine, revealing more similarities than differences. In Part IV, studies of the course taken by psychiatric illnesses in different cultures are reviewed and some surprising findings encountered. Possible explanations are put forward and the available evidence for each of them is evaluated.

Finally, in Part V, the psychiatric problems of migrants are considered. An interesting aspect of immigrants is that they bring much of their culture of origin with them, often providing a dramatic contrast with the culture of their hosts. This makes it relatively easy to relate differences in the expression of psychiatric illness to differences in culture. Immigrants are almost always found to have higher rates of severe psychiatric illness than their hosts. A number of possible explanations for this finding are proposed and explored in relation to immigrants to English-speaking countries.

Julian Leff

Preface to the second edition

In the seven years since this book was first published there have been major contributions to the field of transcultural psychiatry from psychologists, psychiatrists, and anthropologists. Outstanding among these are the international collaborative studies conducted under the auspices of the World Health Organization. The text has been expanded to incorporate the advances in the field, and some of the opinions put forward in the first edition have been modified accordingly.

In particular, the proposed schema for the development of emotional differentiation, which ignored the possibility that bodily complaints might be used symbolically, has been extensively revised. As part of this revision Chapters 4 and 6 have been completely rewritten, taking into account the constructive criticisms made by anthropologists and the wealth of instructive material contained in Kleinman & Good (1985). We believe the book has been improved by these changes, which we trust have rendered it less culture-bound.

Acknowledgements

I am most grateful to my wife Joan Raphael-Leff for putting up with long evenings of writing and for her helpful comments at all stages in the preparation of this book. Doctor Richard Werbner generously gave his professional advice on Part III. Jane Hurry kindly provided data from the Camberwell Register, and Mr J. D. Holden of the Department of Health and Social Security extracted the figures for hysteria used in Chapter 5. My thanks are due to Mrs Rowena Kendal for her immaculate typing of the second edition.

Julian Leff

Introduction

'Ethnocentric' has long been established as a term of abuse in anthropology, and is beginning to filter into the vocabulary of other social scientists and psychiatrists. It refers to the attitude that the beliefs and values of one's own cultural group are the only correct ones, and that any group with different beliefs or values is primitive or at best unenlightened. A clear example of ethnocentricity is provided by uncompromising religious beliefs. The religion into which one chances to be born is presented as the only true faith, and adherents to other religions are labelled as heathens and unbelievers. Historically, a confrontation between different religions has usually led to missionary activity or to holy wars, to which the world is still not immune. Rarely has the outcome been a reassessment of underlying assumptions, including the unique truth of one's beliefs, despite the vast areas of commonality shared by all religions. Fortunately, psychiatrists as a whole are not as fanatical about their beliefs as the religious orthodox, so that a comparison of psychiatric conditions and their treatments in a variety of cultures could lead to a useful questioning of basic assumptions.

Before launching into such a comparison, it is worth attempting to provide definitions of culture and of psychiatry. The latter is by far the easier task, so it will be tackled first. Psychiatry is the branch of medicine that deals with mental illnesses. There can be little disagreement over the inclusion in this category of the organic psychoses, such as senile dementia; the functional psychoses, comprising schizophrenia and manic–depressive illnesses; and the neuroses, such as anxiety and depressive states. However, there are some conditions treated by psychiatrists, such as alcoholism and homosexuality, which do not so clearly qualify as illnesses. There are yet others, such as marital disharmony, which no one would claim to be illnesses but which are treated by psychiatrists in the West. In this book we will be concerned mainly with psychiatric illnesses as such, but will also touch on conditions at the boundaries of psychiatry. These frontier conditions are the very ones in which culture may exert its strongest influence.

In an attempt to define culture, Kroeber & Kluckhohn (1952) discovered over 100 published definitions. We are reluctant to add to this superfluity but feel it is necessary to clarify what is meant by the term. Culture encompasses all those aspects of human society that man has constructed or devised himself as opposed to those characteristics which are inborn. There is of course a massive problem lurking behind this statement, namely the distinction between what is inherited and what is acquired. In the case of some characteristics this distinction has been relatively easy to establish; for instance, eye colour is clearly inherited, whereas language is acquired. In the case of psychiatric conditions, whether we are concerned with schizophrenia, depression, or alcoholism, the degree to which genetic and environmental factors are responsible has proved extremely difficult to determine. It is here that comparison of conditions across cultures is potentially very informative. If a psychiatric disorder is found to have the same manifestation in two different cultural settings, then it must either be the product of genes that are common to man as a species or else the consequence of environmental features which are shared by the two cultures. The more diverse the cultures are, the more likely are genes to be the cause of illnesses which take an identical form. On the other hand, differences in the manifestation of an illness in a number of cultures can lead to the identification of environmental features which may exert an influence on the form of the illness.

Features of an illness that do not vary from culture to culture have been designated 'culture-free', whereas those characteristics that do vary with culture have been termed 'culture-bound'. This is a useful shorthand, with the proviso that invariant features may still be the result of environmental characteristics shared by a number of otherwise diverse cultures. It may be helpful to give an example here. Suppose schizophrenia were found to take the same form in a matriarchal and a patriarchal society. We could then conclude that the sex of the dominant parent has nothing to do with the manifestations of schizophrenia. On the other hand, patients would be brought up in some form of family in both cultures, so that other family factors might still be influential in shaping the illness.

Before being able to study the relative frequency of a particular illness in a variety of cultures, it is necessary to be able to identify the illness wherever it appears. This in itself argues for at least a core of culture-free symptoms, sufficiently characteristic to allow the illness to be differentiated from other similar illnesses. The first part of this book deals with this issue in relation to psychotic illnesses, neurotic conditions, and behaviours that may be socially unacceptable. The influence that culture has on the expression of symptoms is considered, as well as the effect of patients' and doctors' expectations of each other.

It is concluded that certain psychiatric conditions can be recognised in a variety of cultural settings, so that it is possible to address ourselves to the second question: do psychiatric conditions have the same frequency in different cultures? In order to appreciate the attempts that have been made to answer this question, it is necessary to grasp the basic epidemiological concepts of incidence, prevalence, and sampling. These are explained in the introduction to the second part of this book, which includes the small number of studies that compare the frequency of psychiatric illnesses in more than one culture. The reasons for the paucity of relevant work are also examined.

The third question to engage our attention is whether psychiatric conditions are treated in the same way in different cultures. It is possible that treatments have been devised in one culture which are unknown in another culture, but which may still be effective. Apart from this potential therapeutic benefit, inquiry into the treatments given for psychiatric illnesses inevitably leads on to an ascertainment of the local views about aetiology and classification. Lay views about the definition of mental illness, its aetiology, and treatment are usually embedded in a total cosmology, and it is helpful to gain a comprehensive picture of this in order to appreciate the place of mental illness in relation to other aspects of the culture. This is an area of knowledge usually investigated by anthropologists and we draw extensively on their contributions in this section of the book.

In the fourth part of the book we inquire whether psychiatric illnesses run the same course in different cultures. There are a number of advantages to be gained from answering this question. First, course of illness is widely used in the West as one criterion for establishing diagnostic categories. Thus, in general, schizophrenia is expected to have a more protracted and deteriorating course than manic–depressive psychosis. If this were found to be true in a variety of cultures, it would underpin the validity of distinguishing between these two conditions. On the other hand, if the course of schizophrenia were found to vary widely across cultures, this would provide clues to the environmental features responsible for perpetuating the condition. The identification of those would lead to strategies for improving the outlook in schizophrenia.

The fifth and final part of this book deals with immigration and migrants. Our interest in migrants lies in the fact that they transport with them the experience, customs, and values of one culture and bring them into juxtaposition with another culture. The dramatic contrasts that often result from this process can be very illuminating, but it is important to take into consideration a complicating factor. The migration itself and the pressures leading up to it are social events which are likely to produce profound changes in the migrants. Thus we need to be cautious in our interpretation of differences found between migrants and their sedentary new neighbours. Nevertheless, migrants often present unique opportunities for transcultural comparisons and have been the subject of a number of fruitful inquiries. The findings from these and the issues they raise round off our discourse.

I. Are psychiatric conditions manifested similarly in different cultures?

1 The cultural relativity of delusions and hallucinations

Imagine that two butterfly collectors have started to correspond with each other. One lives in London and the other in Ibadan, Nigeria. The Londoner writes that the most common butterfly in his area is the Battersea Beauty, while the Ibadan lepidopterist writes that his most common butterfly is the Ibadan Imperial. Unfortunately, specimens are too delicate to be sent through the mail and neither can obtain photographs, so they decide to exchange verbal descriptions. The Londoner writes that his butterfly has a wingspan of 3 in and that the wings are crenelated. It turns out that the Ibadan Imperial has the same wingspan, but the Ibadan lepidopterist is baffled by the word *crenelated*. The Londoner explains that he uses the term for a wavy edge to the wing, and in return asks his colleague to elaborate on his use of the word *mululu* for the markings on the wings. Back comes the reply from Ibadan that *mululu* is a target used for spear-throwing practice and consists of a central spot with two concentric rings around it in contrasting colours. Once they have clarified the descriptive terms they use, the two lepidopterists realise that they are talking about the same butterfly, which has been given different local names.

Applying this parable to psychiatry, the local names for the butterfly are equivalent to diagnoses, while the descriptive terms for the form of the wings and the colour markings correspond to definitions of symptoms. Unless psychiatrists can agree on their definitions of symptoms, it is impossible to know whether they are talking about the same condition, even if they use the same diagnostic label. Agreement on the definitions of symptoms is an essential prerequisite to studying variations in the appearance of an illness in different cultures. In defining a symptom, it is necessary to make a distinction between *form* and *content*. Symptoms in psychiatric conditions are what patients tell you about their abnormal experiences. The form of a symptom comprises those essential characteristics that distinguish it from other, different symptoms. The content may be common to a variety of symptoms and is derived from the patient's cultural milieu. Thus, severely depressed patients may hear voices telling them they are either criminals

3

or sinners. The religious patient is more likely to hear the latter, and the non-religious, the former. What they both experience in common are auditory hallucinations of a derogatory nature, and it is this that gives the symptom its distinctive character. To give another example, the paranoid patient in a Western city is likely to complain that the police are 'after him', whereas a patient with the same form of symptom in an African village is likely to identify his persecutors as being sorcerers. The essence of the symptom is the incorrect belief that someone is trying to harm you, and this defines the form of a paranoid delusion.

The content of psychiatric symptoms obviously reflects both the place and time in which the patient is living. Thus, the favourite of the cartoonists, the lunatic who believes he is Napoleon, is actually an anachronism. No psychiatric patient today would assert that he is Napoleon; instead Churchill and Hitler are popular. Although as dead as Napoleon, they loom large in modern European culture. More contemporary statesmen rarely figure in patients' mental schemata, probably because they lack the necessary stature as heroes or villains. One patient who had been incarcerated in the back ward of a psychiatric hospital for 40 years, continued to maintain that she was Sexton Blake, a fictional detective popular in the 1930s. This character was unknown to the 1970s' psychiatrists; her delusions had become frozen in time by her isolation from the world outside her institution.

The content of people's beliefs, be they mentally healthy or sick, stems directly from their life experience, and hence is inevitably influenced by their culture. This fact is recognised in the generally accepted definition of a *delusion*; namely, a false belief which the person holds to firmly, despite argument or proof to the contrary, and which is inconsistent with the information available to the individual and with the beliefs of his or her social group. This qualification is essential, since in every culture, people are brought up to believe things for which there is no evidence (for example, the existence of a god), but which are held to with unshakable conviction. To label these beliefs as *delusions*, with the implication of severe mental illness, makes nonsense of the term. The use of this qualification avoids ludicrous propositions such as "all religious people are mad", but requires us to make complex judgements. Clearly, it is necessary to know in great detail the cultural matrix in which individuals are embedded before being able to decide whether their beliefs are inconsistent with those of their culture. This should not be particularly difficult when a person belongs to the same cultural group as the psychiatrist, but the judgement may be nearly impossible when the patient is an immigrant from an alien culture. As a last resort, it may be necessary in such cases to ask normal people from the same culture as the patient whether the patient's ideas are acceptable to them. To return to an example given above, in many traditional rural societies, witchcraft is not only believed in as a potent force by most people, but is often practised, both to enhance their own success and to affect others adversely. Field (1968) reports that in Ghana "people are strikingly paranoid. Houses, lorries, canoes, workmen's tool-boxes and tailors' sewing machines are decorated with such legends as 'Trust no man', 'Enemies around me', 'Fear men and play with snakes', 'Black man trouble' ''. She reports that a successful carpenter, into whose eye a foreign body blew when he was bicycling, made no attempt to have the particle removed but rushed to a diviner to find out who sent it. Similar attitudes are found among the Ganda, who categorise illnesses as those that occur spontaneously and those that are sent by witchcraft (Orley & Leff, 1972). Gillis *et al* (1982) report that many Xhosa patients consult the traditional healer or *isanuse* before seeing a psychiatrist. The *isanuse* will have told the patient that his symptoms are caused by someone directly or through the use of mystical power. A patient who originates from such a culture, expressing to a Western psychiatrist the belief that witchcraft is being used against him or her, could easily be labelled as deluded. This could well be a mistake, resulting from the psychiatrist's ethnocentric assumptions that the beliefs and practices in his or her own culture can be extrapolated across cultural boundaries. This kind of error is most likely to be made with immigrants to Western countries from traditional societies. However, it must be recognised that in Britain today there are small groups of native-born British people who believe in witches and who practise witchcraft rites in covens. It is no more sensible to call these British witches deluded than it is to apply the term to devout religious people. This example does raise the issue of eccentric or outlandish beliefs. The further they are from the mainstream of the prevailing culture, the fewer people are likely to share them, until at the extreme we reach very small subcultures such as personal religious cults formed around a charismatic individual.

Ultimately we are faced with a decision about numbers: how many people are required to adhere to an unusual idea before it can be regarded as constituting a subcultural belief rather than a shared delusion? Certainly, one other person is not enough. When two people share a very unusual belief, it is often the case that one of them is mentally ill and has imposed his or her delusion on the other. An example is the woman suffering from schizophrenia who believed she was in grave personal danger from bombardment with cosmic radiation. She persuaded her husband to line their car with sheets of lead and the two of them drove around the country to escape the radiation. (It is ironical that they may yet be the only survivors of a nuclear holocaust!) This situation is known as *folie à deux*, and similar cases involving up to six people have been recorded. When more than half a dozen people share an unusual belief, it is likely to be subcultural and within the range of normal behaviour, rather than a delusion originated by one person and adopted by the others.

There is a further issue to be considered in the case of small sects or subcultures, and that is that they may sometimes provide an accepting environment for people who are suffering from a psychiatric illness. Miller (1942) has pointed out that people with paranoid delusions choose a variety of ways of acting on them, with differing degrees of social acceptability. The paranoid person may throw a stone through a window or assault a supposed enemy, either of which will elicit a prompt and often punitive reaction from society. Some paranoid people choose to redress their imagined wrongs through the legal system, and become the litigious clients that are the bane of lawyers' lives. Yet others join minority political or religious groups in which the prevailing ethos is the struggle against the hostility of the rest of society. The leaders of such groups are sometimes the proponents of an overtly paranoid ideology, the most striking and horrific example in recent times being Hitler. A parallel example of a religious group on a smaller scale is the sect of Jim Jones in Guyana. There is evidence that Jones himself was suffering from schizophrenia, at least in the final years of his life, but nevertheless he retained such a strong hold over his followers that over 900 of them committed mass suicide at his instigation.

Minority religious sects not only provide a potential haven for the paranoid, but may encourage beliefs and behaviour that are close to those exhibited by psychotic patients. The Rosicrucians value experiences of merging with the cosmos and dissolving the boundaries of the self, which are very reminiscent of the way some schizophrenic patients describe their symptoms. The Pentecostals encourage 'speaking in tongues', a stage of religious ecstasy in which believers gabble in meaningless syllables as a manifestation of inspiration by the divine spirit. This again is very similar to the extremely disjointed speech exhibited, rarely, by schizophrenic patients. This similarity prompted St Paul to discourage speaking in tongues. In his Epistles to the Corinthians, he cautioned that "if tongues must be heard in the public assembly, then let not more than three of the saints exhibit the gift, and they only in succession. Nor let them exhibit it at all, unless there is someone present who can interpret the tongues and tell the meeting what it all means. If the whole congregation be talking with tongues all at once, and an unbeliever or one with no experience of pneumatic gifts come in, what will he think. Surely that you are mad". He further wrote that the gift of tongues was suitable to children in the faith rather than to the mature. From St Paul onwards, there has been a strong tendency for such exuberant manifestations of religiosity to be discouraged. Mary Douglas (1973) considers that symbolic forms of inarticulateness and bodily dissociation are relinquished as rituals lose their function of social control. Both processes are a consequence of an increasing focus in Western societies on inner experience, contemplation, and the internal evolution of the self. These tendencies are exhibited clearly by the established churches, but the older style of religious expression remains alive in the fundamentalist and evangelical sects. The more unconventional the beliefs of such sects, the more likely they are to attract people who are on the fringe of society, either because they are recent immigrants who have not had time to assimilate, or because they have personality difficulties that make it difficult for them to fit in. Both kinds of people are more susceptible to psychiatric illnesses, so that it would not be surprising to find an unusually high frequency of such conditions among adherents to these sects. In fact, there are very few studies on this topic. Spencer (1975) examined in-patient admissions to West Australian psychiatric hospitals and found that Jehovah's Witnesses were admitted twice as often with neurosis and four times as often with paranoid schizophrenia, as the rest of the population. There are problems in interpreting these figures, since Spencer did not distinguish between first admissions and re-admissions (see p. 86), and he used an estimate from Jehovah's Witnesses' official agency for the number of adherents in the general population. Nevertheless, his results are striking enough to indicate the need for further research in this neglected area.

It should be recognised that not all societies provide a large variety of ways in which people can find acceptance for paranoid and other psychotic beliefs and experiences. Many societies are intolerant of minority groups that express viewpoints at variance with the cultural norm. One would anticipate that in such monolithic societies the psychotic patient, finding no sympathetic group in which to express ideas, would be identified all the more rapidly and ascribed a patient role. Unfortunately this interesting proposition has received scant attention.

Having discussed the ways in which the definition of delusions depends on a careful consideration of cultural factors, we shall now turn to another key symptom of the psychoses, hallucinations. A hallucination is a perception that lacks sufficient basis in external stimuli, the origin of which the patient nevertheless locates in the outside world. Hallucinations can occur in any sensory modality, but most commonly affect hearing. Hallucinations are generally considered to be rare in normal people, although they are not infrequently experienced in that twilight state between waking and sleeping. It is therefore usual to stipulate that they should occur in a state of clear consciousness, before being taken to indicate the presence of a functional psychosis such as schizophrenia or manic–depressive illness. However, Rees (1971) has shown that as many as half of all bereaved people experience hallucinations of the dead person for years after the loss. These commonly take the form of a visual image of the dead person, often sitting in a characteristic attitude in a favourite chair. The image has all the qualities of reality, but vanishes as soon as the subject remembers that the other person is dead. Bereaved people may also hear the voice of the dead person, or even feel the dead person as a physical presence lying next to them in bed. While discussing these phenomena with medical students, one of them reported to me that after her pet dog died she would hear its footsteps outside and then hear it scratching at the door. The experience was so real that she would get up and open the door. Rees points out that bereaved people are very reluctant to talk about these experiences for fear of being thought mad, and none of his subjects had spoken about them to a doctor. Their understandable reticence strengthens the professional view of the malign significance of hallucinations.

Once it is recognised just how common these bereavement phenomena are, the possibility is raised that hallucinations may be much more frequent in the general population than we suspect, but that people are inhibited about reporting them. It is possible that the stigma attached to hallucinations in our society not only has an effect in suppressing reports, but may actually alter the threshold for the experiences themselves. There are still many parts of the globe where belief in the existence of spirits flourishes, and normal people readily report seeing a variety of manifestations of the spirit world. Al-Issa (1977) comments that in some traditional societies the experience of hallucinations is actually sought by a variety of methods. He considers that "cultural conditions in such cultures seem to be conducive to positive attitudes and a low threshold in the perception of hallucinations". Cheetham & Cheetham (1976) report that among the Xhosa people of South Africa, auditory and visual hallucinations appear to have status value, particularly as the speech or image is usually that of an ancestor, and related to propitiation or other ceremonies. As a consequence, people who talk to themselves or to imaginary voices are not taken to the traditional healer. This observation is supported by Gillis *et al* (1982) who caution that "one has to bear in mind that ancestors live in the same psychic world as the individual and their influence can be tangible. It is commonly believed, for instance, that they call him by name and the voice may be extremely difficult to distinguish from an auditory hallucination".

In such a milieu, accounts of hearing or seeing things that we would regard as non-existent cannot be given the same pathological significance as in our own sceptical culture. Even within Western society, there are subcultural variations in the readiness with which people report hallucinations. At the fringe of the British Isles, belief in fairies is kept alive. The pisky (pixie) still flourishes in Cornwall, and it is not uncommon to meet an Irishman who claims to have seen a leprechaun. Schwab (1977) conducted a survey of reported hallucinations in northern Florida. He drew a random sample of 6.3% of households from the total population and asked individuals, "How often do you see or hear things that other people don't think are there?" He found that the young were much more likely to report hallucinatory experiences than the middle-aged, but that they were also much more likely to take hallucinogenic drugs which probably explains this finding. However, there were other subcultural differences which could not be accounted for by drug-taking, namely that people from the lowest socioeconomic stratum were five times more likely to report hallucinations than those from the highest, and that Blacks were almost twice as likely to report hallucinations as Whites. There was also a link with religious affiliations; the highest proportions reporting hallucinations were found among the black Baptists, black Methodists, and Church of God, while the lowest appeared among the Lutherans, Presbyterians, white Methodists, Episcopalians, and Jews. The extremes were represented by the Church of God, 21% of whose members reported hallucinations, and the Jews, of whom none did. These findings must be partly due to ethnic and socioeconomic differences in the memberships of the various religious groups. But there is probably also an influence of the factor mentioned above, that certain sects encourage and reward visionary experiences.

It is clear that delusions and hallucinations, the main symptoms of psychotic illnesses, can only be judged as present in relation to the patient's cultural milieu. Failure to take this into account can lead to gross errors in diagnosis. These are well exemplified by a group of conditions known as the culture-bound psychoses, which will be given detailed consideration in the next chapter. First, however, it is worth spending a little time on the implications of the cultural relativity of the major psychotic symptoms.

At first, this aspect of psychiatric symptoms would appear to indicate that psychiatry is radically different from all other branches of medicines. In diseases like coronary thrombosis, the underlying pathology, signs, and symptoms are the same whatever country or culture the patient happens to belong to. To identify a coronary thrombosis from the electro-cardiogram, it is unnecessary to know whether the patient is an African, a European, or a Chinese. This would seem to be true of all physical diseases; namely, that to make a diagnosis it is sufficient to confine oneself to the medical aspects of each condition without considering social factors and influences. However, we have only to think about anaemia for a moment to see that even with physical conditions we cannot ignore cultural factors. Any individual in an African village is likely to be suffering from parasitic infestation, and in addition may well be inadequately nourished. As a result, the haemoglobin level of the average African villager is significantly lower than that of his European counterpart (see Carstairs, 1977, for similar findings in Indian villagers). However, he is most unlikely to suffer from any symptoms attributable to his haemoglobin level, since his body has adjusted to this virtually from birth. Should we consider the African villager to be anaemic? Certainly if we apply European standards this must be the conclusion, but not if we apply the norms of his or her own village population. If we took the European norm to be an attainable ideal, we should admit the African villager to hospital, eliminate the parasites, and maintain the villager on a special diet. As a result, his haemoglobin level would rise towards the European average level, but as soon as the African returned to the village, he or she would become re-infested with parasites, the diet would once more be inadequate, and the haemoglobin level would fall back to its original level. To raise the haemoglobin level of the individual villager permanently, it would be necessary to change the social environment drastically, entailing alterations in dietary habits, methods of agriculture, and hygiene, in addition to supplying piped water and sewage disposal. Now the analogy can be drawn with the assessment of delusions and hallucinations, since to equilibrate the threshold for considering beliefs and perceptions to be pathological with that of a European, we should again have to effect drastic changes in the social environment of the individual

African villager. These would include alterations in fundamental and wide-ranging beliefs.

We would not venture to claim that all physical illnesses have as large a social component determining the threshold for pathology as anaemia does. However, this example suffices to indicate that psychiatry does not stand apart from the other branches of medicine on this account. The cultural relativity of delusions and hallucinations represents a difference in degree, but not in kind, from symptoms of physical illnesses.

2 The culture-bound syndromes

The term *culture-bound*, referring to features of illness that are confined to a particular culture, has already been encountered. The implication is that such features are determined by cultural factors and are not part of the common heritage of human beings. That certain conditions only occurred in specific cultures, would have far-reaching implications for the aetiology of those conditions. The term *psychosis* has up until now been used freely, but it is now necessary to define it having first grasped the meaning and implications of the terms *delusion* and *hallucination*, as these are integral to the definition of psychosis.

Psychosis has been defined in a number of ways, none of which is completely satisfactory. A common definition is that it comprises conditions in which the patient has lost insight, i.e. does not realise that his experiences are part of an illness. However, a great range of degrees of insight, from fully present to totally absent, is found in patients suffering from psychoses, so that insight alone cannot be relied on as a touchstone. Furthermore, there are conditions included among the psychoses, such as catatonia, that render the patient inaccessible to questioning, so that the degree of insight cannot be determined. The presence of insight is usually considered to distinguish neuroses from psychoses, but there are some patients with neurotic conditions, notably chronic obsessional states, who fail to show insight into the pathological nature of their symptoms. A related definition includes losing touch with reality, and certainly this could be true of patients with fully fledged delusions and hallucinations. But it is a very elastic notion, which can easily be applied in neurotic conditions.

A complicating and controversial issue is the division between psychotic and neurotic depression, some people relying on the presence of delusions and/or hallucinations to differentiate the two, while others use the severity of associated somatic symptoms such as insomnia, anorexia, and loss of libido. This latter practice clearly undermines the customary usage of the term *psychosis*.

11

Instead of trying to find a comprehensive definition, I prefer the more pragmatic approach of enumerating the symptoms and signs that qualify conditions for inclusion as psychoses. First and foremost are delusions and hallucinations, which are characteristic of the organic psychoses, such as those caused by drug intoxication and pellagra, in which there is a known physical cause of brain dysfunction, and also of the functional psychoses, such as schizophrenia and manic–depressive psychosis, in which no such cause has been identified. There are other symptoms, consisting of disturbed behaviour, that indicate the presence of a psychosis even though the patient's state of mind cannot be explored because of an inaccessibility to questioning. These include mutism, the absence of speech, and stupor, the absence of both speech and movement occurring in a state of full consciousness. Both these latter symptoms may also be exhibited by non-psychotic patients suffering from hysteria, but a distinction between the conditions is usually possible and will be discussed in a later chapter. Other disturbances of behaviour indicative of a psychosis are seen in a type of schizophrenia known as catatonia. They include standing in strange and often uncomfortable positions for periods of time (posturing), holding awkward positions of the limbs and body imposed by the examiner (flexibilitas cerea), imitating movements made by other people (echopraxia), performing exactly the opposite action to what is asked (negativism) and wavering between two opposing movements (ambitendency). Stupor is also a feature of catatonia and may alternate with periods of wild excitement in which the patient is physically overactive, and can be violent and destructive. These symptoms have been given in some detail, since they will play an important part in our discussion of the culture-bound syndromes.

A number of these syndromes are now well known and carefully described, including koro, wihtigo, amok, latah, and possession states. An account of each of them will be given, and the classification dilemmas they pose considered. Koro affects individuals, but occasionally takes an epidemic form. It is virtually confined to a particular geographical area, south-east Asia, where it is seen most commonly among Chinese people. The affected individual, nearly always a male, becomes convinced that his genitals are withdrawing into his abdomen. This throws him into a state of panic, since he believes that when the last vestige of them disappears he will die. He takes remedial action and may tie his penis to a post or rock with string or even wire. Alternatively, he may induce his relatives to hold on to his penis to prevent the dreaded occurrence, which they will do in relays for long periods of time.

An epidemic of koro occurred in Singapore, fuelled by a rumour that the condition could be brought on by eating pork from inoculated pigs (Ngui, 1969). At its peak, 100 cases were seen in a day, the majority being Chinese. Among those affected were eight women. The epidemic was contained within a month with the aid of reassurance and education. A similar outbreak came to the attention of Harrington (1982) during a visit to Thailand. Known as *rok joo* in Thai, it affected more than 50 tapioca-plantation workers, both male and female, who blamed the shrinkage on the consumption of tinned sardines. The local press reported that a member of parliament visited the afflicted and stated, "I am fascinated; it did shrink." Another epidemic was observed in Assam, in north-east India, in June 1982 (Dutta, 1983). Again, both men and women were affected. The men often arrived at a clinic with their penis securely tied with broad ribbons or elastic bands. There was no local term corresponding to koro, and the condition was labelled *jinjinia bemar*, which means a tingling sensation of the body. The word *jinjinia* is used to refer to a tingling that arises from extreme anxiety. The harmlessness of the condition was widely proclaimed through the mass media, the intensity of the panic subsided, and the epidemic petered out in 3 months.

The belief that a man's genitals can shrink into his abdomen with fatal consequences is unknown in the West, which must have led to this symptom being classified as a delusion, and hence the condition as a psychosis. However, a moment's reflection reveals this as a basic error resulting from a failure to appreciate the cultural relativity of delusions. The fact that relatives are prepared to take action to forestall the disappearance of the patient's penis informs us at once that this is a shared belief and hence, by definition, not a delusion. The belief that this occurrence is possible is widespread throughout the area in which koro is found. Furthermore, there is a feature of Chinese mythology that explains the patient's fear of dying when his penis disappears, namely the belief that ghosts have no genitals. Once we become aware of these background beliefs in the patient's culture, his fear becomes comprehensible and there is no longer any support for viewing koro as a psychosis. Instead, as Yap (1965) pointed out, it is a neurotic condition similar to hypochondriacal conditions commonly seen in the West. The closest parallel is probably with cardiac neurosis, a form of anxiety state in which the patient concentrates on the beating of the heart and becomes convinced that it is about to stop, resulting in death. The patient's anxiety about the heart speeds and accentuates its beat, causing palpitations, and setting up a vicious circle that leads to a state of panic. In this case, the patient's belief about the heart does not strike us as strange because of widespread knowledge concerning heart attacks. However, the fear that the heart will suddenly stop beating is almost as baseless as the fear of the koro patient that his penis will shrink into his abdomen. As with cardiac neurosis, there is probably a physiological basis to koro. Oyebode *et al* (1986) measured changes in the circumference of the penis of a koro sufferer, with a penile plethysmograph. When the subject was required to imagine situations in which his penis might be experienced as shrinking, a reduction in its circumference was recorded. Anxiety, which is usually extreme in koro sufferers, results in a reduction of blood flow to the periphery and a contraction of the cremaster muscle, both of which physiological processes would reduce the apparent size of the penis. Thus, as the Thai MP observed, "it did shrink".

What still has to be explained is why Westerners focus anxiety on the heart, while in south-east Asia, anxiety centres on the genitals. The generality of this question should not be taken too literally: of course there are Asians who worry about their heart and Europeans who worry about their genitals. In fact, koro-like conditions have been reported in a small number of individuals from outside south-east Asia. By considering these cases, we can deepen our understanding of classical koro. Berrios & Morley (1984) recorded that 15 cases of a koro-like state had been reported in non-Chinese subjects, including a patient of their own. All the individuals concerned expressed a fear of their penis shrinking, seven believed it could disappear into their abdomen, but only two thought that death might ensue. No more than four patients used measures to prevent the feared shrinkage. Thus the majority of these patients, none of whom had any knowledge of the cultural background to koro, exhibited only an approximation to the classical syndrome. It is of particular interest that all 15 cases suffered from a primary psychiatric condition, the commonest being anxiety, depression, and schizophrenia. Subsequently Ang & Weller (1984) reported two cases of koro affecting a West Indian immigrant and a Greek Cypriot immigrant to the UK. The first patient suffered from schizophrenia and the second from manic–depressive psychosis. The case investigated psychophysiologically by Oyebode *et al* (1986) involved a Briton who was diagnosed as having an endogenous depression. Modai *et al* (1986) have reported the syndrome in an Iraqi immigrant to Israel, whose wife had developed schizophrenia and then lost interest in sex. The koro-like symptoms developed by non-Chinese patients inform us that it is possible for any individual, whatever his cultural background, to direct anxiety to his genitals and to initiate the physiologically based spiral of penile shrinkage engendering further anxiety. However, in the absence of a folk belief in asexual ghosts, it is rare for the panic to escalate into a fear of death, or for relatives to be involved in preventive measures.

Each of the non-Chinese patients studied was at the margin of society in one or more respects, either being an immigrant or, more commonly, suffering from a severe psychiatric illness. It can be concluded that where the culture openly acknowledges the existence of anxieties about the genitals, as, for example, in the folk beliefs about koro, relatively normal individuals readily express these anxieties, which are accepted without question by their social circle. In such an accepting environment, genital anxiety can spread rapidly from person to person, taking an epidemic form. On the other hand, in Western cultures, where genital anxieties do not take an explicit form in any widespread folk belief, it is only the marginal individual who will express such anxieties openly, and an epidemic spread is most unlikely. It is of interest that Berrios & Morley (1984) found that 8 of the 15 non-Chinese koro sufferers they identified reported premorbid sexual inadequacies. There was also an evident sexual problem in the case documented by Modai *et al* (1986). This is likely to constitute an added pressure on non-Chinese individuals to focus on their genitals, but may well not be a factor in classical koro. Berrios & Morley (1984) consider that it is only of value to use the diagnosis of koro in "specific cultural niches" in which psychotherapeutic routines that are socially meaningful can be activated. It is true that reassurance and education appeared to halt the epidemics in south-east Asia, but these would make little impact on a patient with koro-like symptoms who also suffered from a psychotic or neurotic condition.

The restriction in the application of the term koro suggested by Berrios & Morley (1984) raises a general issue affecting culture-bound syndromes. Prince & Tcheng-Laroche (1987) consider that loose usage of the latter is progressively undermining its meaning. They propose the following definition: "a collection of signs and symptoms (excluding notions of cause) which is restricted to a limited number of cultures, primarily by reason of certain of their psychosocial features". They express their awareness of an inherent contradiction in this statement, since the clause concerning "psychosocial features" is phrased vaguely enough to encompass a notion of causality. In the discussion following their paper, Simons argues that aetiological considerations cannot be avoided in any classification. Indeed, I maintain that the prime purpose of classification in medicine is to determine aetiology eventually. Beiser, in his contribution to the discussion, comments that a dependence on psychosocial features for classification is very difficult to put into operation. Additionally, he reminds us that it has proved extremely difficult to establish the cause of any condition in psychiatry. In the absence of a reasonably watertight definition of culture-bound syndromes, it seems most practical to consider a number of other conditions conventionally included under this rubric, and to return to the problem of definition at the end of this chapter.

Our reasons for stating that koro cannot be considered a psychosis apply equally to wihtigo, or windigo as it is sometimes spelled. This is a condition reported to occur among the North American Indians of the Cree, Ojibway, and Salteaux tribes. They experience very severe winters with extreme cold and scarcity of food. Under these harsh conditions, death from starvation is a distinct possibility, and leads to a fear of cannibalism which is expressed in at least two ways: a rigid taboo on cannibalism, and a belief in the wihtigo, a cannibalistic ice spirit of giant size. The initial phase of what has been called the wihtigo psychosis (Hallowell, 1934) is characterised by a distaste for ordinary types of food, nausea, and perhaps vomiting. If these symptoms continue for several days or more, anxiety develops and, if they fail to subside, rapidly reaches a climax. The sufferer construes the repugnance for food as evidence that he or she is turning into a wihtigo. The anxiety is compounded by the general fear of cannibalism which is shared by everyone in the community. Sufferers are usually considered to have been bewitched and a traditional healer is consulted. If no improvement results, the person with wihtigo often asks to be killed to thwart the cannibalistic urges. Such is the fear of the community that in the past they would follow this wish. As with koro, it is necessary to view the behaviour of the wihtigo sufferer against the cultural background. It is quite clear that they are in complete accord with those of the community, to the extent that fellow members of the tribe are prepared to kill the sufferer in order to avert the danger from the ice spirit. Hence, there is no question of wihtigo being a psychotic condition. Rather, its form is that of an anxiety state, in which the anxiety becomes focused on antisocial urges which are feared by the whole community and expressed in their mythology. Neutra *et al* (1977) express doubts about the actual occurrence of cases of wihtigo. They note that the same description of the syndrome has been copied from one author to another, and that accounts of affected individuals are lacking in the literature. They emphasise the social importance of what may be closer to a myth than a reality and conclude: "like witch-possession in our Middle Ages, it was an issue for major concern and occasional community action, even though the actual condition rarely if ever existed."

Amok presents rather different classificatory problems, since no unusual belief is involved. The condition occurs in the area of the Philippines and Malaysia. However, it is not confined to the indigenous population, as cases have been described in Europeans who have settled in the area. The characteristic story is that a male villager receives a real or a fancied insult. He leaves the village and goes off into the wilds where he nurses his injured pride for several days. During this time he eats nothing and is socially isolated. He then returns to his village in a blind fury, and using a kris, he kills or attempts to kill every living thing he encounters. His murderous anger is vented on relative, friend, enemy, and stranger alike; even domestic animals are not immune to attack. His frenzy is halted only when he himself is killed or else caught and securely bound. This exotic condition has of course given rise to the familiar English phrase 'running amok'. Its only resemblance to a psychosis is to the violent excitement occasionally shown by catatonic patients emerging from a stupor. However, catatonic excitement, unlike amok, has no understandable link with a preceding social situation or with the patient's emotional state. The essence of amok is blind murderous violence arising out of extremely heightened emotions. We encounter this state elsewhere in the world, notably among the Norsemen, who deliberately cultivated it before a battle for obvious reasons. They termed it *berserker* which has also left the English language a legacy in the phrase 'going berserk'. The English seem to need to borrow terms for violent emotions from other languages! Another parallel with amok is the *crime passionnel* in France, which refers to the hot-blooded murder by a husband or wife of his or her spouse and/or lover on surprising them *in flagrante delicto*. In this case the violence is not indiscriminate, but there is an interesting similarity in the legal aspects. In the French legal code, the penalty for *crime passionnel* is considerably less than for other forms of murder, while in the traditional societies concerned, the man who has gone amok, if not killed during the period of violence, is not held responsible for his murders and is not punished. However, some subjects exhibiting amok have been admitted to psychiatric hospitals, as revealed in a study by Tan & Carr (1977). They reviewed the diagnoses on admission, of the patients occupying the male security ward in a psychiatric hospital in West Malaysia. Of the 134 patients, 21 had been labelled 'amok' on admission, after being found guilty, but insane in court. Ten of these, all Malays, were familiar with the folk concept of amok, and their behaviour prior to admission fitted the classical description. Six patients, Chinese or Indian, were totally unfamiliar with the term that had been imposed on them by the civil system, and their murders differed in a number of respects from those in traditional amok. The remaining five patients were severely psychotic at the time of the study and could not be interviewed. Of the 16 patients who could be interviewed, all but two had been given a diagnosis of schizophrenia. These two suffered from manic–depressive psychosis and general paresis respectively. Six of the Malays, who were familiar with the concept of amok, showed no abnormality of behaviour subsequent to admission, although they remained in hospital an average of 15.6 years. Tan & Carr considered that these six were true examples of amok, and therefore wrongly diagnosed as schizophrenic. The remaining patients showed symptoms characteristic of psychotic illnesses, but had been labelled 'amok' by the Malay police who arrested them, because they had committed or attempted homicide in a manner consistent with the amok tradition. They conclude that the majority of cases currently labelled 'amok' involve universally recognisable psychiatric disorders in which violence is a prominent feature, while there is a small cohort of older patients with a single episode of violence and no other evidence of pathology who conform to classical descriptions of amok. They consider that their findings support the view put forward by Murphy (1982) that the traditional form of behaviour is being replaced by a new variant in which a variety of psychopathological conditions are increasingly evident.

Murphy (1982) invokes European colonisation of south-eastern Asia as a major force in altering public attitudes towards amok. Traditionally it was "accepted by the community and expected of any male individual who is placed for some reason or other in an intolerably embarrassing or shameful situation . . . . The Amok must reestablish himself in the eyes of his fellow man and proceeds to do so by a 'violent assertion of his power' – the only court of appeal known to his fathers for countless generations" (Tan & Carr, 1977). When the European powers imposed relative peace on the area, they also brought their own concept of justice to bear on amok. In the 1840s a British judge in the Straits Settlements, in a widely publicised judgement, pointed to the amok tradition as evidence that the Malays were savages and not worthy to associate with civilised people. Murphy contends that, from then on, the rate in European-influenced territories dropped sharply, while the cases that came to medical attention there increasingly exhibited signs of chronic psychosis. It certainly appears from Tan & Carr's study that some patients exhibiting traditional amok were labelled as schizophrenic and incarcerated in a psychiatric hospital for decades, even when free of all symptoms. We cannot tell whether other traditional-amok patients were dealt with differently, but psychiatric relabelling of the behaviour would certainly rob it of its erstwhile function of reinstating a man in public esteem.

A parallel with koro is evident. When koro occurs in a culture that sanctions the expression of genital anxiety, it affects relatively normal individuals and resolves rapidly. When it occurs in cultures that do not tolerate the open expression of this form of anxiety, it is shown by individuals who are psychiatrically ill, or otherwise peripheral to society. This contemporary cultural difference in respect of koro is echoed by historical changes in the cultural attitudes towards amok. As it has become progressively devalued in south-east Asian culture, amok has ceased to be the means of redress of ordinary citizens, and has become restricted to the behavioural repertoire of the mentally ill. The emergence of these same patterns is traced when hysteria is considered in a later chapter.

Latah is found in much the same parts of the world as amok, but similar, if not identical, syndromes have been described in Burma (*yaun*), Thailand (*bah-tsche*), Philippines (*mali-mali*), Siberia (*myriachit*), Lapland (Lapp panic), among the Ainu of Japan (*imu*) and French Canadians of Maine (Jumpers) (Simons, 1980). It differs from amok in predominantly affecting women. It consists of imitative behaviour, the sufferer copying movements made or speech uttered by other people, apparently without being able to help herself. There is also an automatic response to commands, and less commonly the utterance of obscenities apparently without the sufferer's intent. The behaviour may be set off by various stimuli ranging from unexpected gestures by another person or unexpected physical contact with severely frightening events such as the sight of a snake. Chiu *et al* (1972) looked for cases of latah in a large-scale survey of three main ethnic groups in Sarawak, the Chinese, Malay, and Iban. To elicit a latah response, the interviewer would purposely drop a hat or a pencil. The researchers found that children who came to listen to the interviewers would frequently tickle the subjects to bring out the phenomena, this behaviour being quite acceptable socially. It is noteworthy in this respect that the word latah means ticklish in Malay.

These workers found similar numbers of cases among the Malay and Iban subjects, but not one among the Chinese population. The initial attack of latah is believed by the Malays to be the result of a dream during which the *latah antu* or spirit enters the subject; they also believe that dreams maintain the condition. The Malay latah subjects frequently reported dreams with a manifestly sexual content, mostly images of penises. The latah subjects were examined by psychiatrists, but only 10% of the Malays and 23% of the Ibans were considered to be suffering from an identifiable psychiatric illness. These comprised three women with depressive neurosis, two with hysterical neurosis, one with schizophrenia, and one with what is labelled as an adjustment reaction. This accords well with the local views of latah, since none of the Iban heads of household or interviewers regarded latah behaviour as unusual or odd, while the Malays identified only between 11 and 22% of the latah subjects as showing unusual behaviour. Gilmore Ellis, who was medical superintendent of the Government Asylum in Singapore, wrote in 1897 that ''cases of latah are never sent to lunatic Asylums, and the Malays themselves draw a very distinct line between latah and insanity.''

In deciding how to categorise latah, it is worth considering parallels between behaviour of latah subjects and people suffering from formal psychiatric illnesses in the West. The imitation of other people's movements or speech also occurs in catatonic schizophrenia, when it is termed echopraxia or echolalia. Chapman (1966) has recorded an illuminating account of this given by a patient: ''I get shaky in the knees and my chest is like a mountain in front of me, and my body actions are different. The arms and legs are apart and away from me and they go on their own. That's when I feel I am the other person and copy their movements.'' This subjective description vividly conveys the experience of the disintegration of normal psychological processes that underlies many of the symptoms of schizophrenia. Unfortunately we have no subjective account of latah to compare with this. Indeed, some of the latah subjects claim to be unconscious of what is happening at the time of an episode. However, few latah subjects suffer from an identifiable psychiatric illness. We have presented evidence for a physiological basis to koro (Oyebode *et al*, 1986). A similar approach to latah has been taken by Simons (1980). He worked on the assumption that latah represents a physiological hyperstartle response, which is culture-free. He advertised for easily startled subjects in American local newspapers. The respondents described behaviour in which the phenomenology of the experience was strikingly similar. They used phrases such as: ''When I'm alone somewhere and not expecting to be anything but alone and someone comes behind me or into where I am, I have a physical reaction. I jump''. ''People think its amusing when they find out they can startle you; they often do try to startle you.''

Simons then made audiovisual records of startle phenomena in a variety of cultures. He found that startles were most easily elicited when subjects were either intensely monitoring their immediate environment or when they were drowsy or lost in thought. He postulated that latah subjects become extremely aroused when startled, and can then be induced to exhibit imitative behaviour or obedience. He considered that the presence of an audience, the improper nature of the commands, and the presence of higher-status persons, all increase arousal and hence vulnerability to having one's attention captured and one's will imposed on. He noted that whereas the Malays do not exploit latah subjects for any ritual purpose, among the Ainu of Japan, imu subjects attend certain feasts with the object of performing imu behaviour. Whereas Simons views the passivity of latah subjects as a quality that renders them vulnerable to exploitation, Chiu *et al* (1972) stress the advantages of abrogation of responsibility for their actions. They see latah as ''a female attention seeking response involving one of the few permissible overt excitable aggressive and/or sexual demonstrations in a male dominated culture.'' Simons believes that hyperstartlers exist in every society, representing the extreme end of a range of physiological responses to unexpected stimuli. However it is only in a handful of cultures that these responses are recognised and made use of in one way or another.

By contrast, the physiological susceptibility of some individuals to develop possession states has been exploited almost universally, since they are found in 90% of traditional societies (Bourguignon, 1976). They are characterised by certain beliefs as well as by dramatically altered behaviour. The subjects (we shall not refer to them as sufferers, as this term prejudges the issue of whether this is an illness) assert that they are possessed by a spirit, which may be a god, a demon, or a lesser member of the pantheon. They may then run about in a frenzied way, their voice may change out of all recognition, for instance a woman may seem to talk with a man's voice, or they may shout nonsensical words (see Chapter 1, p. 6). They may express unusual desires; e.g. women in the Zar cult may demand whisky and cigars. All these alterations in behaviour are attributed by the subjects to the spirit possessing them, either at the time or later, since they are sometimes in a trancelike state that precludes ordinary communication.

These manifestations are virtually indistinguishable from one of the first-rank symptoms of schizophrenia, delusions of control, the significance of which will be explored in detail in the next chapter. Briefly, delusions of control are used by psychiatrists throughout the world as one of the defining characteristics of schizophrenia. The form of the symptom is the experience that one's will is wholly or partly replaced by some external force, so that bodily movement and actions, including speech and desires, no longer appear to be under one's control. The patient develops a belief that control is exerted by some outside force or power. The content of this belief, as we have learned, reflects the patient's cultural milieu, so that the controlling force may be conceived of in modern technological terms as electricity, laser beams, computers, and so on, or in spiritual terms such as god, the devil, or any other spirit in which the patient's people believe. In the latter case, almost invariably in the setting of a traditional society, many patients assert that the controlling spirit has entered their physical body so that they are possessed. The patient's description of a delusion of control in these terms cannot be distinguished from possession states.

However, there are other distinguishing features. Possession states in traditional cultures almost always develop in the context of a ritual which is specifically designed to induce them. Possession states are valued experiences, which confer a variety of advantages on the possessed. The nature of the rituals, and the functions of possession states will be described in Part III of this book. Furthermore, possession states are transient, seldom outlasting the ritual of which they form a part. They may continue for minutes or hours, but rarely extend for several days. In a study in Thailand, it was found that more than half the possession states investigated lasted 1 h or less, and only

2% lasted more than 8 h (Suwanlert, 1976). By contrast, delusions of control do not develop in the setting of a ritual, and they usually last for at least several days, often persisting for weeks or months.

These two aspects, the social setting and the duration, should be sufficient to prevent confusion between those different states of mind. Unfortunately, though, mistakes can occur. A good example is described in the International Pilot Study of Schizophrenia (World Health Organization, 1973). One of the patients in the series collected was a Taoist priestess. At the age of 37 she developed restlessness and insomnia, refused food, knelt on the bed to worship, and talked to herself. She felt she had the power of receiving ghosts and believed that God had removed her soul and used her body and voice to speak his will. She suspected she was possessed with her foster-father's spirit. She sat on the bed the whole day pretending to be Buddha and refused to get off the bed or to eat. She was admitted to hospital in a state of extreme physical exhaustion as a result of almost continuous "episode of communication with God for nearly 15 days". She was rated by a centre psychiatrist as exhibiting delusions of control and given an overall diagnosis of hysterical psychosis. The duration of her experiences is very unusual for possession states; on the other hand, it was an integral part of her job as a priestess to become possessed by spirits. Without this talent she would lose her occupation. This cultural aspect of the case makes it clear that she was suffering from a prolonged possession state and not a delusion of control.

This case, and the preceding argument, suggest that we should not consider possession states to be a symptom of an illness at all. The possessed do not suffer from these states of mind, but rather gain advantage from them – sometimes including an occupation. It can be argued that hysterical dissociative mechanisms are responsible for possession states and that certain personality types are more prone to develop them. By itself, however, this is not a convincing argument for regarding them as symptoms of a psychiatric illness, and they are better viewed as the manifestations of a psychological discovery, made by the vast majority of traditional societies, and integrated into each culture in different ways.

All the culture-bound syndromes considered so far originate in developing cultures and are rarely seen in Westerners. Is there any condition which shows the reverse distribution? The obvious candidate is anorexia nervosa. This syndrome comprises a revulsion for food, self-induced vomiting, a denial of thinness despite pronounced weight loss, and emaciation which may lead to death. It most often affects women in their late teens and early twenties, in whom it is accompanied by amenorrhoea, but is occasionally seen in young men. It was first identified in Europe during the 17th century and appeared to be comparatively rare until recent decades, during which there has been an explosion of interest in the condition – three of the professorial psychiatric departments in London currently specialise in anorexia nervosa! The increasing incidence in the West has not been paralleled in developing countries, from which a minute number of cases has been reported. Crisp

(1980) has noted the appearance of some patients with this condition in Arab states, while Buchan & Gregory (1984) have described what is probably only the third case in a Black African recorded in the literature. The patient in the latter was extensively exposed to European cultural values, as she was placed with White foster parents in the UK between the ages of 2 and 4, and subsequently received her education in White boarding schools.

What is the nature of this condition that can readily end in the death of a young person? There are undoubtedly bodily changes in anorexia nervosa, such as alterations in hormone levels and the new growth of hair, but these are the consequences of an inadequate food intake, not the cause. For instance, menstruation ceases when weight drops below a certain level and resumes when it exceeds that level again. The primary cause is a set of attitudes about food, and body size and shape. Although embedded in the psychology of the individual, these are obviously susceptible to cultural influences. In the West, immensely strong pressures are exerted on women to become slim, through advertising in the mass media and role modelling by 'stars'. This manipulation of women's self-image has been attacked by feminist writers (e.g. Orbach, 1978). Social pressures in the developing world appear to be in the reverse direction. Where food is a scarce commodity, being plump is a visible sign of success and security. In Tonga and Samoa the nobility are expected to grow to a vast size, while in Shona society a fat wife is traditionally regarded as an important manifestation of her husband's affluence (Buchan & Gregory, 1984). These different polarisations of attitudes towards weight in the West, and the developing world, are expressed dramatically and poignantly by the fact that while millions of people die of famine each year, Western consumers are urged by advertisers to buy food and drink on the basis that they contain little or no food value. If society's attitudes towards food and weight are indeed the main determinant of anorexia nervosa, the incidence ought to rise with increasing affluence and Westernisation of developing countries. The oil-producing Third World countries would be the obvious sites for this postulated effect.

Having considered a diverse sample of culture-bound syndromes, we are in a better position to formulate a more precise definition. The common thread running through these examples is that *some characteristic of humankind, that might otherwise remain ignored, unexpressed or even buried in the depths of the unconscious, is brought into overt expression by a particular culture in which it fulfils a function for the individual or his social group.* In koro, a physiological reaction to fear becomes the cultural focus for sexual anxieties, which can then be openly expressed and elicit help and support from the sufferer's social group. In latah and possession states, a physiological vulnerability of a proportion of the community is transmuted by culturally prescribed procedures into behaviour that allows women the expression of otherwise forbidden wishes, among a variety of other benefits. The institution of amok sanctions (or used to do so) the expression of the murderous rage of which any human being is capable under provocation. Wihtigo is a myth or near-myth that expresses and contains anxieties about starvation, while anorexia nervosa is the consequence of a set of attitudes about food, and body image, that are driven by the culture to a pathological level in individuals whose psychosexual development renders them vulnerable.

In order to understand culture-bound syndromes fully, we need to be able to identify the substrate on which cultural influences operate, be it physiological or psychological. We also need to define the functions that the syndrome fulfils for the individual and/or his social group. Additionally, and this has proved most difficult to date, we should attempt to specify the forces within a culture that lead to an emphasis on certain human propensities and not on others. We have already noted in the case of amok and wihtigo that culture-bound syndromes are no more static than the cultures themselves. As cultures alter, the functions that these syndromes fulfil can become obsolete, although the behavioural patterns may persist in attenuated forms, as the mode of expression of marginal individuals rather than those in the mainstream of the culture.

3 The universality of the functional psychoses

In 1893, Emil Kraepelin published a textbook in which he distinguished a syndrome for which he used the name *dementia praecox*, from an undifferentiated pool of patients regarded as suffering from madness. Eugen Bleuler (1911) later changed the name of this syndrome to *schizophrenia*, but he did not improve on his predecessor's masterly clinical description. The breadth of Kraepelin's vision was such that he realised the importance of demonstrating that his new syndrome could be recognised in non-Western cultures. Consequently, he made a trip to the Far East and reported that he could identify cases of dementia praecox in Java, a culture as different from that of his native Switzerland as could be imagined. Since Kraepelin's pioneering transcultural investigation, psychiatrists from the West have worked in many non-Western cultures and have invariably been able to identify schizophrenia wherever they have gone. Of course we are dealing here with the unstandardised clinical impressions of people who were often unfamiliar with the local language and culture. To examine this issue scientifically we need a very sophisticated methodology.

What occurs in the clinical psychiatric interview? From the moment psychiatrists meet patients they have ample opportunities to observe their behaviour. Abnormalities in this may be signs of illness, equivalent to the physical signs in other branches of medicine, such as altered heart sounds, or a patch of numbness on the skin.

However, psychiatrists do not have to use special techniques, such as listening to the chest through a stethoscope or pricking the skin with a pin, to elicit clinical signs. It is sufficient to sit in a chair and observe the patients carefully, with the proviso that they need special training to know what to look for and how to interpret what they see and hear. We add *hear* because the vocal aspects of speech – tone, volume, rate, and quantity – are also signs, as well as the form of speech, which includes relevance and coherence. The patients' complaints, which form part of the content of speech, are the symptoms. Patients express some, but by no means all, of their symptoms spontaneously. They may never have formulated certain of their abnormal experiences in words until expressly asked to by the psychiatrist. The interviewer therefore has considerable latitude as to how far he or she will probe to elicit and clarify the patient's symptoms. The psychiatrist's theoretical orientation will determine the focus of the questions; for instance, an interviewer working within a psychoanalytic framework will spend a lot of time attempting to define the nature of the patient's relationships with his or her parents and relatively little time on the phenomena of illness. A phenomenologist will reverse the emphasis, cross-examining the patient intensively about the symptoms and skimming over emotional relationships. Hence, if we wish to compare the symptoms of psychiatric illnesses in different cultures, we must make sure that the psychiatrists involved are inquiring into the same areas.

Furthermore, as we learned from the parable of the butterfly collectors, in Chapter 1, it is essential for psychiatrists engaging in international studies to agree on the definitions of signs and symptoms. These two problems, defining the area of inquiry, and agreeing on the definition of signs and symptoms, have been solved by the construction of semistructured clinical interviews, of which the Present State Examination (PSE, Wing *et al*, 1974) is a widely accepted example. This consists of a series of stipulated questions that cover the major areas of psychiatric symptomatology. The questions have to be asked in the form in which they are written down, but each question is in the nature of a probe. If the response to the probe suggests to the interviewer that the symptom concerned may be present, he or she then embarks on a series of cross-questions, which interviewers are free to make up themselves, to establish the presence of the symptom beyond reasonable doubt. If the phrases we have used convey the atmosphere of the courtroom rather than the clinic, this is intentional, since the procedure is a matter of sifting through the available evidence to establish 'the truth'. In the case of a patient, the truth is a matter of matching the patient's description of experiences with a standard definition of the symptom, which the interviewer carries in his head. For each symptom in the PSE, there is a standard definition included in a glossary, which has to be learned by the interviewer as part of training in the use of the interview. Only when these definitions have been mastered is the interviewer able to generate the appropriate cross-questions to establish the presence or absence of each symptom.

The procedure may sound like a rigid structure that is imposed on the patient, and which departs considerably from the usual free-ranging clinical interview. This is not so, since the interviewer is free to vary the order of the questions, so that once he is thoroughly familiar with the PSE, it can be used to follow wherever the patient leads. Furthermore, the semistructured nature of the interview allows the interviewer considerable flexibility in the cross-questioning routines, so that he or she can introduce something of a personal flavour into the procedure. An example of a cross-questioning routine taken from a live interview of the author's may better convey to the reader the style of a PSE. This example illustrates an attempt to determine the possible presence of a delusion of control, a symptom which is described on p. 20.

> Interviewer: Do you ever feel controlled from outside like a puppet or robot?
>
> Patient: Yes, oh yes, definitely. I get the impression that there are people who are greater than I am who are therefore controlling me. It is true. People are controlled. I don't think there's much argument about this really.
>
> I: Of course some people are controlled by money or by force of character, but do you ever get the feeling that your arms and legs are being moved for you or your voice used?
>
> P: Nothing like that. Only an indirect control.
>
> I: Do you ever feel completely possessed by another person?
>
> P: Not possessed, no. Influenced more. People with more power than you can influence you.
>
> I: How do they exert this influence?
>
> P: By giving you their views.

This patient does not have a delusion of control. He feels somewhat weak willed and can be influenced externally by people of stronger character, a common human frailty, but he does not experience his will being replaced from inside, which is the essence of this symptom.

The use of a semistructured interview such as the PSE avoids a number of problems bedevilling comparisons of patients interviewed by different psychiatrists, but obstacles of considerable magnitude remain. Some of these relate to the influence that preconceptions can exert on perception. This topic has been extensively investigated by social psychologists, who have demonstrated that subjects' preconceptions or prejudices can cause them to misperceive things presented to them as visual or auditory stimuli. A classical example of this is provided by the elegant study of Bruner & Postman (1949).

They presented to university students a series of playing cards shown in very brief exposures. Some of the cards were normal, while others were trick cards, with the colours of the suits reversed, e.g. a black three-of-hearts, a red six-of-spades. If subjects failed to recognise any card, it was shown again with progressively longer exposures, up to 1 s. If the card was still incorrectly recognised at this duration of exposure, the experimenters went on to the next card in the series. It is not surprising to find that the subjects required longer exposures to recognise the trick cards than the normal cards. However, even with an exposure of 1 s, 10% of the trick cards were incorrectly recognised. Some subjects reported the colour of the trick cards as being altered, e.g. the red six-of-spades was described as a purple six-of-hearts or a purple six-of-spades. Bruner & Postman comment that "the subjects often perceived colour in such a way as to make it more in keeping with, or to bring it nearer to, normal expectations".

The psychiatrist is just as liable to misperceptions as the naive subject of a psychological experiment, since the former's perceptions of a patient's symptoms are moulded by what he wants to see and expects to see. Psychiatrists, like anyone else applying a classification scheme, prefer to encounter phenomena that fit neatly into one or other of their categories, rather than straddling the boundaries between categories. Phenomena that do not fit neatly into pigeon-holes raise awkward questions about the validity of the classification scheme. Psychiatrists encountering symptoms in a patient that do not fit with the diagnosis that has already taken shape in their minds are likely to ignore such symptoms, or even to misperceive them. A theoretical example of this was put forward by Shepherd *et al* (1968). They point out that a patient whose face is relatively immobile could be assumed to be exhibiting the blunting of emotion that is typical of schizophrenia, or the masklike face of severe depression, depending on the diagnosis chosen by the interviewer. This theoretical example received confirmation in a study by Katz *et al* (1969), who showed films of interviews with psychiatric patients to audiences of psychiatrists. The psychiatrists were asked to note the presence of symptoms using a standardised rating scale. For two of the patients, audiences showed significant variations in their ratings of apathy. Psychiatrists who made a diagnosis of schizophrenia for the two patients were more likely to record high ratings of apathy than those who made other diagnoses. The expected association between schizophrenia and apathy, or between other diagnoses and the absence of apathy, had influenced the psychiatrists' perception of the patients' behaviour.

Another example of the way in which psychiatrists' preconceptions can influence their perception of symptoms is provided by this author's work on ratings of unpleasant emotions (Leff, 1973, 1974). This will be explored in more detail in Chapter 4, but it demonstrates that even the use of a standardised interview technique, in this instance the PSE, does not eliminate this source of bias. It is unrealistic to expect psychiatrists (or any other kind of doctor) to clear their minds of diagnostic expectations while interviewing patients, and the only precaution that can be taken against this bias is to make interviewers aware of its existence and potential distorting effect while they are being trained.

There is another, more subtle, problem raised by the use of standardised interviews, and that is the danger of incorporating into them an ethnocentric stance. This is generally remediable for individual symptoms, if they are defined in terms of their form as opposed to their content. However, this strategy does not touch the issue of the choice of symptoms for inclusion in the instrument. In virtually all the standardised clinical instruments that exist, symptoms have been included if they occur reasonably frequently in populations of psychiatric patients. Inevitably, each instrument has been constructed in the context of a particular culture, almost always a Western technological society. As we shall see later on in this chapter, the symptoms included in such instruments have proved to be identifiable among populations of psychiatric patients in developing countries. However, in such countries, the psychiatric services have been closely modelled on Western facilities, and still only deal with a small fraction of the psychiatrically ill. It can be argued that they screen off only those clients who fit the Western stereotype of the psychiatric patient, and that the rest are excluded. Hence, the Western stereotype, embodied in one of the standardised psychiatric interviews, is never challenged by the indigenous psychiatrically ill who depart from it.

There is a way to avoid this bias and that is to build up a psychiatric interview from scratch in a developing country. To do this, it is necessary to study people who have been designated as mentally ill by the local population. Most of these would be treated by traditional healers in the first instance, so that one could sample the clientele of a representative selection of traditional healers. It would be vital to get these clients to state their complaints in their own words, rather than use a structured interview with its own built-in assumptions. From a large number of accounts of complaints of clients and their relatives, it should be possible to derive common symptoms expressed in the local language and to use these to construct a questionnaire. There is still a snag, and that is that the person crystallising symptoms from a large number of anecdotal accounts is applying a process of selection that could reflect an inherent bias. Therefore, it would be preferable for someone without a Western psychiatric training to carry out this task in the first instance. It is the kind of job that would be within the compass of an anthropologist. In the past, anthropologists have been interested in identifying concepts of illness, including mental illness, in traditional cultures (see Chapter 10), but have not embodied these in standardised interview schedules.

There have been several attempts to construct indigenous psychiatric interviews, although they have not included all of the above precautions to avoid a Western bias. Carstairs & Kapur (1976) constructed the Indian Psychiatric Interview Schedule in Kannada, a South Indian language. They examined the case records of 285 patients who had attended out-patient clinics, and used the array of symptoms recorded to prepare a provisional interview schedule. This schedule was then tried out on two new series of out-patients, and revised in the light of the experience gained. This procedure fails to eliminate the biases resulting from the selection of patients attending a Western-style facility, and from the use of complaints recorded by professional staff. It is not surprising, therefore, that the Indian Psychiatric Interview Schedule, when translated into English, looks almost identical to questionnaires developed in the West.

A more genuinely indigenous interview has been constructed by Verma & Wig (1976). They derived items for a questionnaire on neurotic symptoms from two sources. First, the heads of specialist departments in a general hospital were contacted. They were asked to give five symptoms, in Hindi or Punjabi, which adult neurotic patients attending their clinics commonly complained of. The complaints were supposed to be couched in the patient's own language, but the use of doctors to report patients' symptoms in a secondhand way is no advance on Carstairs' & Kapur's approach. Second, they noted the complaints of a large number of neurotic patients attending a psychiatry department. The patients' complaints were recorded in their own words in Hindi and Punjabi, thus avoiding possible distortion by a professional intermediary. Over half the patients came from rural areas, but nevertheless they were selectively included, by virtue of the fact that they attended a Western type of medical facility. The items from the two sources were combined and any overlap reduced, leading to 74 in all. From these, the 'best' 50 were selected. The authors do not give any details about the criteria involved in choosing the 'best' items, although they acknowledge "that there would be some subjectivity involved in this". Indeed, there is plenty of scope for the imposition of Western stereotypes in the elimination of one-third of the original items. Nevertheless, the (PGI) Health Questionnaire N-2 does differ in important respects from Western equivalents. At least 20 of the 50 items refer directly to physical symptoms, and some of these would be heard very rarely from neurotic patients in the West. Examples of such items are: "I often get watering of the eyes"; "I belch a lot after eating"; "I feel very thirsty"; "I often have to go to the toilet straight after meals"; and "I find difficulty in passing water".

Somatic complaints of this type made by Nigerian psychiatric patients impressed Ebigbo (1982) so forcibly, that he decided to develop a schedule exclusively concerned with eliciting them. Like Verma & Wig (1976), his starting-point was the complaints of the patients of a psychiatric hospital. He reviewed the case-notes of patients admitted to Enugu Psychiatric Hospital, and abstracted their somatic complaints to construct a questionnaire. In the completed version, 23 items referred to the head and 42 to the body. He then administered the questionnaire to a sample of psychiatric in-patients and out-patients and to a group of students. Many items discriminated between the patients and the healthy control subjects, of which the following are some examples: things like ants keep on creeping in various parts of my brain; occasionally I experience heat sensation in my head; something like worms live in my body, crawling at times to different parts of my body; I experience itching sensations in different parts of my body. The emphasis on bodily symptoms illustrated by the questionnaires devised by Verma & Wig (1976) and by Ebigbo (1982) will be given detailed consideration in the next chapter.

Beiser *et al* (1972) have taken an approach very similar to that we have argued for above. They wished to conduct a full-scale survey of the mental health of the Serer people of Senegal. As a first stage, they built up a native lexicon of disease terms and determined the patterns of behaviour to which they referred. They achieved this by conducting extensive interviews with family chiefs and other authorities in five Serer villages, with seven native healers and two European priests who had worked in the area for 20 years, and who spoke the Serer language well. They identified seven categories of disorder, which were described by the Serer as "illnesses of the spirit". These included: *O Dof* – people who became mad as a result of spirit attack, and who show hostile, excited, and destructive behaviour; and *Pobouh Lang* – people who eat earth. It was considered normal for pregnant women and for children prior to weaning to eat earth, but in other circumstances this behaviour was deemed pathological.

Having elucidated these native categories of illness, Beiser *et al* interviewed a sample of 50 people identified as suffering from one or more of them. Each person was interviewed on two occasions, once with a Western psychiatric questionnaire and once with an unstructured clinical interview carried out by psychiatrists who were working in Senegal. This is an interesting method of comparing native ideas of disturbance with Western psychiatric concepts embodied in standardised and unstandardised interviewing techniques. These workers were able to classify each item of disorder in the Serer system by means of a category in the Western scheme, with the exception of *Pobouh Lang*, earth eating, which may qualify as a culture-bound syndrome and clearly demands further study.

We have now considered the problems that standardised psychiatric interviews solve and the ones they do not, and can go on to review the international studies in which they have been used. This field of research is dominated by two large-scale international programmes, the US:UK Project (Cooper *et al*, 1972) and the International Pilot Study of Schizophrenia (World Health Organization, 1973). Before presenting these, it is worth considering one of the earliest and simplest international comparisons of diagnostic entities, which did not employ a standardised psychiatric interview. Rawnsley (1968) approached the problem by circulating short summaries of case records of psychiatric in-patients to psychiatrists in different countries and asking them to make a diagnosis in each case. The summaries of no more than 400 words were first sent to 205 psychiatrists in England and Wales. The 30 summaries on which these psychiatrists were in broad agreement were then sent to 260 psychiatrists in America, 30 in Denmark, 28 in Norway, and 18 in Sweden. Thus, all the psychiatrists were assessing the same material, and in 22 of the 30 cases there was fairly close agreement in the international panel, if broad diagnostic categories were employed to subsume the individual labels. However, there was a marked tendency for American psychiatrists to diagnose schizophrenia in cases to which European psychiatrists assigned diagnoses of depression, obsessional disorder, and paranoid psychosis. This observation foreshadows the findings of the two major international studies mentioned above. The Scandinavian psychiatrists, in particular the Norwegians, exhibited an idiosyncratic use of the term *psychogenic psychosis*, which was hardly ever employed by American and British psychiatrists, who tended to call the same cases neurotic. Apart from these local variations, this study demonstrates a broad agreement in diagnostic categories among an international group of psychiatrists.

However, it must be remembered that the presentation of clinical material in the form of case summaries eliminated a major source of variation in diagnosis, namely the preliminary stage of observation of symptoms.

This stage was an integral part of the US:UK Project, which employed the PSE for assessing patients' clinical state. This instrument in the hands of trained interviewers can be used with a high degree of reliability (Wing *et al*, 1974), so that the assessment of symptoms was standardised as much as possible. A different approach was taken to standardising the diagnostic procedure. This was a vital part of the aims of the project, which was stimulated by striking differences between the mental-hospital statistics from England and America. For instance, Kramer (1961, 1969*a,b*) found that the first-admission rate for manic–depressive illness in the age group 55–64 years was 20 times as high for England and Wales as for America. If these figures represented a true difference in the incidence of manic–depressive illness in the two countries, an excellent opportunity to investigate possible causes of this condition would be provided. Before embarking on this course, it would be essential to make sure that psychiatric diagnoses were being made in the same way on both sides of the Atlantic. The US:UK Project was set up to study this issue. The strategy chosen to compare American and British diagnostic practices was to build up a project team of research psychiatrists who would be trained to assess symptoms with the PSE and to apply, as far as possible, the same diagnostic framework to the symptoms. The diagnostic procedure was not standardised in the sense that a set of rules was specified and had to be learned by the team members, but great care was taken to ensure diagnostic uniformity. This was achieved by holding regular discussions between project members on diagnosis, by exchanging interviewers between the centres in London and New York, and by numerous statistical checks on consistency. This resulted in a team of psychiatrists who could be assumed to be interchangeable in the matter of diagnostic practice. Four of the six members of the project team had received their psychiatric training in the UK, so that it could be anticipated that project diagnoses would approximate to British rather than American practice. This might appear to introduce a source of bias into the study, but a consideration of the following analogy should dispel that impression. Suppose one wished to compare the height of Nelson's Column in Trafalgar Square with the height of the Empire State Building in New York. One could use a ruler calibrated in either inches or centimetres. It is immaterial which measuring system is employed as long as it is standardised and the same ruler used in London and New York. The project team acted as just such a transportable ruler, which happened to be calibrated in British units.

The first cross-national comparison in the project was made by interviewing 250 recently admitted patients in Netherne Hospital, near London, and the same number in Brooklyn State Hospital, New York. In order to avoid contamination of the diagnosis either way, there was no communication on the cases between project psychiatrists and hospital staff. The project

TABLE I

A comparison of the hospital and project diagnoses of the Brooklyn and Netherne patients[1]

	Brooklyn patients		Netherne patients	
	Hospital diagnosis	Project diagnosis	Project diagnosis	Hospital diagnosis
Schizophrenia	65.2[2]	32.4	26.0	34.0[2]
Depressive psychosis	7.2[2]	20.0[3]	28.0[3]	32.8[2]
Mania	0.8	6.8	3.6	1.6
Personality disorder	0.8[2]	2.4	4.4	8.4[2]

[1] The figures represent percentages of the total sample. Significance levels relate to comparison of the two sets of hospital diagnoses with each other, and the two sets of project diagnoses with each other.
[2] $P < 0.01$.
[3] $P < 0.05$.
From Leff (1977).

psychiatrists were constrained by the design of the study to use for their diagnoses the ICD–8 (World Health Organization, 1967). The hospital diagnoses of the Brooklyn and Netherne patients were taken from the official returns and were combined into 10 broad groupings. Table I shows a comparison of the most important diagnostic categories.

It can be seen that the hospital diagnoses differ in distribution highly significantly for three of the four categories shown. Schizophrenia, in particular, appears to be almost twice as common among Brooklyn patients as among Netherne patients, whereas depressive psychosis is diagnosed more than four times as frequently by the Netherne psychiatrists. By contrast, the project diagnoses for the two hospitals are much more similar, only the difference in proportion of depressive psychosis reaching significance. As anticipated, because of the British bias in the project team, the project diagnoses are much closer to the diagnoses of the Netherne psychiatrists than to those of the Brooklyn psychiatrists.

These striking results were obtained from a comparison of only two hospitals. It was considered necessary to broaden the study to include a representative sample of newly admitted patients from the whole of New York and the whole of London. This was achieved by randomly selecting between 150 and 200 admissions to all nine psychiatric hospitals serving New York, and nine representative hospitals serving the London area. The procedures were exactly the same as in the Brooklyn–Netherne comparison. The main findings are presented in Table II.

The results are very similar to the Brooklyn–Netherne comparison, although perhaps even more remarkable. The distributions of all four major diagnostic groups differ significantly when the hospital diagnoses are compared. All these significant differences disappear when the project diagnoses are compared, and in fact, the project diagnoses on both sides of the Atlantic are remarkably similar in their distribution.

TABLE II

A comparison of the hospital and project diagnoses of the New York and London patients[1]

	New York patients		London patients	
	Hospital diagnosis	*Project diagnosis*	*Project diagnosis*	*Hospital diagnosis*
Schizophrenia	61.5[2]	29.2	35.1	33.9[2]
Depressive psychosis	4.7[2]	19.8	22.3	24.1[2]
Mania	0.5[2]	5.7	6.3	6.9[2]
Personality disorder	1.0[3]	4.2	2.9	4.6[3]

[1] The figures represent percentages of the total sample. Significance levels relate to comparison of the two sets of hospital diagnoses with each other, and the two sets of project diagnoses with each other.
[2] $P < 0.01$.
[3] $P < 0.05$.
From Leff (1977).

This work confirms and underlines previous findings that the American diagnosis of schizophrenia is much broader than the British diagnosis. It includes most of what the British psychiatrists would call mania, which is hardly recognised at all by the New York psychiatrists. It also encompasses substantial parts of what the British psychiatrists would regard as depressive illness, neurotic illness, and personality disorder.

It is evident from these results that if British diagnostic practice is applied to American patients, or if American diagnostic practice is applied to British patients, the striking transatlantic differences in frequency of the various psychiatric conditions disappear. One problem is solved, but is replaced by another; namely, that schizophrenia is a very different condition in New York compared with London. Although the same term is being used, it refers to two quite different diagnostic concepts. This is a serious blow to transatlantic communication in psychiatry and means that the findings of the great mass of studies done on schizophrenia in America cannot automatically be assumed to apply to schizophrenia in the UK.

The findings of the US:UK Project also represent a partial answer to our initial question: schizophrenia does *not* look the same in America and the UK. Does this mean that schizophrenia varies from country to country, or is there some unusual hiatus between British and American views? This question is answered by the other major international study of diagnostic practices, the International Pilot Study of Schizophrenia (IPSS) (World Health Organization, 1973).

The IPSS is a transcultural psychiatric investigation of 1202 patients in nine countries: Colombia, Czechoslovakia, Denmark, India, Nigeria, China, USSR, UK, and USA. It was designed as a pilot study to lay scientific groundwork for future international epidemiological studies of schizophrenia and other psychiatric disorders. Its main aim was to investigate whether schizophrenia as diagnosed by the psychiatrists in each of the participating centres would have the same pattern of signs and symptoms. It was therefore necessary, as in the US:UK Project, to train an international group of psychiatrists to observe signs and symptoms in a standardised way. Once again, the PSE was chosen as the interviewing tool, but whereas this English instrument could be used as it stands in both New York and London, it had to be translated into seven other languages for the purposes of the IPSS. By and large, few problems were encountered in translating the items in the PSE schedule that deal with psychotic symptoms. More serious difficulties arose with the questions relating to neurotic symptoms, and these will be explored in detail in the next chapter. However, for the purpose of studying the diagnosis of psychotic conditions in a diversity of cultures, the PSE appears to be suitable.

Whereas in the US:UK Project, the research team acted as a transportable diagnostic standard, the aim in the IPSS was to study and compare the diagnostic habits of the research psychiatrists themselves, on the assumption that they were representative of psychiatric practice in their respective countries. Hence, it would have defeated the object of the IPSS to make any attempt to standardise the diagnostic practice of the research psychiatrists. Therefore, they were trained in the use of the PSE and were then instructed to continue making diagnoses on the research patients just as they would in their usual clinical work. They used the translated versions of the PSE to interview a consecutive series of more than 100 psychotic patients admitted to their local psychiatric facilities. The screening criteria for 'psychosis' were deliberately chosen to represent broad limits in order to include a wide variety of patients who might receive a local diagnosis of schizophrenia.

A total of 1202 patients from the nine centres were included in the study as satisfying the screening criteria for psychosis, and 77.5% of them were given a diagnosis of schizophrenia by the research psychiatrists. A straightforward way of comparing schizophrenic patients in the various centres is to construct symptom profiles, using the percentage of patients exhibiting each symptom. As the signs and symptoms rated with the WHO version of the PSE amounted to 360, it was necessary to reduce them to a more manageable number before constructing profiles. This was done by grouping them into 27 clusters, which were named *units of analysis*, on the basis of clinical judgement and statistical tests of association of items within each cluster.

Fig. 1 shows the symptom profiles of all patients diagnosed as schizophrenic from three of the centres: Aarhus in Denmark; Ibadan in Nigeria; and Washington in the USA. It can be observed that the profiles for Aarhus and Ibadan are closely similar across all the units of analysis. The profile for the Washington schizophrenic subjects approximates to the other two profiles on many of the units of analysis, but diverges on a number of them. In particular, the Washington schizophrenic subjects showed lower proportions than the other two groups on lack of insight (10) and auditory hallucinations (13), and higher proportions on affect-laden thoughts (5), and

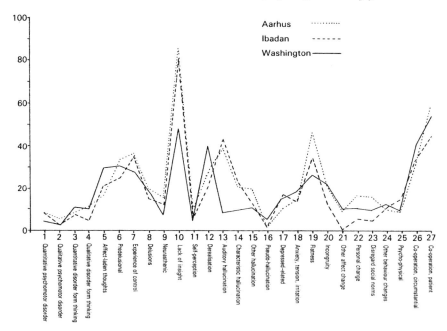

Fig. 1 – Symptom profiles of all patients diagnosed as schizophrenic in the studies at Aarhus, Ibadan and Washington.

derealisation (12). One could infer from this comparison that as a group the patients diagnosed as schizophrenic in the Washington centre were less psychotic and more neurotic than those from Aarhus and Ibadan. This is in accord with the finding of the US:UK Project that a group of patients diagnosed as schizophrenic in New York included a proportion of cases that would be given a diagnosis of neurosis in London. The construction of symptom profiles allows one to see at a glance whether patients given the same diagnosis from all centres have similar patterns of symptoms, but it is more difficult to grasp from this kind of display the nature of the diagnostic process. To do this, it is necessary to have some kind of ruler against which diagnoses made in various centres can be measured.

As we saw in the US:UK Project, the diagnostic ruler was constructed from the project team members by rendering their diagnostic habits as uniform as possible. A different approach was taken in the IPSS, namely to compile a standard set of diagnostic rules that could be applied to the data obtained from the PSE. This procedure has obvious advantages; if the rules can be made explicit, then the diagnostic process can be studied in fine detail; furthermore, the rules can be embodied in a computer program to ensure that their application to the clinical data is free from human error.

The question is, whose rules should be used? Given the current state of knowledge of psychiatric illnesses, this decision must be arbitrary, since we have no criteria for choosing one person's diagnostic scheme rather than another's. All that one can stipulate is that the scheme chosen should preferably represent the mainstream of a major diagnostic tradition, in order that it may be familiar to as many psychiatrists as possible. In practice, the scheme chosen lies in the mainstream of British diagnostic habits and is firmly based on the principles of Kurt Schneider (1957). The rules were formulated and incorporated in a computer program, Catego, which can be used to process the items included in the PSE (Wing *et al*, 1974). It should be noted that the combined use of the PSE and the Catego program represents standardisation of both the assessment, and translation into a diagnosis of symptoms.

It is worth digressing for a moment to consider how the Catego program operates. It is divided into several stages, the first of which consists of the condensation of the large number of PSE items into more manageable groupings. This is done on the basis of clinical judgement that certain items often occur together, and also on account of the diagnostic significance of particular items. Thus, all Schneider's first-rank symptoms are grouped together in a cluster named Nuclear Syndrome. The condensation process of the early stages of Catego results in the reduction of the 360 items of the WHO version of the PSE to 35 syndromes. From then on, another procedure comes into operation, namely a differential weighting of syndromes. This conforms to some extent to a hierarchical model of psychiatric symptoms in which they are organised in the form of a pyramid (Sturt, 1981).

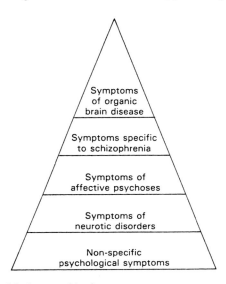

Fig. 2 – The hierarchical pyramid of symptoms.

As can be seen from Fig. 2, patients with organic brain disease exhibit symptoms from all layers of the pyramid. Patients with schizophrenia do not show the disturbances of consciousness typical of patients occupying the top layer, but may have symptoms from all lower levels; and so on down the pyramid. People with only the very lowest layer of symptoms, such as worrying and tension, are quite common in the general population and would not be considered as suffering from distinct psychiatric illnesses. Foulds (Foulds & Bedford, 1975; McPherson *et al*, 1977; Bagshaw & McPherson, 1978) has put forward a similar hierarchical model and has shown that it fits the observed patterns of symptoms for all acute psychiatric illnesses, with the possible exception of mania. Other workers have tested the assumptions of Foulds & Bedford's model, and have found that it accounts for the symptom patterns of between 75% and 96% of patients studied. The research has included patients in Turkey (Gilleard, 1983) and in America (Morey, 1985). The Catego program is by no means unique, and other diagnostic programs constructed on similar principles have been designed in Denmark and the USA.

The PSE findings on all the patients from the nine centres were fed into a computer and processed by the Catego program. The diagnoses resulting from the application of the standardised set of rules can be compared with the centre diagnoses to throw light on the diagnostic process in each centre. This comparison is shown in Table III. The Catego classes S, P, and O are equivalent to clinical diagnoses of schizophrenia and paranoid psychoses, class M to mania, and classes D, R, and N to depressive psychoses and neuroses. The bottom line of the table shows the total discrepancy in diagnosis between Catego and the centre psychiatrists for each centre.

The total discrepancy between Catego classes and centre diagnoses is smallest for the London centre. This is readily explicable, since I made virtually all the diagnoses on the London patients, and am a colleague of Wing, who was largely responsible for the construction of the Catego program. Such an explanation cannot account for the remarkably small discrepancy between Catego and the Taipei psychiatrists, complete agreement being achieved on schizophrenia. It should be noted that since the Catego procedure is a complex one, the likelihood of such close agreement being reached by chance is negligible, and it is safe to assume that the Taipei psychiatrists were using diagnostic rules very similar, if not identical, to Catego.

Consideration of the nine centres reveals that only in Moscow and Washington is the discrepancy large enough to indicate a substantial difference from Catego in diagnostic procedure. If these two centres are excluded, the overall agreement between the seven remaining centres and Catego is 95.5% on schizophrenia and 86.2% on affective psychoses and neuroses. For Moscow and Washington combined the agreement with Catego is only 70.5%. It can be seen from Table III that this discrepancy is largely accounted for by broad definitions of schizophrenia in both these

TABLE III

A comparison of centre diagnosis and Catego classes

Catego classes	Aarhus	Agra	Cali	Ibadan	London	Moscow	Taipei	Washington	Prague
Centre schizophrenia and paranoid psychoses									
S, P, O	73	92	97	117	100	52	107	75	73
M	—	5	4	5	1	10	—	11	8
D, R, N	4	3	1	—	—	21	—	10	7
Centre mania									
S, P, O	4	2	—	1	1	1	1	—	—
M	18	18	3	3	6	—	5	4	9
D, R, N	—	—	—	—	—	2	—	1	—
Centre depressive psychoses and neuroses									
S, P, O	4	6	2	7	3	4	4	3	2
M	5	2	1	1	—	1	1	1	—
D, R, N	15	9	6	9	16	20	13	16	25
Total patients	123	137	114	143	127	111	131	121	124
Percentage discrepancy	13.8	13.1	7.0	9.8	3.9	35.1	4.6	21.5	13.7

From Leff (1977).

centres, with substantial proportions of centre schizophrenics being assigned by Catego to mania or depressive psychoses and neuroses. The results for Washington echo the findings of the US:UK Project. While the Moscow psychiatrists also have an unusually broad concept of schizophrenia, this stems from a different approach from that of American psychiatrists. American diagnostic practice has been strongly influenced by the psychoanalytic movement, with considerable emphasis being placed on intrapsychic processes such as *projection*, and notions such as *weak ego-strength*. These abstractions are conceived as underlying a whole range of symptoms, and are used as criteria for the presence of psychosis. This reliance on inferring the presence of non-observable abstractions apparently leads to a broad definition of schizophrenia.

In Moscow the departure from symptomatology as a basis for diagnosis is not a consequence of psychoanalytic theories, which are held in low esteem, but of an emphasis on the course of psychiatric conditions. All the Moscow centre psychiatrists came from the same institute, headed by Professor Snezhnevsky. A school of psychiatry developed under his leadership in which the description of the course taken by the illness and the level of social adjustment between episodes of symptoms were given greater importance than the symptoms themselves. This did not result in a neglect of the phenomena of symptoms, as generally occurred in the USA. The symptoms occurring in each episode of illness are carefully described, and the clinical pictures that emerge are instantly recognisable to a British psychiatrist; it is the significance given to the episode that is different. The Moscow psychiatrists identify three main varieties of course of illness that characterise schizophrenia (see Fig. 3). Periodic schizophrenia consists of

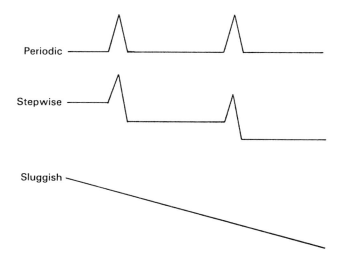

Fig. 3 – Varieties of schizophrenia in the Moscow school.

recurrent acute episodes of symptoms, many of which would be diagnosed by British psychiatrists (and Catego) as manic or depressive, following which the social adjustment of the patient returns to the premorbid level. In stepwise schizophrenia, the social adjustment following each episode of illness is lower than it was before the episode. In sluggish schizophrenia, there are no discrete episodes, but an inexorable downhill course. This entity seems to correspond to British chronic schizophrenia. We saw in Chapter 1 that psychiatric diagnosis incorporates a substantial social component. However, in the Moscow school, this is considerably greater than elsewhere because of the emphasis placed on social adjustment between episodes of symptoms. This practice takes on a particular significance in a society that is relatively intolerant of deviations from a cultural norm. Thus, eccentric or rebellious individuals may be viewed as 'suffering' from deterioration in their social adjustment. The diagnostic practice of the Moscow school does not necessarily represent the whole of Russian psychiatric practice. It appears that in Leningrad psychiatric diagnosis is much closer to that in the United Kingdom and Germany.

For the seven centres other than Washington and Moscow, it is clear that the diagnostic rules operated by the centre psychiatrists must be very similar to those incorporated in Catego. Schneider's first-rank symptoms ought to be of central importance in the diagnosis of schizophrenia. One can calculate the probability that a centre psychiatrist will make such a diagnosis when a particular first-rank symptom is present. The probabilities are as follows: third-person auditory hallucinations, 95%; voices commenting on the patient's thoughts or actions, 95%; thought broadcast, insertion, or withdrawal, 97%; delusions of control, 96%. Only in a tiny minority of cases is a diagnosis other than schizophrenia made when a first-rank symptom is present.

These findings prompt us to ask why Schneider's first-rank symptoms, elaborated from his experience with German psychiatric patients, should be in regular use by psychiatrists in such a diversity of cultures. One of the reasons must be his claim that these symptoms are pathognomonic for schizophrenia. That means that if one first-rank symptom is present, the patient should automatically receive a diagnosis of schizophrenia. Schneider's proposition is an attractive one as it seems to put diagnosis on a solid basis, but in the absence of any confirmatory test for schizophrenia, it is virtually impossible to evaluate the truth of his assertion. Nevertheless, it is apparent that the psychiatrists involved in the IPSS were using first-rank symptoms in the way he recommended. It is also evident that they have not each made this discovery independently, but that Schneider's doctrine has spread around the world within the psychiatric community. Another reason for its popularity is likely to be that the descriptions he gives of first-rank symptoms are culture-free and hence applicable in any language and cultural setting. This would be supported by the experience of the psychiatrists in the IPSS.

It must be emphasised that psychiatrists throughout the world are willing to make a diagnosis of schizophrenia in patients who do not exhibit any first-rank symptoms. It is these patients who give rise to most diagnostic disagreements among psychiatrists. The proportion they make up of all patients diagnosed schizophrenic varies considerably from place to place. For example, first-rank symptoms were present in 68% of patients labelled schizophrenic in the London centre of the IPSS, but in only 25% of a recent sample of schizophrenic patients examined in Sri Lanka (Chandrasena & Rodrigo, 1979). Such a marked difference could be due to the contrast between a narrow and a broad definition of schizophrenia. However, it could also result from differences in the kind of patients attending psychiatric facilities. These possibilities will be explored later in the book.

These two major international studies, the US:UK Project and the IPSS, were carefully planned and carried out over a number of years with detailed consideration being given to standardisation of research techniques. They revealed that psychiatrists in the USA and in Moscow had different operational definitions of schizophrenia from those in many other parts of the world. However, the patterns of symptoms exhibited by psychotic patients in all the places studied were remarkably similar. It is not that completely different kinds of patients were being called schizophrenic in the USA and Moscow compared with elsewhere. Patients diagnosed as schizophrenic in countries as diverse as India, Nigeria, and Nationalist China would have been given the same diagnosis in the USA and Moscow. However, in the latter two places, patients with other kinds of symptom pictures were included under the rubric of schizophrenia. Since the publication of these two studies, American diagnostic practice has been dramatically altered, at least officially, by the production of DSM–III (American Psychiatric Association, 1980). Unlike its predecessors, this edition of the manual advocates the use of operationally defined phenomenological criteria to arrive at a diagnosis. Furthermore, one of the criteria specified for a diagnosis of schizophrenia is a duration of illness of at least 6 months. By contrast, the criteria for affective disorders have been considerably broadened and include Schneider's first-rank symptoms if these occur during a full affective syndrome. The diagnostic pendulum has swung in the USA with remarkable velocity. The official diagnostic category of schizophrenia is now somewhat narrower than its European counterpart instead of being twice as broad. However, official policy is one thing and clinical practice quite another. As Mukherjee (1983) points out, it will be necessary for American psychiatrists to adjust from a psychodynamic to a phenomenological paradigm if they are to assimilate DSM–III into their everyday practice.

At present, we have no way of deciding whether a broad or narrow definition of schizophrenia is more valid. This decision will have to await the discovery of some index other than symptoms – one capable of differentiating between the major psychoses. However, in the mean time, we can confidently state that both schizophrenia and manic–depressive psychoses appear symptomatically similar across a wide variety of cultural settings. Psychoses do indeed seem to be universal.

We have to record two reservations about this broad statement. One is that, as discussed above, the instruments used in these studies were constructed in the West and may have imposed a cultural stereotype on the patient populations examined. It is necessary to repeat these kinds of international comparisons with clinical instruments developed in non-Western cultures. The second reservation is that none of these studies included a pre-literate culture such as is found in New Guinea or among South American Indians.

4 The language of emotion

Turning from the psychoses to the neuroses, two startling facts that have to be accounted for by any broad theory concerning cultural variation in neurotic conditions are faced. One is the marked and rapid decline in the prevalence of hysteria in the West compared with its persistence in the rest of the world. This forms the topic of the next chapter. The other is the absence from a number of languages of verbal equivalents of anxiety and depression. This gap in certain vocabularies first came to our attention when the PSE was translated from English into the seven other languages included in the IPSS. Difficulties in finding words for various unpleasant emotional states were encountered when translating into Yoruba, a Nigerian language, and Chinese. In particular the words *depression* and *anxiety* seemed to have no direct equivalents in Yoruba. Instead, two phrases equivalent to them were found that were later respectively back-translated as "the heart is weak" and "the heart is not at rest". The problem with Chinese was that only one word could be found to stand for *anxiety*, *tension*, and *worrying*, these being well-differentiated items in the original English version of the PSE. No such difficulties were found in translating the PSE into the other five languages, Czech, Danish, Hindi, Russian, and Spanish, which belong to the same family as English, namely the Indo-European group.

Translation of a word from one language to another is not a simple matter of finding as exact an equivalent as possible. Even at this basic level, it is possible to commit howlers that are not shown up by back-translation. Swartz *et al* (1985) translated the PSE into Xhosa and used the term *inimba* for 'emotions'. They subsequently discovered that although *inimba* does denote emotions, it does so specifically as a feeling-state that cannot be experienced by men. Consequently they had to reword an apparently adequate translation. This example emphasises the importance of context in understanding the usage of words, a point made strongly by Beeman (1985), who wrote, "The question of the pragmatic use of language is in fact central to the study of the meaning of any linguistic complex". In order to determine the meaning of non-Western terminology used to describe emotional disorder,

43

he advises thorough study of the way the terms are actually used in natural interaction contexts for describing emotional distress. He makes a distinction between everyday social interactions and ''those that pit physician against patient in Western fashion'', which he states do not exist in many places in the world. This is obviously correct, but in the absence of Western physicians, and often alongside them as well, traditional healers perform a similar role. The process of negotiation of emotional distress between client and healer, whether traditional or Western, plays a crucial role in the definition of emotionally based symptoms, and will be considered in a later chapter. For the present discussion, it is sufficient to bear in mind Beeman's point that emotional distress may be presented very differently to the person's social circle and to the healer.

There is considerable evidence that words that denote pathological emotional states in European lexicons are lacking in many non-Indo-European languages. Marsella (1979) reviewed cross-cultural studies of depression and noted that research on indigenous categories of mental disorders in Malaysia, Borneo, Africa, and among American Indians, revealed that there were no concepts that represented depression as either a disease, symptom, or syndrome. However, that does not preclude the existence of words or phrases that convey sadness in ordinary social intercourse. Morice (1978) studied the Pintupi tribe of aborigines in Western Australia and found a rich and varied lexicon in the areas of fear and anxiety, and grief and depression. The Pintupi make many fine distinctions, for instance between a sudden frightened feeling that makes the person turn around, *kamarrarringu*, and a sudden fear that causes a person to stand up to see what is causing it, *nginyiwarrarringu*. An example from the area of depression is provided by the contrast between *minyirrpa*, a serious mood with no talking or laughing, often caused by sadness or loneliness, and accompanied by worry and bad dreams, and *mirrpanpa*, a serious mood with reduced speech, often associated with anger.

Even when an extensive vocabulary in the area of emotion is lacking, it does not follow that speakers of the language cannot express emotions in other ways. Henry (1936) studied Kaingang, a Brazilian Indian language which has a restricted vocabulary for emotions. He noted that, ''By means of changes in pitch and force of articulation, through modification of sounds, by unconscious contraction of the pharynx and unconscious changes of the vowels; by means of changes in facial expression and bodily position, Kaingang achieves a richness of color and flexibility, which could never be inferred from the manifest content of the language''. Henry's observations prompt us to consider the variety of means whereby emotions may be experienced and expressed. This is an entire field of study in itself which is currently undergoing a theoretical reappraisal, but it is necessary to make some forays into it, as it is fundamental to our concerns.

In a theoretical analysis of the role of cognition in emotion, Leventhal & Scherer (1987) came to the conclusion that all childhood and adult emotional behaviour patterns reflect complex integrations of subjective feeling, auto-nomic responses, expressive motor responses (gesture, posture, speech), and cognition. The cognitive component partly involves the development of schemata, which are created in emotional encounters with the environment and are conceptualised as memories of emotional experience. Schemata are "concrete representations in memory of specific perceptual, motor (expressive, approach-avoidance tendencies and autonomic reactions), and subjective feelings each of which were components of the reactions during specific emotional episodes". In other words, past experiences of emotional encounters with other people shape one's current emotional repertoire. This formulation allows the operation of a major cultural influence in determining the individual's experience of emotion. Leventhal & Scherer cite the example of an infant whose parents regularly tickle it or swing it in the air when it smiles at them. This infant will associate strong autonomic and skeletal motor reactions with its smiling response: its memory schema of happiness might be described as 'excited'. By contrast, an infant whose parents respond to smiles with coos and endearments will develop a different type of schema, which might be termed 'calm happiness'. One can add that an infant whose father and mother respond differently to smiling will develop at least two varieties of happiness schemata.

Research into neonatal psychology has blossomed in the last decade and has produced some surprising findings. Very young babies have proved capable of much finer acts of discrimination than was believed possible. Field *et al* (1982) have shown that smiles, frowns, and expressions of surprise, can be elicited in day-old infants in response to the same facial expressions adopted by adult experimenters. This indicates that the newborn have a built-in capacity to discriminate between at least three basic emotional expressions. How each culture shapes this ability is still a matter for surmise, but by reviewing emotional expressiveness in a variety of cultures, we can gain some idea of the process.

It is a truism that we behave differently in public from the way we behave in private. However, there may be a surprisingly large discrepancy in some cultures. Shweder (1985) studied Oriya Brahman families in Bhubaneswar, India, and discovered that "the husband–wife relationship is scripted for mild avoidance. Spouses may not eat together. They do not address each other by name. They never touch or display affection to each other in public. They move through social life separately . . . . Husband and wife rarely present themselves or appear in public as 'a couple' ". Nevertheless, the Oriya Brahman feels close to his or her spouse, even though a public display of this is out of the question. Shweder warns of the danger of assuming that "choreographed displays of avoidance or aloofness" reveal the underlying private feelings of the actors.

Among the Balinese, the split is not so much between public and private displays of feeling, as between the external signs of emotion and inner events. The inner self contains feelings that are not expressed in gesture or action but are dealt with by meditation. Gesture occupies a separate domain from inner feelings and is regularised by etiquette (Lutz, 1985). The Kaluli, a forest people of Papua New Guinea, provide a striking contrast with the Balinese, since they conceive of emotions in terms of action. Kaluli words for affects are not nouns describing types of feelings, but verbs (Schieffelin, 1985). Affect is displayed openly and often dramatically, and is in part aimed at influencing others. Kaluli have at least seven expressions for states of anger, one of which, *ilib nagalub*, literally translates as 'chest hurts'. There are two expressions for grief or sadness: *nofolab*, to feel sad, feel compassion, and *kuwayab*, to grieve (wail) for death or misfortune. Kaluli society is operated through an evenly balanced system of reciprocity. If a thief steals a pig, the owner may steal a pig from the thief or demand money in compensation. The same concepts are applied to emotional expression. Kaluli anger almost always contains the implication that the angered person has suffered a loss of some kind, and the sufferer expects to be compensated. The extent of a man's rage is in proportion to the loss he has experienced. Grieving is a response to devastating loss and represents an appeal for retaliation and compensation. Grief is publicly expressed and worked through in weeping and song, not just at funerals but on many occasions in ceremonies where it evokes social support.

I referred above to the interlinked components of emotional states: subjective feeling, autonomic responses, expressive motor responses, and cognition, which largely relates to social interactions. Any particular culture may choose to highlight and encourage the development of one or more of these components and to discourage others. In Western cultures there has been an increasing emphasis on subjective feelings, one index of this being the construction and development of psychoanalysis. The aim of the Balinese is to calm and smooth over inner feelings, while for the Kaluli, the value of inner feelings is that they are expressed through action, which operates on the social environment to bring about change. The Oriya Brahman does his best not to express feelings in public, but may do so in the intimacy of his closest relationship.

The autonomic component of emotional states has not been discussed so far. This does emerge as a conscious experience in some cultures, particularly the accelerated pulse and stronger beat of the heart that accompany emotional arousal. We noted above that one of the Kaluli terms for anger literally means 'chest hurts'. Ebigbo (1982), in studying the somatic experiences of Nigerian students, found that 40% of them complained of *obi-ilo-miro*, which is translated literally as 'melting of the heart'. Among Turkish-speaking peoples in Iran, the heart provides an idiom for expressing emotion, for example, *qalbim narahatdi* – 'my heart is upset, uncomfortable, distressed' (Good, 1977). The Xhosa of South Africa use the word *mbilini* to refer to sensations of palpitation, throbbing, discomfort, or pain in the epigastric region. *Mbilini* is associated with increased sensitivity and emotional instability (Cheetham & Cheetham, 1976). Ben-Tovim (1987) explored the use of the phrase *pelo, pelo y tata* by the Tswana. The literal translation is 'heart, heart too much' and the phrase is used to express a variety of forms of distress, including that occasioned by physical pain. Ben-Tovim interviewed a group of Tswana about their concepts of the sites of thinking, worrying, and being angry and sad. He found a widespread belief, particularly among those with no more than a primary education, that the heart was the organ where feelings were generated and controlled.

The above descriptions apply to the emotional experiences of everyday life. Is it safe to assume that pathological emotions are simply exaggerations of these experiences? A study by Yanping *et al* (1986) conducted in China suggests that it is not. They used depressed patients to generate indigenous Chinese phrases or words for key symptoms of depression in the West. From these they constructed a Verbal Expression Style Investigation Schedule (VESIS). This was administered to samples of psychiatric patients with affective illnesses and to a group of normal control subjects. Responses to the VESIS were categorised as psychological, somatic, neutral (a mixture of both), and deficient (no response). 'Depression' was frequently expressed in either a somatic or a neutral mode, a commonly used term being "it is uncomfortable inside my heart". However, it was more frequently expressed somatically by depressed patients than by normal control subjects. Yanping *et al* concluded that patients who have actually experienced pathological depression place greater emphasis on somatic symptoms in their expression of depression than do normal subjects. This could result either from a heightened awareness of autonomic activity in those with emotional disorders, or from actual quantitative or qualitative changes in the autonomic accompaniments themselves. These findings suggest a disjunction between patterns of emotion in everyday interactions, and those exhibited by people who have sought medical help.

Thus differences in the personal descriptions of emotion in pathological states compared with normal, everyday fluctuations may arise from alterations in the nature of the experiences themselves. Additionally, they may be produced by the shaping of experience through the mutual interaction of client and healer, a process which will be explored in a later chapter. Finally, it is conceivable that some cultures have developed means of averting or containing emotional responses that prevent them reaching pathological levels. Some evidence for this intriguing possibility is now presented.

As stated above, the immediate Kaluli response to loss is anger and an expectation of being adequately compensated. Blame over loss is not personally accepted, but is always turned outward as a sense of feeling wronged and owed. Of course, some losses cannot be adequately compensated for, such as death of a loved person, in which case the aggrieved person appeals for social support, which is always forthcoming. In Western cultures, the predominant emotion evoked by loss is depression, in which self-blame is often a major constituent. Brown & Harris (1978) have shown that the support of a confidant is an effective buffer against the impact of loss, but if this is lacking, the person experiencing loss is liable to develop depression. The cultural expectation of the Kaluli is that loss will evoke anger, that blame will be externalised, and that social support will be provided for the individual suffering loss. These may well be effective means of preventing the development of depression. Indeed, Schieffelin (1985) notes that the Kaluli do not recognise depression or have a term for it in their vocabulary.

Iranians certainly do not lack words for depression. Indeed, sadness, grief, and despair are central to the Iranian ethos (Good *et al*, 1985). Secular literature, both classical poetry and modern novels, is filled with melancholy and despair. Tragedy, injustice, and martyrdom are central to Iranian political philosophy and history. Iranian culture ascribes a positive connection to sadness, which is viewed as a mark of personal depth. The ability to express sadness appropriately and in a culturally proscribed manner is an integral component of social competence. Most children first learn to grieve in the context of religious ceremonies for Iranian martyrs. Thus from an early age, experiences of loss, grieving, and sadness are assimilated into the suffering of the wider community. By this means, personal losses are put into the perspective of national tragedy, and no bereaved individual grieves alone. In this culture, the response to individual loss is submerged in the sea of communal consciousness of historical tragedy. This may not be as effective a way of dealing with depressive reactions to loss as the Kaluli employ, since there is a lexicon in Iranian languages for such experiences. The formal Persian word for depression – *afsordegi* – is not commonly used in popular discourse, which instead favours the term *nârâhat*. This means 'not comfortable, upset, or in distress' and includes a range of mixed and undifferentiated anxiety and depressive phenomena. *Narhati-e-qalb* (distress of the heart) refers to palpitations, pressure on the chest, and a sensation of the heart being squeezed, and is often associated with feelings of sadness, dysphoria, and anxiety.

A different way of dealing with loss is employed by the Buddhists of Sri Lanka (Obeyesekere, 1985). In Buddhism, everyone's lot is seen as hopeless. Hopelessness lies in the nature of the world, and salvation lies in understanding and overcoming that hopelessness. This is achieved by recognising the illusory nature of the world of sense, pleasure and domesticity. As in Iran, those afflicted by bereavement and loss can generalise their despair from the self to the community (in this case the whole of humankind) and can invest their experience with a religious significance. Buddhism, however, does not ennoble individual suffering. Instead, the intention is to minimise the sense of loss. The commonest form of meditation practised in Sri Lanka is probably meditation on revulsion, the aim of which is to induce a sense of disgust for sense pleasure, which will emphasise the transitoriness of the body. The body is imagined as "a clay pot, polished on the outside, but full of faeces". This image is extended to include people close to the meditator, such as parents, spouse and children, and eventually to encompass the whole of humanity. Thus a sense of loss may be assuaged by the attenuation of emotional bonds to individuals. Obeyesekere cites the instances of a woman who began such meditation when her father died, and of an elderly man whose regular observances began when the head monk of his village, whom he loved, died. He states that it is almost impossible for a Sinhala person to employ words expressing sorrow without invoking Buddhist concepts. Thus ''words used for personal emotional states resonate with the hopeless dilemma of mankind''.

These three examples suggest that what Obeyesekere calls ''the work of culture'' may be more or less successful in resolving emotional responses to loss. Evidently, longitudinal studies of individuals experiencing loss in a variety of cultures are needed to determine the long-term effectiveness of such cultural resources. Obeyesekere views the definition of painful emotions in terms of a disease known as depression as a Western cultural resource. This 'new definition of human suffering' leads to a different method of coping with loss, namely, the provision of a variety of treatments for the consequent emotional distress, when it is brought to a doctor.

It was noted above that Western cultures have focused increasingly on the subjective feeling component of emotional states. The historical consequences of this have included the relative eclipse of bodily experiences and an increasing differentiation of unpleasant feeling states. Murphy (1982) studied the accounts of melancholia written by Burton in 1621 and Baxter in 1673 and concluded that over that period there was a major shift in the mode of expression from somatic to psychological symptoms. Murphy ascribes it to a number of influences: the rise of Protestantism with the development of a guilt-ridden relationship between man and God, a change in child-rearing patterns towards more consistent parent–child relationships, and the effect of capitalism in increasing economic individualism and a reduction in close social ties. Whatever the causes, the effects on the expression of emotion can be traced through a study of the historical development of English words for unpleasant emotions.

Take the word *anxiety*, which derives from a Greek root αγχω, which meant to press tight or strangle (Lewis, 1967). There are a number of Latin words with the same root, *angustus*, *ango*, *angor*, *anxius*, *anxietas*, and *angina*, angina being the technical term for chest pain caused by ischaemic heart disease. All these words contain the notion of constriction and discomfort. The French word *angoisse*, from which *anguish* is derived, was defined in the 19th century as a feeling of constriction in the epigastric region with difficulty in breathing and great sadness. So far, it is clear that words like anger, anguish, and anxiety have a common root, and embody (literally) some of the somatic accompaniments of unpleasant emotion. A surprising fact is uncovered if the historical development of these words in the English language is considered. In Old English, a language which was current up to the middle of the 12th century, the word *ange* meant to be in trouble and to suffer affliction, while *anger* had a now obsolete meaning of trouble or sorrow. It is of interest in this respect that the modern Icelandic word *angr* means grief or sorrow. It appears that the words we now consider distinct in meaning, anger, anxiety, and sadness, at an earlier stage in the development of English were much closer in meaning, if not interchangeable.

Before trying to account for these interesting observations, we need to introduce two further items of evidence. Modern German exhibits much the same relationships as Modern English; the word *eng* means narrow, and in its superlative form becomes *engste*. This has a close phonetic relationship to *angst*, the word employed regularly by Freud and translated as *anxiety*. The phrase *enge auf der Brust* is used for angina, and the word *enghertig* refers to someone without many feelings. The second piece of evidence is the origin of the word *depression*, which is derived from the Latin root *depremere*, meaning to press down. Many depressed patients complain of a feeling of pressure on the head, the two words being linguistically related.

It seems likely that at some stage in the development of the English vocabulary for unpleasant emotions, one word phonetically similar to the root *angh* denoted a range of relatively undifferentiated feeling states. As the focus shifted from the somatic to the psychological experience of emotion, the root word split up into a number of phonetically related variants. This process, which may well have occurred in other languages of the Indo-European family, led to an overshadowing of the bodily experiences of emotion. Of course, English still offers a profusion of words and phrases that refer directly to the somatic experience of emotion, as is evident from the following passage.

> My heart was in my mouth as I strode up the driveway. Although I hated his guts, my stomach turned over as I approached his house. I knocked on the door and my heart leapt as I heard his footsteps inside. Shivers went down my back as he fumbled with the catch, then as he flung open the door my skin crawled at the sight of him. "I speak from the heart when I say I can't stomach you," I blurted out. He laughed sneeringly and I felt my gorge rise. "You're a pain in the neck," he growled. His retort stuck in my throat. "I am here because of the woman whose heart you have broken," I asserted, and the thought of Amanda brought a lump to my throat. He turned his back on me so suddenly that I almost jumped out of my skin. My brain reeled as I reached for my . . .

These references to bodily experiences are no longer taken at their face (or body) value. They have become metaphors, as they have been supplanted by the extensive range of words for the psychological experience of emotion that has developed in the English language. We often speak of certain patients as 'somatising' their emotions. This reflects our ethnocentric and contemporary bias in disregarding the direction of the historical process that has taken place. We should more properly describe other patients as 'psychologising' their emotions.

The ability to differentiate between unpleasant emotional states can be tested by examining the symptoms of psychiatric patients. Data from the

IPSS, described in the previous chapter, provided an opportunity to compare the degree of differentiation of emotions exhibited by patients from a variety of cultures. A technical problem arose in deciding on a measure of the degree of emotional differentiation shown by a particular patient. The problem was tackled in the following way. It is possible to summate the scores on individual items of a section of the PSE. Thus, one can easily calculate total scores on depression, anxiety, and irritability, the three sections representing major unpleasant emotions covered by the PSE. It is then possible to calculate the correlation coefficient between any pair of total scores. A high correlation between two sections, e.g. depression and anxiety, means that when the patient complains of a great deal of depression, he will also complain of a great deal of anxiety. A low correlation indicates that there is little or no connection between the patient's complaints of anxiety and depression. If patients are able to report that they are depressed, but not at all anxious, it is reasonable to assume that they are making a clear distinction between these emotions. On the other hand, if they always report feeling anxious at the same time as feeling depressed, it is likely that their ability to differentiate between the two emotions is low. Hence, the correlation coefficient between two section scores was used as an index of emotional differentiation, high values representing poor differentiation, and low values, good differentiation (Leff, 1973).

The correlation coefficients between the emotions for the different centres in the IPSS are shown in Table IV. The level of statistical significance of the values is also indicated. The most common pattern of correlations for anxiety:depression, depression:irritability, and anxiety:irritability was high, low, low, respectively, shown by Aarhus, Agra, Moscow, and Prague. This indicates that, in these centres, depression and anxiety were both well differentiated from irritability, but not from each other. The two centres that showed the highest overall correlation were Ibadan and Taipei. These were also the two centres in which the patients speak non-Indo-European languages, which gave rise to difficulties in translating from English some of the emotional symptoms in the PSE. Even within the centres where Indo-European languages were spoken, the patterns were not uniform. For instance, although the patients from London showed the lowest correlation and hence the clearest differentiation between anxiety and depression, they experienced more difficulty in distinguishing depression from irritability than the patients from Agra. The patients from Cali, although speaking Spanish, an Indo-European language, had difficulty in distinguishing anxiety from irritability, despite making a sharper differentiation between depression and irritability than patients from Washington. These findings indicate that the existence of an extensive vocabulary of emotion does not in itself guarantee that patients will be able to make clear distinctions between unpleasant feeling states. The use of the vocabulary is bound to be influenced by the value placed by each culture on the expression of the different feeling states, an area we have surveyed above.

TABLE IV
Correlation coefficients between the emotions for the IPSS centres

Centre	Number of patients	Anxiety: depression	Depression: irritability	Anxiety: irritability
Aarhus, Denmark	129	0.39[1]	0.05	0.13
Agra, India	140	0.51[1]	0.05	0.05
Cali, Colombia	127	0.33[1]	0.16	0.36[1]
Ibadan, Nigeria	145	0.50[1]	0.43[1]	0.26[3]
London, England	127	0.23[3]	0.25[2]	0.18
Moscow, USSR	140	0.32[1]	− 0.10	− 0.01
Prague, Czechoslovakia	122	0.56[1]	− 0.13	− 0.17
Taipei, Taiwan	137	0.62[1]	0.29[2]	0.39[1]
Washington, USA	132	0.37[1]	0.34[1]	0.21[3]

[1] $P < 0.001$.
[2] $P < 0.01$.
[3] $P < 0.05$.
From Leff (1973).

Where an extensive vocabulary of emotion is lacking, it is possible to express a variety of emotions in paralinguistic and non-verbal ways. In respect to these alternative modes of expression, it is of interest to consider recent research on the autonomic expression of emotional distress. For some time it has been assumed that patterns of autonomic activity cannot be utilised to distinguish between emotional states. The prevailing concept has been of a generalised state of arousal, which heightens the subjective experience of emotion, but does not inform the subject which particular emotion has been elicited. Recent work by Ekman *et al* (1983) suggests that this view has to be modified. They measured five physiological parameters in subjects who were asked to perform a non-emotional expression, an emotional expression, and to relive a past emotional experience. The emotions simulated were surprise, disgust, sadness, anger, fear, and happiness. When performing the emotional expression, subjects were told precisely which muscles to contract and were helped by a coach and by observing their own face in a mirror. Ekman *et al* found that these directed facial expressions produced more clear-cut differences than the relived emotions. In particular, the heart rate was significantly higher in 'fear', 'sad', and 'anger' than in 'happy', 'disgust' and 'surprise'. Skin temperature was significantly higher in 'anger' than in 'fear' and 'sad'. This finding is echoed in the popular expressions – red with rage, and white with fear. 'Sad' showed significantly larger decreases in skin resistance than other negative emotions. Ekman *et al* consider the possibility that subjects produced these patterns of autonomic activity by viewing their own face in the mirror or the coach's face. They discount this as unlikely, but the work of Field *et al* (1982) quoted above, showing that the new-born have an innate ability to discriminate facial expressions, supports this explanation. On this basis, it would be social interaction with other people expressing emotion that produces the most differentiated autonomic responses. Whatever the mechanism, it now appears that bodily experiences can be used to discriminate between emotions. The next chapter considers a condition that, more than any other in psychiatry, comprises the bodily representation of emotional distress: hysteria.

5 The history and geography of hysteria

Before considering changes in the distribution of hysteria over time and around the world, it is necessary to discuss the nature of the condition. Hysteria has been known from ancient times, and according to Plato was due to the womb coming adrift from its moorings and wandering all over the body causing symptoms in a multiplicity of organs. The word hysteria derives from the Greek for womb. It is used for at least two different presentations of symptoms. One consists of a large variety of bodily symptoms complained of by a single patient in the absence of organic disease. This appears to correspond to the Platonic description of hysteria, and has been labelled Briquet's syndrome (Briquet, 1859). The other presentation is usually confined to a single organ or part of the body. It is characterised by a loss or disturbance of function which does not conform to what is known about the anatomy and physiology of the body. Thus, the patient loses the ability to speak, but can still sing or whisper. If the loss of speech is due to damage to the vocal apparatus or to the part of the brain controlling speech, singing and whispering would also be affected. Another example of this discrepancy is afforded by hysterical anaesthesia, in which the area of numbness usually affects a body part like the hand or arm, rather than following the distribution of a particular nerve to the skin. Any function of the body can be involved in hysteria – sight, hearing, touch, movement, balance – and organic diseases can be imitated, for instance, epilepsy. Henry Head (1922) commented that "no branch of medicine is free from the puzzling manifestations of hysteria". He felt, however, that the distinction from organic disease should be simple for the experienced clinician. He wrote that "hysteria is sometimes said to 'imitate' organic affections; but this is a highly misleading statement. The mimicry can only deceive an observer ignorant of the signs of hysteria or content with perfunctory examination". This confidence was not shared by Janet (1965) who commented on "the distinction between the epileptic and the hysterical fit, which was a long time considered impossible". How can we reconcile this difference of opinion between two experts?

The answer lies in the fact that the form of a hysterical symptom is determined by the patient's concept of disordered function. Hysterical anaesthesia involves the whole hand, and stops abruptly at the wrist, because the patient thinks of the hand as being a functional unit, and is unaware of the distribution of nerves to the skin of the hand. Janet (1965) wrote that the hysterical phenomena "are the result of the very idea the patient has of his accident". He went on to emphasise the unique character of hysteria: "There is not any organic disease nor even any other mental disease in which matters go in this way. Nobody will maintain that in a maniacal fit the patient is agitated because he is thinking of agitation". Once it is acknowledged that the patient's own idea of pathology is translated into a physical disability, it follows that the degree to which a hysterical symptom mimics organic disease depends on the level of medical sophistication of the subject. Thus, someone who has witnessed an epileptic fit is more likely to produce a hysterical fit that looks like the real thing than a person who has not. To carry this argument further, the patient who has experienced an epileptic fit is likely to throw the most convincing hysterical fit of all. This is not just a hypothetical conjecture. Hysteria can complicate epilepsy, and the distinction between true and hysterical fits in such cases can puzzle the most experienced clinician. The most difficult cases of hysteria to diagnose correctly are those occurring in members of the medical profession, who have the expertise required to mimic organic disease perfectly.

A recent instance of this diagnostic dilemma is provided by what has become known as Royal Free Disease. This was an epidemic of neurological, psychiatric, and other miscellaneous symptoms, which swept through the staff of the Royal Free Hospital in London between July and November 1955. A total of 292 members of staff were affected and 255 were admitted (Medical Staff of the Royal Free Hospital, 1957). The earliest symptoms of the condition were malaise and headaches, frequently associated with disproportionate depression and emotional lability. Characteristic of the fully developed syndrome were pain in the neck, back, or limbs, and dizziness. At times the pains were severe enough to require the strongest analgesics for their control. Patients frequently complained of hypersomnia, nightmares, panic states, and uncontrollable weeping. Motor weakness was found more commonly than sensory disturbance and was noted in 69% of cases. A facial palsy was found in just under one-fifth of the patients, bulbar palsy occurred in 11 cases, and one patient developed a total paralysis of the eye muscles with ptosis. There was a tendency for day-to-day variation in the intensity of symptoms and signs. The condition was found more often in women staff than men, more commonly in resident than in non-resident staff, and affected a disproportionate number of those under the age of 35. In the Medical Staff Report, it was concluded that an infective agent was responsible, because of the explosive character of the outbreak. However, none was found despite careful and extensive investigations, and fewer than 5% of the sufferers developed a fever of over 100 °F. Nevertheless, the report presented the epidemic as an outbreak of encephalomyelitis caused by an unknown virus.

McEvedy & Beard (1970) were not impressed with this interpretation of the data and put forward an alternative suggestion that Royal Free Disease was in fact an epidemic of hysteria. They re-examined the neurological findings and discovered from the charts of sensory loss that this almost always affected a whole limb, and if part of a limb was involved there was invariably a horizontal upper limit to the anaesthesia. Thus the pattern of sensory loss rarely, if ever, followed the distribution of nerves to the skin: instead it was characteristic of hysteria. They went through the clinical notes of individual cases and found descriptions of 'fits' that were hysterical in nature rather than resembling epilepsy. Indeed, the clinicians who had witnessed them recorded their impressions that these were hysterical phenomena. McEvedy & Beard also pointed out that the spread of the symptoms, predominantly affecting young female resident staff, is characteristic of epidemics of hysteria, which usually occur in populations of segregated females, e.g. in girls' schools (Moss & McEvedy, 1966), convents (Huxley, 1952), and factories (Kerckhoff & Back, 1968).

McEvedy & Beard's interpretation of the Royal Free epidemic elicited irate letters in the *British Medical Journal* (1970, i, pp. 170–171), in which correspondents declared themselves to be "incredulous" and "upset", and the interpretation to be "nonsense". McEvedy & Beard clearly anticipated this kind of response, as they wrote in their paper: "Many people will feel that the diagnosis of hysteria is distasteful". It is true that hysteria has a pejorative ring in our society, but that should not prevent doctors from weighing the evidence dispassionately. McEvedy & Beard (1973) later followed up the patients involved in the epidemic and compared them with members of the medical staff who had not been affected. They found that the patients had higher scores on the neurotic questions of a personality inventory than unaffected staff, and had been admitted to hospital more often than the control subjects before the epidemic. On follow-up examination, two of the patients indicated that they had faked a high temperature at the time of the epidemic.

In retrospect, it is very difficult to decide between a viral infection of the central nervous system and an epidemic of hysteria. It might have been somewhat easier at the time if the clinicians involved had been more willing to consider hysteria as a possibility. However, the main lesson to be drawn for the purpose of our argument is that distinguishing hysteria from organic disease in a population of medical professionals is exceedingly difficult.

Having progressed some way towards defining the nature of hysteria, we may now consider its history and geography. It is difficult to determine changes in the frequency of occurrence of hysteria over time accurately because of the paucity of adequate records prior to the last 30 years. However, anecdotal evidence is available from social documents, and fairly detailed figures were produced by military hospitals during the two world wars. We know from novels of the era that Victorian ladies were inclined to swoon when their emotions were aroused. So prevalent was this behaviour that most women carried a bottle of smelling salts in their handbag. It was believed that the wandering womb disliked the pungent odour and would return to its place, allowing the woman to recover consciousness. This hysterical mode of reaction to emotionally arousing situations now rarely occurs in individuals, although it may still be seen among massed teenage girls at concerts of pop music. A set of data is available from Victorian Britain which provides some estimate of the relative frequency of hysteria. The District Surgeon for Glasgow was responsible for compiling an annual report of domiciliary visits to the poor. This included a breakdown by diagnostic category, of the number of patients seen and treated outside the hospital. In 1828 the number of patients with hysteria was 38, about one-third the number with fever (116), and more than double the number with bronchitis (15). Hysteria was certainly common enough in Europe at the end of the last century to attract considerable attention from neurologists such as Charcot and Freud. Ernest Jones reports that ''Freud's studies under Charcot had centered largely on hysteria, and when he was back in Vienna in 1886 and settled down to establish a practice in nervous diseases, hysteria provided a large proportion of his clientele'' (in Breuer & Freud, 1956). Since that time, hysteria has become excessively rare in psychiatric practice, but we have to rely on the medical records of the two world wars to document its decline during the first half of this century.

Hysteria attracted the attention of military doctors because of the obvious secondary gain – it invariably led to soldiers being taken out of the front line, and because of the need to develop rapid means of curing the physically healthy men affected (Hurst & Symms, 1918). It was initially labelled *shell shock* in World War I and *battle neurosis* in World War II, but these conditions are readily identifiable as hysteria from the clinical descriptions given at the time. Under battle conditions, the way in which hysterical symptoms provide a solution for emotional conflicts is particularly clear. A soldier torn between fear of facing death and shame at being thought a coward may develop a hysterical paralysis of his arm, sickness being a legitimate way out of the conflict. An amusing instance of the transparency of such symptoms is given by Forsyth (1920). He describes a soldier who was zealously obedient but ''at heart a red-hot revolutionary''. He had nearly recovered from his wounds and was allowed to go into town for the first time. ''But as luck would have it, this was the very day when there arrived from London that famous order of the War Office requiring even wounded soldiers to salute officers in public. This seems to have stirred mixed emotions. In the event, as he reached the town and saw the first officer approaching, he straightened himself in soldierly fashion and at the correct moment began to raise his right arm in salute. But . . . when his arm got half-way up it stuck, the three middle fingers curled into the palm, and with thumb and little finger stiffly extended – thumb at the tip of the nose, little finger to the officer – he walked past. From that moment, his arm has never gone higher than the level of his nose, and no hand of marble could have retained its expression more faithfully''. The soldier was discharged from the army on an invalid pension.

Several authors have recorded their impressions of the frequency of hysteria during World War I. Hurst & Symms (1918) commented that hysterical symptoms formed one of the largest classes of war neuroses, while Head (1922) wrote that "disorders of speech were amongst the commonest hysterical affections due to the strain of war''. Actual figures are given by Culpin (1920), who obtained 415 records of cases of psychoneurosis from military hospitals. Unfortunately, he gives no details regarding the method of selecting cases, so that one cannot assess whether his series is representative of patients admitted to military hospitals. He identified the primary diagnosis as being hysteria in 115 cases (28%) whereas anxiety state was the primary diagnosis in 205 cases (49%). These figures may be compared with those given by Hadfield (1942), who commented that the most striking change in war neurosis from World War I to World War II was "the far greater proportion of anxiety states in this war, as against conversion hysteria in the last war''. Unfortunately, he does not quote figures from World War I, but records that of the patients suffering from psychoneuroses admitted to a neuropathic hospital from the army in World War II, 371 (64%) out of 577 were diagnosed as having anxiety neurosis, which included depression, compared with 170 (24%) with a diagnosis of hysteria. It is impossible to determine whether these figures are comparable with those given by Culpin, but they do indicate a higher ratio of anxiety neuroses to hysteria than in Culpin's data.

World War II not only afforded comparisons with World War I in terms of patterns of neurotic symptoms, but also provided the opportunity for cross-cultural comparisons between troops from widely differing cultural backgrounds. Abse (1950) studied hysteria in India during World War II. He tabulated the number of patients admitted to the Indian Military Hospital in Delhi during the year 1944. Of a total of 644 patients, 370 (57%) were diagnosed as suffering from hysteria and 80 (12%) with anxiety states. He also collected data from a British Military Hospital in Chester for the months of June–October 1943. The distribution of diagnoses was 161 (24%) out of 669 suffering from hysteria, and 331 (50%) with anxiety states. The figures for the British hospital are very similar to those given by Hadfield (1942) and are markedly different from the Indian hospital data. For ease of comparison, the available figures are presented in Table V.

It is evident that the difference between the British figures over time is trivial compared with the reversal of proportions shown by the Indian soldiers. These data are supplemented by a study conducted by Williams (1950) of British and Indian soldiers fighting in Burma. His figures relate to consultations rather than admissions, so are not directly comparable with the data in Table V. Nevertheless, the patterns of distribution of neurotic

TABLE V
Distribution of hysteria and anxiety states in military hospitals

	British soldiers (%)			Indian soldiers (%)
	World War I	World War II		World War II
	Culpin (1920)	Hadfield (1942)	Abse (1950)	Abse (1950)
Hysteria	28	24	24	57
Anxiety states	49	64	50	12

conditions are very similar. Williams, who spoke Urdu, was a psychiatrist appointed to an Indian division from 1944 to 1945, during which there was a period of fighting in Burma with jungle battles and an opposed landing. Throughout the 18-month period, there were six times as many Indian as British troops in the area. The referral rate to the psychiatrist was two-and-a-half times more frequent in all British than in all Indian troops. Over 50% of the British troops referred presented with an anxiety state compared with less than 10% of the Indians. Hysterical reactions were shown by 32% of Indian patients compared with 7% of the British. Here we see the same reversal of the hysteria:anxiety state ratio in the Indian soldiers when compared with the British as appeared in Abse's data. Williams makes the additional point that Indian hysterical patients were often of high morale and were of all grades of intelligence, whereas among the British, gross hysterical reactions were the breakdowns of men with low stability and morale and usually of low intelligence. This contrasts vividly with Hurst's (1919) experience during World War I that "many cases of gross hysterical symptoms occurred in soldiers who had no family or personal history of neuroses, and who were perfectly fit."

The data presented suggest that from World War I to World War II there was a small relative decline of hysteria among British soldiers, which was paralleled by a relative rise in anxiety states. Clinical observations suggest that as hysteria declines in frequency, it tends to be found among soldiers of relatively low morale and intelligence. By contrast, hysteria was still the most common form of neurosis among Indian soldiers in World War II and affected those of good morale and normal intelligence. The contrasting patterns shown by British and Indian soldiers suggest that hysteria and anxiety neurosis bear a reciprocal relationship to each other, so that the decline of the former is compensated for by a rise in the latter. This reciprocity is not so absolute as to preclude the coexistence of the two conditions in the same patient. As Head (1922) commented: "In a large number of cases, especially in civil life, removal of hysterical symptoms is only a prelude to the discovery of an anxiety neurosis".

This chapter has so far concentrated on military records, because they yield more readily comparable data than civilian records for the first half of this century. They involve the disadvantage of recording the responses of a restricted age group of men under extreme stress. It could be argued that the kind of stress encountered under battle conditions is particularly conducive to the precipitation of hysterical symptoms. This argument would not explain the differential frequency of hysteria in British and Indian troops fighting in the same area under the same conditions (Williams, 1950).

Centralised records for the civilian population of England and Wales came into being with the establishment of the National Health Service in 1948. It proved possible to extract from them, with the assistance of the Statistics and Research Unit of the Department of Health and Social Security, the number of admissions for hysteria to psychiatric hospitals in England and Wales from the year 1949 onwards. There is a gap in the records from 1961 to 1969 inclusive when the information for hysteria as a separate neurotic condition was not available. In Table VI, we present the number of cases of hysteria admitted each year, the percentage they make up of all admissions

TABLE VI

Annual admissions for hysteria to psychiatric hospitals in England and Wales

Year	Number of admissions with hysteria	Percentage of neurotic conditions	Percentage of all admissions
1949	1628	19.77	2.92
1951	1766	18.95	2.98
1953	1970	18.35	2.92
1954	2016	16.03	2.81
1955	2091	16.21	2.66
1956	2152	16.43	2.56
1957	2172	16.06	2.44
1958	2005	14.20	2.13
1959	2226	13.90	2.11
1960	2425	14.19	2.12
1970	2402	9.30	1.31
1971	2333	8.97	1.27
1972	2056	7.89	1.11
1973	1958	8.08[1]	1.06
1974	1870	7.86[1]	1.03
1975	1759	7.21[1]	0.95
1976	1639	—	0.86
1977	1530	—	0.82
1978	1459	—	0.80

[1] Figures available for England only. Percentage has been scaled up to give estimate of figures for England and Wales.

These figures are derived from tables in the Registrar General's Statistical Review – Mental Health Supplement, 1949–1970, and the Mental Health Enquiry, 1970–1978, Crown copyright, HMSO, London.

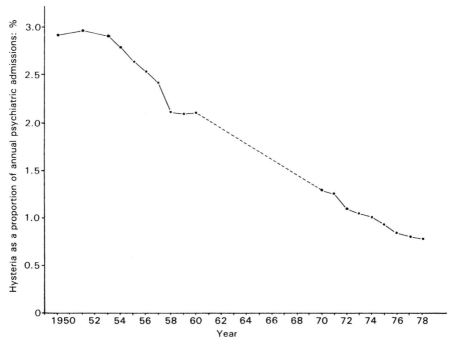

Fig. 4 – Hysteria as a percentage of annual admissions to psychiatric hospitals in England and Wales, 1949–1978.

for a neurotic condition, and the percentage of all admissions regardless of diagnosis.

It is evident that in the 30 years covered by these records, hysteria as a proportion of admissions for neuroses and of all psychiatric admissions has diminished by nearly two-thirds. The decline of admissions for hysteria is presented graphically in Fig. 4. After a plateau during the early years of record-keeping, the graph begins to descend in 1954 and continues to do so thereafter in an almost linear fashion. A possible explanation for this is that, over this period, the responsibility for treating patients with hysteria shifted from psychiatrists to neurologists. This can be checked by analysing data for non-psychiatric hospitals. Unfortunately the figures available for these do not relate to admissions but to discharges and deaths. However since discharges plus deaths must equal admissions over a period of time, and since death from hysteria is virtually non-existent, they can be treated as equivalent to admission figures. In Fig. 5, the data for discharges and deaths from non-psychiatric hospitals have been expressed as cases per million population. They demonstrate a steady reduction over time to the extent that the rate for 1982 is less than one-third of that for 1958. Consequently, when these figures are added to the admission rate for psychiatric hospitals to constitute the upper graph in Fig. 5, the linear decline of Fig. 4 is reproduced. This reduction, documented on a national scale, is also evident in microcosm when data from the Camberwell Register are examined, allowing us to study the phenomenon in finer detail. This advantage stems from a methodological advance in the maintenance of records, namely the setting up of psychiatric case registers, which record all contacts with the psychiatric services made by people living in a particular geographical area. The Camberwell Register (Wing & Hailey, 1972) was established in 1965 to cover the old London borough of Camberwell, a predominantly working-class area in the south-east of the city. It is possible to determine the number of patients from the catchment area who make contact with the psychiatric services, either out-patient or in-patient, each year. The total number of episodes of contact each year labelled as cases of hysteria are shown in Table VII, together with the overall total for all diagnoses.

A marked decline in the proportion of psychiatric contacts diagnosed as hysteria occurs from 1971 onwards, after which time the condition virtually disappears. These figures are somewhat misleading, since they do not distinguish between individuals and occasions; i.e. the same individual making contact three times in a year is recorded as three separate episodes of contact. It is more satisfactory to count each individual only once and, furthermore, to credit only their first-ever contact with a psychiatric service. The figures are standardised even further if out-patient contacts are excluded, leaving only admissions to hospital to be counted. This is known as the first-admission rate or incidence, and is given for hysteria in Table VII. The decline in the incidence of hysteria occurs more gradually than the decline

TABLE VII
Hysteria in Camberwell

| Year | Camberwell contacts with psychiatric services | | First admissions with hysteria |
	Hysteria	All diagnoses	
1965	9 (1.6%)	555	4
1966	10 (1.9%)	520	3
1967	9 (1.6%)	564	0
1968	11 (1.8%)	624	2
1969	6 (0.9%)	642	0
1970	12 (1.8%)	653	1
1971	3 (0.5%)	638	0
1972	1 (0.1%)	691	1
1973	0	620	0
1974	1 (0.1%)	628	1
1975	1 (0.1%)	755	0
1976	2 (0.2%)	777	1
1977	0	729	0
1978	0	NK	0

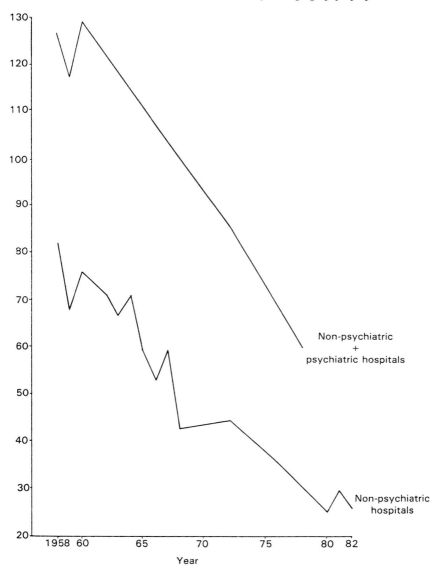

Fig. 5 – Admissions, discharges, and deaths with hysteria in NHS hospitals in England and Wales.

in proportion of psychiatric contacts, and becomes apparent several years earlier. One can readily calculate the average incidence of hysteria over the 14 years covered by the Camberwell Register and relate it to the average population of Camberwell over the same period. The figure that results from this is an annual incidence of 0.6 per 100 000 population. This can be compared with the annual incidence of schizophrenia for Camberwell of 12 per 100 000, indicating that schizophrenia is twenty times as common as hysteria in Camberwell in an in-patient population. Freud would have been hard pushed to make a living out of hysteria if it had been so rare in 19th-century Vienna.

Another interesting fact is the number of cases of hysteria in this series that are complicated by other diagnoses. Eight out of the thirteen were assigned one or more additional diagnoses, comprising depression (3), schizophrenia (2), epilepsy (1), cerebral palsy (1), personality disorder (1), and schizoid personality (1). The coexistence of hysteria, which is classed as one of the neuroses, with organic disorders of the nervous system and functional psychoses is predicted by the hierarchical model of psychopathology described in Chapter 3. However, the paucity of uncomplicated hysteria in this series requires an explanation. A clue is provided by Eliot Slater's changing view of hysteria over time. During World War II, he studied over 2000 soldiers admitted to the neuropsychiatric wards of a British emergency hospital. He found that 384 (19%) were given the diagnosis of hysteria. There is no mention of any complicating conditions, and Slater (1943) records that complete recovery was most frequently seen in these men, an unlikely outcome if they had also suffered from schizophrenia or organic brain disorders. Twenty years later (Slater, 1965), he published an influential article in which he argued that the diagnostic category of hysteria was a nonentity. As part of the evidence, he cited a personal series of 'hysterics', many of whom on follow-up examination proved to be suffering from schizophrenia, manic–depressive conditions, organic psychoses, and neurological diseases. It is our contention that the alteration in Slater's attitude towards the diagnosis of hysteria from acceptance during World War II to rejection in 1965 was brought about by a genuine change in the presentation of the condition. During the war, although diminishing, it was still a relatively acceptable mode of expression of distress, utilised by men who may have been of somewhat lower intelligence than average (Slater, 1943; Williams, 1950), but who had no other complicating disease. Figs 4 and 5 showed that hysteria in Britain began a steep decline in frequency after World War II. By the 1960s, it had ceased to be a common form of neurosis, and consequently its manifestation became restricted to people who were in other respects marginal; afflicted with schizophrenia, epilepsy, or other organic brain disorders. The same argument was applied in Chapter 2 to the culture-bound syndromes of amok and koro.

The picture of hysteria as a disappearing condition in England and Wales as a whole and in Camberwell is duplicated by a study in Athens. Stefanis *et al* (1976) studied the records of Egnition Hospital, which is situated centrally in Athens and draws patients from an extensive geographical area and a wide social spectrum. They reviewed the records of all out-patients who attended during three 2-year periods, 1948–1950, 1958–1960, and

1969–1971. They enumerated the patients who satisfied their criteria for hysteria and found that they constituted 6.0%, 3.0%, and 3.1% of the total out-patients for each of the three periods, respectively. The decrease in proportion from the first to the second period is statistically significant, and indicates that a substantial reduction in the frequency of hysteria presenting to psychiatrists occurred during the decade following World War II.

Having charted the decline of hysteria in the West from its heyday in the 19th century and during the world wars, we can inquire if the same process has occurred in non-Western cultures. Elsarrag (1968) reports that conversion hysteria is common in northern Sudan: "hysterical blindness, mono-ocular diplopias, paralysis, monoplegia, diplegia or hemiplegia, fits and comas, are seen every day of the week in the Clinic of Nervous Disorders. In general terms, the less educated or sophisticated the patient, the more gross his features." It was reported from a psychiatric clinic in Tonga that "most cases have taken the form of a dissociative state or hysterical conversion syndrome. Paraesthesia, pseudo-paralysis, pseudo-epilepsy and hyperventilation are all to be encountered, just as if one were with Charcot a hundred years ago" (Murphy & Taumoepeau, 1980). Actual figures are available from Ain Shams University Psychiatric Clinic in Cairo (Okasha *et al*, 1968). This clinic is situated in the centre of Cairo, but its catchment area extends over the whole of Egypt. Okasha *et al* give the diagnoses for the first 1000 patients attending the clinic from the beginning of 1966. Of these, 112 cases (11.2%) were suffering from a hysterical illness. This figure represents 23.8% of all attenders given a diagnosis of any form of neurosis. A very similar figure was obtained from Lebanon, where Katchadourian & Racy (1969) conducted a point prevalence survey (see Chapter 7 for explanation) of all patients attending the available psychiatric facilities on one particular day in 1964. They found that conversion hysteria amounted to 22.4% of all neurotic disorders. A more recent study in Eastern Libya produced a figure for hysteria of 8.3% of all first attenders at an out-patient clinic (Pu *et al*, 1986). Figures are also available from the Department of Psychiatry of the Postgraduate Institute of Medical Education and Research in the city of Chandigarh in North India (Wig & Pershad, 1975, 1976, 1977). This is the only in-patient psychiatric facility for the city and surrounding rural areas, although there are one or two other out-patient clinics. The Triennial Report for the years 1975–1977 gives figures for out-patient contacts and in-patient admissions, but does not distinguish between first and subsequent contacts or admissions. Therefore, the data are comparable with the figures in Table VII for Camberwell contacts, but not for first admissions. They are displayed in Table VIII.

It can be seen that at a time when hysteria has virtually disappeared from Camberwell, it still accounts for just under 10% of all out-patient contacts and in-patient admissions in Chandigarh. The proportion of out-patient cases diagnosed as depressive and anxiety neuroses over the 3 years amounts to

TABLE VIII
Hysteria in Chandigarh

	Out-patient contacts			In-patient admissions		
Year	Hysteria	Percentage of neuroses	Percentage of all diagnoses	Hysteria	Percentage of neuroses	Percentage of all diagnoses
1975	151	24.4	9.8	17	50.0	8.3
1976	112	21.7	8.6	14	30.4	5.4
1977	171	22.4	8.9	25	54.3	9.2

Adapted from Wig & Pershad, *Triennial Statistical Report, 1975–1977.*

25, 28, and 28%. It is not possible to make direct comparisons with the figures given by Abse (1950) and Williams (1950), since they were dealing with military groups, comprising men in early adult life who had been screened for mental and physical health. With this proviso, one can tentatively note that hysteria forms a similar proportion of out-patient and in-patient cases in Chandigarh today as it did in Indian soldiers during World War II. One study has been conducted that involved a direct comparison of the frequency of symptoms of hysteria in two different cultural groups. Gilleard (1983) applied a self-report symptom inventory to 100 English psychiatric patients and 100 Turkish psychiatric patients. Among the neurotic symptoms in the inventory, significant differences were found only for dissociative and conversion symptoms. These hysterical phenomena were reported more frequently by the Turkish patients.

The evidence reviewed so far indicates that, as opposed to the decline in the frequency of hysteria documented in England and Wales and in Athens, it still flourishes in developing countries. There is, however, at least one exception to this pattern: Japan. Fukuda *et al* (1980) reviewed the records of the psychiatric out-patient departments of two general hospitals serving a mixed rural and urban population of 1 million. They calculated the rates over two decades (1952–1973) of all women attending with hysteria. They employed a broad definition: the development of physical symptoms in the absence of physical illness but in the presence of some significant psychological change in life circumstances. Most of the patients complained of breathing disturbances, fits or pain, suggesting that conversion hysteria affected only a proportion of the cases. Fukuda *et al* found that hysteria in women as a proportion of new out-patients fell from 6 to 2%, despite a comparable attendance rate. These figures are remarkably similar to those from Athens over an almost identical historical period. Any explanation for the decline of hysteria in the West has to accommodate the same phenomenon in Japan.

Our understanding of the process that is occurring is aided by a study of hysteria carried out at the National Hospitals, London. Wilson-Barnett

& Trimble (1985) used the Illness Behaviour Questionnaire (IBQ) constructed by Pilowsky (1975) to investigate the way individuals perceive, evaluate, and act in relation to the state of their health. The sample of patients consisted of 79 consecutively referred to the psychiatric service of the National Hospitals. They had presented to the hospital with well-defined neurological symptoms, but all investigations had given negative results. The patients completed the IBQ and their responses were analysed using seven major factors originally identified by Pilowsky. One factor of particular relevance to our discussion of hysteria represents a dimension of somatic *vs* psychological perception of distress. Positive correlations were found between somatisation on this factor and affective inhibition, low acknowledgement of anxiety and depression, and a high tendency for denial of life problems. Thus, these British patients with hysteria demonstrate an inverse relationship between the overt expression of anxiety and depression and the presentation of their distress in a bodily form. Furthermore, they tend to deny the environmental problems that have led to their distress.

The material presented on hysteria can now be summarised and incorporated into an overview of cultural influences on emotional expression. Hysteria was a major form of neurotic illness in the West during the 19th century, and remained so up to World War II. Since then there appears to have been a rapid decline in its frequency and it is now a rare condition. It has been replaced by the now common conditions of depressive and anxiety neuroses. The picture in India provides a vivid contrast; hysteria was the most common form of neurosis among Indian soldiers during World War II, while anxiety states were relatively infrequent. Hysteria remains a prominent condition among Indian psychiatric patients today, as it does among other non-Western nations, although anxiety and depressive neuroses may have gained a little ground. We have seen that hysteria is a response to stress which represents the patient's concept of bodily dysfunction. With an increasing emphasis in the West on subjective feeling states as indicators of distress, patients have altered their mode of presentation from the bodily experiences of hysteria to the psychological experiences of anxiety and depression. The utilisation of the psychological mode has resulted in an increasing differentiation between these emotional states, which is reflected in the use of language.

Hysteria remains a prevalent form of neurosis in many non-Western countries, although it is not the only somatic mode of emotional expression encountered there. The questionnaire developed by Verma & Wig (1976) in Chandigarh to elicit neurotic symptoms contains a high proportion of items relating to physical complaints, such as watering of the eyes and gas in the stomach. Ebigbo's (1982) schedule for Nigerian patients is exclusively concerned with a multiplicity of bodily experiences. The field of bodily expression is a very rich one, and the many body parts and functions can readily be utilised to represent symbolically problems in human relationships, as Freud pointed out (Breuer & Freud, 1956). Furthermore, as we discovered in the previous chapter, even autonomic function can be used to distinguish between emotions. Thus, in transferring from a bodily to a psychological vocabulary of expression, patients are exchanging one differentiated modality of experience for another, the two being equally capable of conveying the vicissitudes of the human condition. The social and cultural influences that lead to this shift in the expression of distress will be examined in the next chapter.

6 The communication of distress

As mentioned previously, Obeyesekere (1985) asserted that Western medicine has redefined human suffering as a disease known as depression. He argues that the power and prestige of the medical establishment is such that people begin to accept the new definition, particularly members of the elite in non-Western societies. Missing from this provocative formulation is the fact that doctors are as much a part of society as their clients, and subject to the same cultural influences. The nature of these influences is examined in this chapter, after first considering the process of consultation to assess the plausibility of Obeyesekere's contention. Here, the generic term 'doctor' includes all types of Western medical practitioners. We have attempted to display diagrammatically the complex processes operating in a consultation in the hope that this will make the text easier to follow (Fig. 6).

The patient brings to the doctor a series of complaints that are his formulation in his own words of "experiences of disvalued changes in states of being and in social function" (Eisenberg, 1977). It is of great significance that Eisenberg includes changes in social function in his definition of

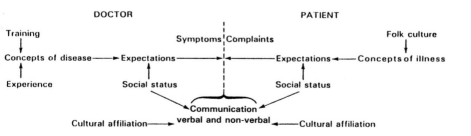

Fig. 6 – Influences on the process of consultation.

complaints. These encompass not only failures to meet social obligations, such as an inability to cope with the housework or with study, but also dissatisfaction with interpersonal relationships. It has become acceptable for patients in Western countries to complain to doctors about their marriages, but not usually about other relationships. It is not conceivable in current practice that a patient would express his presenting complaint in terms of difficulties in getting on with his boss. In non-Western cultures, complaints about relationships are not presented explicitly to doctors or traditional healers, although, as we shall see, they may be translated into a veiled form of communication.

In selecting from his uncomfortable or painful experiences what to complain about, the patient is influenced by his expectations concerning what the doctor is qualified to deal with. To take an obvious example, the sufferer from toothache knows that it is appropriate to consult a dentist rather than a doctor. But what about the person experiencing heartache? Some Western doctors are known to be sympathetic to emotional problems and will deal with them as best they can or refer them to a specialist. Others will have no truck with them. Patients of these doctors quickly learn that such complaints receive short shrift. They either transfer to a more receptive doctor or learn to formulate their distress in physical terms to which the doctor will respond positively.

Patients' expectations of what a doctor should deal with are also moulded by the concepts of illness they hold. These in turn are formed by the folk culture that surrounds them. Anthropologists have studied concepts of illness in a variety of traditional cultures, but surprisingly little attention has been paid to this topic in the West, particularly in the medically most sophisticated cultures of America and Western Europe. In these countries there is a large output of technical knowledge about medicine from the media, but the impact this has had on folk notions of illness is almost unknown. One of the few attempts to probe this area was reported by Helman (1978) who worked as a general practitioner (GP) in a middle-class suburban community in London. He considered that, because of the process of negotiation at the consultation, the operational model of the GPs bears a closer resemblance to the folk model than to the official model of biomedicine promulgated by hospitals, medical schools, and medical textbooks. However, he might have been generalising unjustifiably from his own practice. The folk classification he described was reported mainly by older patients, and comprised two basic polarities: hot and cold, and wet and dry. Wet conditions involved overproduction of fluid – phlegm, sputum, vomit, urine, diarrhoea – while dry conditions were those in which a raised temperature was the sole, or paramount symptom, e.g. in shivering and rigors. Chills and colds were explained as due to the penetration of the environment through the boundary of the skin. Damp or rain was classified as cold/wet, and cold winds and draughts as cold/dry. Night air was considered dangerous by many of the older patients. Some areas of the body were seen as more vulnerable to environmental influences than others, particularly the top of the head, the back of the neck, and the feet. The classification Helman sets out did not include concepts of emotional disturbance, which remain to be explored on the same lines.

On the other hand, the doctor's expectations of what he will be presented with are strongly influenced by his concepts of disease. These theoretical constructs provide a structure within which he can organise the patient's complaints and make sense of them. His initial efforts in a consultation are directed towards making a diagnosis. To this end, he reformulates the patient's complaints in terms of symptoms, neglecting as irrelevant anything that does not fit. The cluster of symptoms is then matched against an array of disease concepts for goodness of fit. These concepts are instilled during the doctor's training, but may be modified by his subsequent experience of clinical practice, as claimed by Helman (1978) with respect to GPs.

In the case of neurotic disorders, textbooks describe anxiety and depression as clearly differentiated conditions. Experienced psychiatrists continue to harbour these idealised disease concepts, despite the fact that patients usually exhibit a mixture of the symptoms considered characteristic of each type of neurosis. The extent of this discrepancy was revealed by an investigation of concepts of anxiety, depression, and irritability held by psychiatric patients and psychiatrists in the same institution. The subjects of the study (Leff, 1978) were 20 patients suffering from neurosis and 10 experienced psychiatrists. They were each asked to rate feelings of depression, anxiety, and irritability on 11 somatic, and 11 psychological, constructs. For instance, they were required to state whether when they felt depressed their heart beat fast (somatic construct), and whether they wanted to die (psychological construct). The patients were asked to rate their own unpleasant emotion, while the psychiatrists were requested to respond as they imagined a typical neurotic patient would do. The material was analysed by calculating the correlation coefficients between anxiety and depression, depression and irritability, and anxiety and irritability, using the ratings on the 11 somatic and 11 psychological constructs. The results are shown in Table IX.

There are striking differences between patients' and psychiatrists' concepts of these unpleasant emotional states. In each comparison, the psychiatrists

TABLE IX
Correlation coefficients between constructs of unpleasant emotions

	Anxiety: depression	Depression: irritability	Anxiety: irritability
Patients	0.62	0.49	0.58
Psychiatrists	0	0.18	0.28

From Leff (1978).

produced a much lower correlation than the patients, indicating that they expect a much greater differentiation between the emotions than the patients experience. In particular, the psychiatrists' stereotypic neurotic patient is capable of making a perfect distinction between anxiety and depression (correlation coefficient of 0), whereas the actual patients conceive of these emotions as overlapping to a considerable degree (correlation coefficient of 0.62). It might be thought that abstract concepts held by patients bear little relation to their actual complaints and to diagnostic usage by psychiatrists. However, there is evidence that the overlap in patients' concepts of unpleasant emotions is indeed reflected in their symptoms and in psychiatrists' rating of them. Snaith *et al* (1976) required patients suffering from endogenous depression or anxiety neurosis to complete a Leeds Self-Assessment of Depression Specific Scale and an equivalent scale for anxiety. Of the patients diagnosed clinically as suffering from anxiety neurosis, only 24% had scores that did not overlap with those of the depressed patients. A similar proportion (26%) of patients with endogenous depression had scores that did not overlap with those of the anxious patients. Of the total group, 73% fell into the middle range of scores and were considered by Snaith *et al* to represent "anxiety-depressions".

These findings indicate that English patients still have a considerable way to go in achieving a clear distinction between anxiety, depression, and anger. On the other hand, psychiatrists have crystallised quite distinct concepts of these unpleasant emotions. It is not surprising to find that they are at the leading edge of this process of emotional differentiation, where they act not only as pioneers, but also as educators. They convey their expectations directly to patients in clinical interviews and indirectly to the general public via the mass media. In a study of popular attitudes to psychiatric illness, Una Maclean (1969) found that the most common source of information for the person in the street was television.

The doctor is inevitably of a higher social status than the majority of his patients, but even when the patient equals or overlaps the doctor's social position, the doctor still wields an advantage by virtue of the power his professional skills and knowledge confer. Thus his expectations are likely to influence the nature of the complaints the patient brings to him.

In non-psychiatric consultations, communication forms only a part of the procedure, the physical examination being a central feature.¹ In psychiatric consultations, communication is everything. Patients who complain directly about unpleasant subjective feelings will usually have no difficulty in making the doctor understand the nature of the immediate problem, although tracing its antecedents requires a psychological sophistication he may not possess. Patients who couch their distress in terms of bodily symptoms are likely to meet a number of hindrances to communication. The first step the doctor will take is to attempt to exclude a physical basis for the symptoms. A careful review of the patient's history in conjunction with a physical examination may be sufficient to put the doctor's mind at rest. If not, then he will embark on a series of laboratory tests, which may appear puzzling and irrelevant to the patient if the doctor has not explained his strategy carefully. When the doctor is satisfied that he has excluded physical disease, he is then faced with the problem of understanding the physical complaints in terms of the patient's life circumstances. This is no easy matter, as the patient is quite often unaware of the links that exist. Furthermore, the patient's concepts of illness may not include the notion that bodily symptoms can result from problems with relationships. Thus the doctor often has to pursue his investigations with the patient as a passive rather than an active partner.

Racy (1980), an Arab-speaking psychiatrist, saw 40 Saudi women during a 2-month period in a psychiatric clinic in Saudi Arabia. His experience is illustrative of the problem. He found that considerable effort was required to break through the barriers of somatisation and passivity in order to obtain a picture of the patient's life, concerns, and troubles. He learned to turn the passivity to his advantage by giving the patient direct commands to reveal specific facts about members of the family, past events, and current difficulties. He was frequently able to discover ordinary human concerns that were coloured by the nature of Arab culture. "Commonly heard themes are those of neglect by the husband in favour of a younger and prettier wife, feelings of loneliness on separation from parents and siblings, lack of money or food, fatigue from prolonged child-rearing, and conflicts with in-laws, since Arab homes tend to house several generations." Racy was in an advantageous position to "break the code of somatization" as he put it. Since he spoke Arabic fluently and had an intimate knowledge of Arab culture, he could ask the crucial questions about the patients' life circumstances.

A thorough understanding of the relevant culture is usually essential to decode the somatic complaint presented. This is highlighted by Nichter's (1981*a*) study of Havik Brahmins in South India. He states that a Havik woman is socialised against the overt expression of emotions within the family. One bodily symptom which commonly signals distress is *tale tirigutade*, which translates as 'head turning' and is interpreted literally by most medical practitioners as giddiness or dizziness. However, the term as used by villagers denotes more than physical dizziness. Nichter studied 22 clients of a traditional healer who presented with this symptom. He identified five cases of impending family partition, four cases of economic crises, four cases of women over 25 years of age anxiously awaiting marriage, two cases of adjustment problems following marriage, and one woman recently widowed who had two daughters but no sons. The common theme he abstracts from the problems presented is that they induce uncertainty and disorientation, which is expressed symbolically by the somatic symptom of dizziness. As indicated in a later chapter, traditional healers are adept at back-translating from bodily complaints to psychosocial problems. If the doctor is perceptive enough to appreciate that the somatic symptoms presented signify emotional distress, but is unable to make the link with the patient's life circumstances, he is likely to provide reassurance and/or psychotropic medication. This may result in temporary relief but is almost certain to lead to the patient returning later or seeking help elsewhere. Racy (1980) in reviewing the case records of Saudi women out-patients found that the same somatic complaints had been presented in the same fashion on previous occasions. Almost invariably pills or injections had been prescribed, leading to mild or moderate relief, which proved transitory.

The dilemma of the doctor faced with complaints formulated in one modality which he interprets as symptoms within a different conceptual framework is vividly conveyed by Kleinman's (1986) work in China. This merits an extended exposition, as it illustrates the whole range of issues discussed above. In 1980, he collected a consecutive sample of 100 patients who attended the psychiatric out-patient clinic of a hospital in Hunan for the first time, and who were given the diagnosis of neurasthenia. This term was coined by Beard, an American physician, in 1869, when it denoted nervous exhaustion. He believed that neurotic symptoms were due to a diminished nervous force. The term spread to Europe, where it was used by Charcot among others (Drinka, 1984). Kleinman believes that the term neurasthenia may have entered China via Western medical missionaries and Japanese medical authorities, who themselves borrowed it from the Germans. Beard's notion of a reduced nervous force is in accord with the concept in traditional Chinese medicine of a decrease in vital energy – *qi*, which is probably why the term found favour. Neurasthenia has lost ground in the West and has been dropped from DSM–III (American Psychiatric Association, 1980), but remains the most common diagnosis for neurotic disorders in China. In traditional medicine, a number of types of neurasthenia (*shenjing shuairuo*) are recognised, depending on the body organs believed to be affected. The type that is due to a decrease of *qi* in the liver gives rise to emotional symptoms associated with chest discomfort, hypochondriacal pain, depression, anxiety, irritability, anorexia, abdominal distension, menstrual irregularities, and a variety of other complaints.

The neurasthenic patients studied by Kleinman were each interviewed for several hours about symptoms, course, illness behaviour, help-seeking, and ethnomedical beliefs associated with the current illness. Data were also collected on psychosocial events and problems. Patients were assessed with the Schedule for Affective Disorders and Schizophrenia, and a DSM–III diagnosis was made. Using Western categories, 93 of the 100 patients were diagnosed as suffering from clinical depression, and 87 of these met strict diagnostic criteria for major depressive disorder. One-third of the latter gave evidence of melancholia, a particularly severe form of the disorder, and in 60%, the depression had lasted for more than 2 years. One-quarter of the sample was diagnosed as exhibiting hysteria, the term covering both conversion disorder and somatisation disorder. There was some overlap between depression and hysteria, particularly conversion disorder.

Forty-four of the neurasthenic patients met the criteria for chronic pain syndrome – pain in a single site or several sites lasting for more than 2 years and causing disability with social impairment in family or work settings.

Of the 100 patients, each volunteered a mean of seven complaints, of which five were somatic, and two, psychological. Of the 93 depressive patients only nine complained of depression, and of the 87 with major depressive disorder 30% complained entirely of somatic symptoms and 70% of a mixture of somatic and psychological with a strong emphasis on the former. Kleinman noted that "nonspecific, undifferentiated, or partly differentiated affects" were expressed in the majority of cases with psychological symptoms, and concluded that patients were more able to differentiate somatic than affective states.

The great majority of patients, 78%, maintained that their disorder was wholly or partly organic, but most ascribed it to work problems (61%) followed in frequency by political problems (25%). Their view of causality was confirmed by the ethnographic interviews conducted, which probed for the significance of illness. In 43% of cases, this was judged to be the communication of personal or interpersonal distress or unhappiness.

The next thing Kleinman did was to attempt to convey to the patients his own, Western, concept of depressive disease, following which he treated all 87 patients satisfying the criteria for major depressive disorder with tricyclic antidepressant medication. At a follow-up examination 6 weeks later, 65% reported that they were substantially improved, and another 17% that they were slightly improved. However, 30% considered their social impairment to be worse, and 37% sought further help from practitioners of traditional Chinese medicine and biomedicine. This is similar to Racy's (1980) experience in Saudi Arabia, and Kleinman came to the same conclusion, namely "Medical treatment for chronic conditions without significant psychosocial intervention exerts only a limited effect on the overall illness".

In order to determine the long-term effects of his Western-style intervention, Kleinman followed up 21 patients with both chronic pain syndrome and major depressive disorder 3 years later. For many of them, depression had become a less severe but very chronic problem, and one-third still met DSM–III criteria for major depressive disorder. The same proportion had experienced no change in their chronic pain. Only two patients had come to regard their illness as depression, while nine still considered they were suffering from neurasthenia. Originally, in 1980, all the patients with pain regarded it as entirely or mainly organic in origin. By 1983, half of them considered it to be chiefly or entirely psychological. This change in attitude was accompanied by a decrease in medical help-seeking. Kleinman views this as the successful communication by the researchers of a psychosomatic stress model of patients' illnesses. Thus he had limited success in indoctrinating the Chinese patients with a Western view of their complaints, although he failed to persuade them to adopt the Western label of 'depression'.

Another of Kleinman's conclusions is worth quoting verbatim: "Not the least of illness's properties is the medium of communication it affords to express distress, demoralization, unhappiness, and other difficult, dangerous and otherwise unsanctioned feelings in terms that must be heard and may lead to change". But if the medicalisation of suffering, as Obeyesekere (1985) formulated it, results in the prescription of medication without attention being paid to the individual's psychosocial problems, how will the suffering be alleviated on a long-term basis? Kleinman's answer is a plea for professionals to be exempt from local systems of social control and to intervene in family-, school- and work-related problems, and at the community level. "Change," he asserts, "must also occur at the macrosocial level." This stance reveals political naivety. Doctors can no more stand outside the social system in which they are embedded than any other member of society. Is it conceivable that doctors could have pleaded successfully with the instigators of the Cultural Revolution in China on the grounds that it was increasing human unhappiness?

There is a close parallel between Kleinman's formulation of depression and that of Brown & Harris (1978). Indeed, the title of his book (*Social Origins of Distress and Disease*) echoes theirs (*Social Origins of Depression*), surely no coincidence. One of Brown & Harris's key findings, that lack of employment is a factor leading to depression in women, can be used to argue for major social changes. However doctors do not have the expertise or power to engineer such changes. Instead, perhaps the answer can be learned from traditional healers who use their position of authority to alter the immediate social environment of their clients to beneficial effect. This is examined in a later chapter.

After gaining understanding of somatic complaints, hysteria, and other neurotic disorders, another dilemma arises. If the disorders represent culturally determined modes of conveying distress that originates in psycho-social problems, how far along the spectrum of psychiatric disorder can this explanation be applied? If the most severe end, which is occupied by the psychoses, schizophrenia, and manic depression, is considered, then there is ample evidence for a genetic basis to both these conditions. Psychosocial factors undoubtedly influence their course, a matter that we will consider later, but they cannot account entirely for the origins of these psychoses. Where along the spectrum do biologically based disorders give way to psychosocially determined ones? This has been debated often with respect to depression. Opposing factions still disagree over whether there is a continuum from reactive to endogenous depression, or whether two distinct diseases exist. It is not appropriate to rehearse the arguments here, but it is worth emphasising that cross-cultural studies could illuminate this area.

I have just stated my conviction that schizophrenia has a biological basis, but that does not preclude cultural forces from shaping the form of this disorder. One type of schizophrenia, catatonia, varies in frequency among cultures, and over time. Catatonia used to be seen commonly in the back wards of psychiatric institutions in the West. Over the past 100 years, it has progressively disappeared, and is now a rarity. For instance, the records of the Bethlem Royal Hospital, London (the original Bedlam), show that catatonia accounted for 6% of all admissions in the 1850s, but only 0.5% in the 1950s. The same decline has been documented in the United States by Morrison (1974), who studied the records of Iowa State Psychopathic Hospital from its opening in 1920 up to 1966. He calculated incidence rates and found that the proportion of catatonia dropped from 14.2% of all schizophrenic patients during the years 1920–1944, to 8.5% during the years 1945–1966, a highly significant decrease. He considered that this dramatic change was unlikely to be attributable to alterations in diagnostic habits, since the motor symptoms of catatonia are readily identifiable. It certainly could not be accounted for by the introduction of the major tranquillisers, since a sudden decline in catatonia was noted at least 20 years earlier, around 1930. For the same chronological reason, Ödegaard's (1967) explanation in terms of the social changes that have occurred in the care of chronic patients is unlikely to be correct. Furthermore, neither the introduction of innovative pharmacological nor social treatments could influence the *incidence* rate, i.e. the number of new cases coming into hospital from the community for the first time, which was the focus of Morrison's study.

The Camberwell Register (Wing & Hailey, 1972) can be used to assess the situation regarding catatonia in this area of south-east London. By 1965, when the register was started, catatonia was already a rarity, and accounted for only 1 case out of 28 first admissions for schizophrenia. In the following year, a single case was also recorded out of a total of 18 schizophrenic first admissions. In 1976, not one case of catatonia was diagnosed among the new admissions.

As with hysteria, the disappearance of catatonic schizophrenia in the West has not occurred in non-Western countries. Okasha *et al* (1968) studied the first 1000 patients attending Ain Shams University Clinic in Cairo from the beginning of 1966. They found the proportion of catatonia among all schizophrenic patients to be 14.4%. Chandrasena & Rodrigo (1979) examined every patient with a functional psychosis admitted to a psychiatric unit in Kandy, Sri Lanka, over the course of 2.5 years. The proportion of catatonic schizophrenia, at 21%, was even higher than in the Egyptian sample. A direct comparison of the frequency of catatonia in developing and developed countries is possible from the IPSS data (World Health Organization, 1973), although one must have reservations, as the samples were not epidemiologically based. Catatonic schizophrenia was diagnosed in 22% of schizophrenic subjects in the Agra sample of patients, 13% in Cali, and 8% in Ibadan, while it comprised no more than 4% of the schizophrenic patients from any of the other six countries in the study. It is of interest that of the three catatonic patients in the London sample, two were West Indians, suggesting that the Caribbean belongs with the developing countries in this respect.

The recently completed WHO incidence study (Sartorius *et al*, 1986) probably provides the most reliable data available on the cross-cultural incidence of catatonia. Catatonia was diagnosed in 10% of the cases of schizophrenia from developing countries, but in only a handful of cases in developed countries. The extinction of catatonic schizophrenia in the West, and its current survival in the developing countries so closely mimic the history and geography of hysteria as to suggest that the same forces are responsible. I have argued that hysteria is a bodily expression of distress. Is it possible that catatonia is the bodily form of schizophrenia? The principal symptoms of catatonia were enumerated on p. 12, and their possible equivalents among the psychological symptoms of schizophrenia can now be considered. There is a group of bodily symptoms that appear to have a common basis: waxy flexibility, *mitgehen*, echopraxia, and echolalia. These represent the passive adoption of posture and movement by patients in response to the examiner's manipulation of their bodies, or else the imitation of the examiner's own movements and speech. These can be viewed as the bodily equivalent of delusions of control, in which patients believe their actions and speech are being controlled by some external force or person. The subjective account by a catatonic patient of his pathological experiences recorded on p. 19 confirms this interpretation. Posturing and mannerisms are stances and gestures exhibited by the patient that appear to have some private symbolic meaning for him which is not shared by others. These can be interpreted as the bodily expression of delusions. Catatonic excitement, which often leads to attacks on people and objects, is to be seen as a non-verbal expression of fear and anger, emotions that are common in schizophrenic illnesses. A few major catatonic symptoms cannot easily be absorbed into this scheme, namely negativism, ambitendence, grimacing, and stereotypes. Nevertheless, the correspondence between the somatic symptoms of catatonia and the psychological symptoms of other subtypes of schizophrenia is close enough to give credence to the speculation that the disappearance of catatonia in the West is a consequence of the general shift among the populace from bodily to psychological modes of expression. Murphy (1982) quotes a study by Piedmont (unpubl. *PhD thesis*, 1962) that supports this suggestion. Piedmont compared German-American with Polish-American schizophrenic patients in two hospitals in New York in the early 1960s. The German immigrants were better educated than the Poles, and came from an urban culture, whereas the Poles had migrated from a peasant society. There were 30 patients in each group: 23 of the Poles exhibited marked somatic and hypochondriacal symptoms compared with 10 of the Germans, a highly significant difference ($P < 0.001$). Moreover, significantly more Poles (18) were catatonic than Germans (8).

It has been shown that in the West an increasingly psychological mode of expression has been adopted by patients to communicate their distress, whereas, in developing countries, complaints are predominantly couched in bodily terms. What are the possible explanations for this difference?

Doctors, and psychiatrists in particular, play some part in channelling complaints into a psychological form, but, like their patients, they are subject to larger societal forces, which are impelling this change. The suggestions made by Murphy (1982) may be reconsidered in the light of the studies we have reviewed. The rise of Protestantism could hardly account for the same phenomenon being observed across Europe. In particular, we have documented the decline of hysteria in Greece, a country unaffected by Protestantism. His second suggestion, a change in child-rearing patterns towards more consistent parent–child relationships, is also difficult to generalise to all Western cultures. Furthermore, we noted a decline in hysteria in Japan, comparable in magnitude to that recorded in Greece. Japan's being one of the most rapidly industrialising nations in the world supports Murphy's third suggestion that capitalism increases economic individualism and leads to a reduction in close social ties. I favour this last suggestion and will devote the rest of this chapter to its consideration.

In traditional societies, the group overshadows the individual in importance, and is the reference point for the culture. This difference in emphasis is reflected in a whole variety of activities as well as in the structure of society. Differences between traditional and modern societies are presented in Table X in the form of polar attributes for dramatic contrast. However, it is recognised that no single society will conform to either stereotype, and that in reality a continuum exists between traditional and modern cultures

TABLE X

Polar attributes of traditional and modern societies

Traditional society	Modern society
Group-oriented	Individual-oriented
Extended family	Nuclear family
Income-producing linked to kinship ties	Income-producing independent of kinship ties
Economic functions non-specialised	Economic functions specialised
High mortality, high fertility	Low mortality, low fertility
Status determined by age and position in family	Status achieved by own efforts
Relationships between kin obligatory	Relationships between kin permissive
Relationships determined by role and position in family	Relationships determined by individual choice
Arranged marriages	Choice of marital partner
Individuals can be replaced by others filling same roles	Individuals unique and irreplaceable
Extensive classification terminology for distant relatives	Restricted classification terminology for close relatives only
Behaviour to specific kin prescribed	Great variation in kin behaviour

(Miner, 1952). Any particular culture may exhibit both traditional and modern features concurrently.

In traditional societies, the family tends to be extended rather than nuclear, three or four generations live under the same roof, and within each generation, siblings remain in the household after marriage, bringing their spouse to join the family. This latter practice varies with sex; in some cultures, women move into their husband's household on marriage, but in others, it is the new husband who is integrated into the family. Within such extended families, a system of mutual obligations exists between members, which acts to enforce the cohesion. If one member becomes disabled through sickness or infirmity, the other members support the individual without question. The activities which produce an income for the family tend to be performed by family members working in co-operation. This applies as much to a family business as to agricultural pursuits. Whereas it is acceptable in Western society for a family to run a farm, it is generally frowned on when relatives are appointed to positions in a business or professional institution. The boss's son or daughter is never popular with other employees, and nepotism is a pejorative term. By contrast, in non-Western societies, any family member occupying a position in an organisation is expected to find jobs in it for relatives.

In the economic sphere, traditional societies are relatively unspecialised. This is particularly true of rural subsistence economies, and as we shall see later on has important implications for the rehabilitation of psychiatric patients. For the moment, it is sufficient to note the consequence – that one worker can be readily replaced with another. Individual qualities are of relatively little importance. We encounter the same phenomenon in family roles in the extended family, in which there are likely to be several substitute fathers, mothers, and children. In general, family roles are more important than the individuals who fill them. The roles confer important properties on their occupants, and status is automatically associated with certain roles, such as the oldest male, or the first-born. The precedence of roles over individuals is reflected in the custom of arranged marriage.

Each role involves certain obligatory forms of behaviour towards other family members, according to the roles they occupy. Behaviour to particular members may be specified in considerable detail. For instance, in strict Muslim families, a man may not speak to his wife while in the presence of a senior male, while among Orthodox Jews a widow is expected to marry her deceased husband's brother. Among Australian aborigines, a man cannot approach, speak to, or deliberately look at his mother-in-law, and if he recognises her footprints, he carefully erases them with his foot (Meggitt, 1974). Forms of behaviour may be laid down for quite distant kin, so that it is important to be able to distinguish varieties of distant relatives. Thus, the lexicons used in traditional societies for kinship differentiate clearly between, for example, maternal and paternal uncles, whereas the English word *cousin* covers a multitude of relationships. Languages not only provide evidence of the relative importance of kinship ties, but also chronicle in a more direct way the emergence of the individual. Schlauch (1943) considers that "there is a reason to believe that the first person (singular) was a comparatively late development in some languages. This is vivid grammatical testimony to the relative unimportance of the individual as opposed to the tribe! It seems to imply that in such tribes men could conceive of themselves only as part of a larger social whole."

In societies in which a person's behaviour to kin is specified in considerable detail, a greater emphasis is placed on maintaining harmonious relationships than on introspection. For instance, among the Ifalak of Micronesia, a person who experiences a longer than optimal period of mourning for a dead loved one is not viewed as having a primarily intrapsychic problem. Rather the problem is defined as that of an inadequate replacement of the lost relationship with another (Lutz, 1985). Among the Chinese, 'ego-centred intrapsychic experience' is seen as potentially disruptive to social relationships and the open verbal expression of distress outside close family relatives is viewed as embarrassing and shameful (Kleinman, 1986). As a society moves from the traditional to the modern on the dimensions enumerated above, the unique qualities of the individual become prized above the value of group cohesion, and introspection consequently flourishes. The effect of these changes on the emotional life of the individual is to shift the focus of emotional experience from the body towards the psychological mode. It could be argued that introspection is practised to a high degree in Buddhist cultures in the form of meditation. However the purpose of meditation is to dissolve the sense of self, not to emphasise it, as in the West.

An increasing emphasis on the individual weakens the interpersonal bonds that are so evident in traditional societies. The high value placed on introspection in Western cultures has led substantial numbers of people to experiment with so-called 'mind-expanding' drugs. It seems likely that if the uniqueness of the individual's inner experience became the dominant value in society, the bonds between people would be so attenuated that such a society would probably not be viable. Already some Western societies seem to be far down that road, since even the nuclear family is progressively being replaced by the single-parent family. However much we may regret what has been lost, the process traced here has an incalculable momentum, and is probably irreversible.

Whatever the scientific status of our speculations about the societal forces responsible may prove to be, the major differences in the modes of expression of distress between cultures represent a massive obstacle to the comparison of rates of illness. We can anticipate considerable problems when it comes to counting numbers of neurotically ill people in various cultures, an endeavour that is examined in the next part of the book.

II.   Do psychiatric conditions
      have the same frequency
      in different cultures?

7 Counting

As concluded in Part I, schizophrenia is recognisable wherever it occurs in the world, and its form is relatively independent of cultural influences. The opposite conclusion was formed in considering neurotic conditions, which are more likely to take a somatic form in developing cultures than in Western technological societies. When the form is that of hysteria, it may or may not be distinguishable from physical disease, depending on the medical sophistication of the patient. However, when the clinical picture is dominated by the autonomic accompaniments of emotional distress, the distinction from physical disease is often very difficult to establish. Hence, it is easier to compare the frequency of schizophrenia than neurotic conditions in different cultures. Even with schizophrenia, considerable problems are encountered, which arise directly from the methods of measuring the frequency of any disease. To appreciate these, the measures involved must be discussed.

If you were asked to determine the number of marbles in a box, you would carry out the obvious procedure dictated by common sense and simply count them. But psychiatric conditions are not objects like marbles, which are easily distinguishable from all other objects, and are persistent immutable states. Once a marble, always a marble; but people who develop depression or schizophrenia often recover and may appear perfectly normal. Thus, psychiatric conditions are constantly arising in members of the public, and are sometimes disappearing forever, sometimes disappearing but recurring after an interval, and sometimes persisting for the rest of the sufferer's life. If we applied the marble-counting procedure to any population at a particular point in time, we would detect the people who had recently developed the condition, but had not yet recovered (b in Fig. 7), and the people who developed the condition some time ago but never recovered (d). We should miss a and c, who were well at the time of counting, but exhibited the condition before and after the counting point, respectively. The counting of people exhibiting a particular condition at a single point in time is known by the technical term *point prevalence*. As previously seen, the figure obtained by this method, which yields the quickest results, includes both chronic

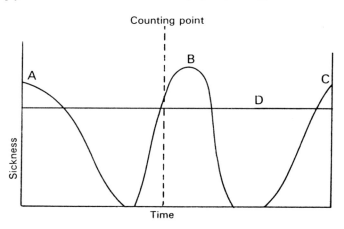

Fig. 7 – Counting sick people.

sufferers and recent acute sufferers. By indicating how many people are suffering from a particular condition at a given moment, the point prevalence is useful for determining the service needs of a population. However, the mixture of acute and chronic sufferers it represents makes it unsuitable for other purposes. The acute sufferers are also a mixed group, including those developing the condition for the first time and those experiencing a recurrence.

The counting of people suffering from chronic and recurrent symptoms indicates the effectiveness, or otherwise, of treatment for a particular condition. The more effective the treatment and management of a condition, the fewer recurrent and chronic sufferers will be detected. The counting of people who have developed a condition for the first time can suggest factors that are contributing to the origin of that condition. The number of people developing a condition for the first time is known by the technical term *incidence*. There is little point in recording the incidence at one moment because, unless the condition is exceedingly common, very few sufferers will be detected. It is usual to calculate the incidence over the course of a year, the *annual incidence*. If the incidence of schizophrenia, for example, were found to be considerably higher in Western societies than in traditional cultures, it would suggest that aspects of urbanisation and industrialisation were implicated in the aetiology of schizophrenia.

It is helpful to return to our analogy of the marbles to illustrate another problem that arises in counting sufferers from any condition. Suppose that, instead of being set the simple task of calculating the number of marbles in a box, you were required to count up the total number of marbles in a room, and were told that a child had been playing with them recently and may not have returned them all to the box. This task would involve you in a thorough search of the room, including other containers, odd nooks and crannies, and the space under pieces of furniture – a much more laborious exercise. The 'counter of ill people', or epidemiologist as he is known, is faced with the latter task, rather than the former, for the following reasons. People who develop sicknesses, whether psychiatric or not, do not necessarily consult a doctor. For this reason we have avoided the term *patient*, since this implies that the person is in contact with a medical service, and have used *sufferer* instead. Patients in contact with medical services, like marbles in a box, can easily be identified and counted; sufferers at large in the community cannot. The search for these sufferers involves a large expenditure of effort and expertise, the magnitude of which will become evident as we consider the practical procedures required. It also involves the demarcation of boundaries. In moving from the box of marbles to the room, there was an implicit limit to the search set by the boundaries of the room. No such obvious boundaries exist in the general population. Instead, one has to construct more or less artificial ones to limit one's search to feasible proportions. One could choose to study the total population of an island or a city, if the numbers were not too large. Alternatively, one could choose a particular sample from a population e.g. all males between the ages of 15 and 25. If one was interested in studying a total population, but it was too large, one could draw a sample of, for example, one in ten people. However, it would be necessary to ensure that the sample was really representative of the whole population.

The issue of the representative nature of any sample studied is of the utmost importance in placing interpretations on the numbers of sick people detected. We need to know, for example, whether the patients attending a medical facility with a particular condition comprise all the people in the population suffering from that condition, or only a proportion of them. If only a proportion, are they representative of the total group of sufferers in the community in terms of age, sex, clinical history, pattern of symptoms, and so on? If not, then what factors are determining the attendance of sufferers at a medical facility, and what kind of bias is introduced into that group? These questions can be illustrated by reference to schizophrenia.

In a Western European country such as the UK, psychiatric services are well developed and comprise a network of facilities, both in-patient and out-patient, covering the whole population. In addition, every person has the opportunity of being registered with a GP who will treat patients with psychiatric disorders or refer them to a specialist service. People developing schizophrenia for the first time are likely to be seen initially by their GP and then referred to a psychiatric clinic, since very few are sufficiently confident of their psychiatric expertise to diagnose and treat first episodes of schizophrenia. Where else might we find people with schizophrenia who are unknown to the psychiatric services? Some people developing the symptoms of schizophrenia may be living solitary lives so that there is no one to notice their abnormality and take appropriate action. People in this situation may remain ill and unknown to the psychiatric services for years, but eventually they usually exhibit some form of antisocial behaviour that brings them to the attention of the police, or else suffer from a degree of self-neglect that results in the social services being alerted. In either case, contact will lead to referral to the psychiatric services, since social workers and the police are trained to recognise psychiatric conditions, and both groups have the legal right to commit patients involuntarily to psychiatric hospitals. It is possible that some solitary schizophrenic people in the community never attract attention to themselves through odd or criminal behaviour, but they are likely to be rare exceptions.

Of course, people suffering from schizophrenia who commit crimes are not always sent to psychiatric hospitals, but committed to prison. However, patients committing crimes that lead to imprisonment have usually been ill for a long time and have previously been admitted to psychiatric hospitals (Rollin, 1965). Hence, one would be very unlikely to pick up new cases of schizophrenia in British prisons. The same argument applies to vagrants. Vagrancy usually occurs at a later rather than earlier stage in the history of someone suffering from schizophrenia, and reflects the failure of aftercare on the part of the psychiatric services. A survey of men entering the largest reception centre for homeless men in England (Tidmarsh & Wood, 1972) revealed that one-third of the newcomers were suffering from a psychiatric illness as their primary problem. However, all of them had a long history of symptoms and had been admitted to a psychiatric hospital at least once previously.

It is evident that surveys of psychiatric in-patient and out-patient facilities in a developed country like England will identify the great majority of first episodes of schizophrenia. This is supported by the fact that the incidence of schizophrenia calculated in this way is very similar in all Western European countries, around 12 per 100 000 population per year. The situation regarding neurotic conditions in developed countries is very different, as only a small proportion of such patients is referred by GPs to psychiatrists; Shepherd *et al* (1966) estimated this proportion at about 5%. Furthermore, there is a substantial number of people in the general population who are suffering from neurotic disorders, but who have not sought treatment from GPs. Such people have been detected by population surveys, and in London amount to as much as 45% of cases arising during the course of 1 year (Hurry *et al*, 1980). Thus, a survey of psychiatric hospitals and clinics in a developed country will detect only a small fraction of people suffering from neurosis, and the size of the problem can be determined only by a population survey.

The problem affecting estimates of the incidence and prevalence of the neuroses in a developed country applies to both neuroses and psychoses in a developing country. A comparison of the situation in developed and developing countries is displayed in Table XI for ease of reference. Where psychiatric facilities are sparse, only a small proportion of people developing first episodes of psychosis or neurosis are likely to be treated in them.

TABLE XI
Where psychiatrically ill people are found in developed and developing countries

	Developed countries	Developing countries
In-patient and out-patient services	Nearly all onset psychotic patients; small proportion of onset neurotic patients	Small proportion of onset psychotic and onset neurotic patients
GPs	Most onset neurotic patients; tiny proportion of onset psychotic patients	Service not usually available
Traditional healers	No onset psychotic patients; small proportion of onset neurotic patients	Many onset neurotic and onset psychotic patients
Vagrants	Chronic psychotic and neurotic patients with previous contact with medical services	Chronic psychotic and neurotic patients without previous contact with medical services
Prisons	Chronic psychotic and neurotic patients with previous contact with medical services	Some onset psychotic patients
General population	Possibly a handful of onset psychotic patients; substantial proportion of onset neurotic patients	Some onset psychotic patients; most onset neurotic patients

Furthermore, those people reaching the psychiatric services are not representative of sufferers in general. Where the nearest psychiatric facility may be several days' journey distant, only the most difficult and disruptive patients are likely to be referred. Orley (1970) has shown for Butabika Hospital in Uganda that patients referred from the nearby town are representative in general of sufferers from psychosis, whereas those travelling from distant rural areas have a disproportionate number showing violent behaviour. In addition to the difficulties posed by long distances from the facilities, it is likely that there is greater tolerance for psychiatric disorders in rural areas. The lesser complexity of village life compared with city life and the smaller number of demands imposed on people favour the retention of the psychiatrically ill person in the community, unless they are very disruptive. Behaviour likely to lead to referral comprises violence to people or property and affronts to public decency.

The different attitude to work in a developing, compared with a developed country also aids the retention of the psychiatrically ill in the community. In the latter type of country, production is geared to making more than is needed for local consumption, whereas, in the former, one often finds a subsistence economy: what is produced is only just enough for the local population, and there is no attempt to create a surplus. As a result, if the climate and soil are reasonably good, an all-out effort by the available work force is not required. People do the minimum agricultural work necessary, and have plenty of free time for other activities. It is not uncommon to find that the women do the bulk of the agricultural work while the men discuss matters of moment. In such a situation, if an individual is rendered unfit for work by psychiatric illness either temporarily or permanently, little or no effect on the economy results. By contrast, in an urban environment in an industrialised country, an inability to work rapidly draws attention to the psychiatric sufferer.

It is also necessary to take account of the public's attitude to psychiatric illnesses and their treatment. In Uganda, for example, 'madness' is considered to be one of a number of conditions which is susceptible only to traditional healing techniques (Orley & Leff, 1972). Hence, there is great reluctance to refer 'mad' patients to Western-style facilities. The same attitude was revealed in a study by Harding (1973), who found that 91% of a random sample of rural Nigerians considered the traditional healer to be the appropriate person to deal with mental illness, whereas only 2% opted for the health clinic. As a confirmation of this, Wyatt & Wyatt (1967) did not record a single case of functional psychosis in over 4000 consecutive patients seen at a Nigerian health centre in a 12-month period.

In developing countries, the scarcity of psychiatric facilities is generally accompanied by an absence of general practitioners. Instead, the primary-care facility in the community is represented by the traditional healer. As shown in Part III, traditional healers deal with a large number of first episodes of psychosis and neurosis. Occasionally they establish a liaison with Western-type psychiatric facilities which enables them to refer difficult cases in the same way as do GPs. More usually, it is the relatives who bring to the psychiatric facility patients who are unsuccessfully treated by the traditional healer. The bias introduced in this process of referral depends, of course, on the measure of success achieved by traditional healers in treating psychiatric disorders. This also is considered in Part III. Treatment given by traditional healers is relatively expensive, some psychotic patients living in the healer's compound for months at a time. If treatment is unsuccessful and the relatives are unable to pay any more, patients are often turned loose to wander where they will. If relatives are unwilling to shelter them, they may die of starvation and neglect or may gravitate to an urban centre to eke out an existence as vagrants. Asuni (1971) examined the vagrants living in the town of Abeokuta, Nigeria, which has a population of 90 000. He identified 35 vagrants suffering from psychosis, which in every case was schizophrenia. The duration of their illness ranged from 6 years to over 25 years. Harding (1973) also identified a number of vagrant psychotics in the area of Ibarapa, Nigeria, with the aid of information from the police and local authority.

In some developing countries, prisons are used as substitutes for psychiatric hospitals, and patients who are violent or disruptive in other ways are incarcerated in them. In Zambia, for example, the director of the psychiatric hospital in the capital city regularly visits prisons in outlying districts to examine possible psychiatric patients and arrange for their transfer to the central hospital if necessary. Some patients, however, are likely to recover and be released before he has a chance to interview them. Hence, prisons in developing countries may well be a source of first-onset psychotic patients who are not known to the psychiatric services.

Finally, we need to consider the general population in a developing country. It is quite likely that it includes people who have at some stage developed an acute psychosis, which resolved after brief contact with a traditional healer. Such people are unlikely to be identified in a survey of the clientele of traditional healers unless it covers a fairly long period of time. We should also expect to find people living on their own or with relatives, who are suffering from chronic psychotic conditions that have failed to respond to traditional healing techniques, but who have had no contact with Western-type psychiatric services. The community also includes the great majority of neurotic sufferers, some of whom may have consulted a traditional healer but never a psychiatrist. Among them will be a large proportion who are not recognised as psychiatrically ill by their neighbours or by themselves, because their symptoms take a predominantly somatic form.

These considerations of the distribution of the psychiatrically ill among the various treatment and containment facilities in a developing country make it clear that any procedure for counting psychoses or neuroses has to be carried out on the general population and in addition must cover all the places listed in Table XI. Only a single study has embodied such a comprehensive approach: an international project carried out under the auspices of the World Health Organization (Sartorius *et al*, 1986).

8 Knocking on doors in Asia

We have seen that, to make valid comparisons of the frequency of psychiatric conditions in Westernised and traditional societies, it is essential to conduct population surveys. These ventures require a considerable expenditure of money and a group of people with relevant experience and expertise. Such resources are rarely found in developing countries, so that it is not surprising to find that few studies of this kind have been carried out, and that the earlier ones were initiated and often conducted by Western psychiatrists. This raises all kinds of problems concerning lack of familiarity with the languages and cultural backgrounds of the respondents, many of which were examined in Part I. Even in a developed country, population surveys represent a considerable demand on resources, and various ways of economising have been attempted.

The most expensive way of conducting a population survey is to use fully trained psychiatrists to interview every person in the sample. This is wasteful, since the majority of respondents will be free of significant psychiatric symptoms. An alternative strategy is to use key people in the community as case identifiers. These people must have the confidence of the populace, so that they act as a channel for information, or else they need to be in a position that brings them into contact with many people. Thus, village chiefs, policemen, and teachers, have been used as key contacts for collecting information about mentally disturbed members of the community. The reliability of this approach clearly depends on developing an excellent liaison with the key contacts and on the degree to which psychiatric conditions are stigmatised and hence kept hidden by sufferers and their relatives. An idea of the efficiency of the key informant approach compared with interviewing the total sample can be gained from a study by Hagnell (1966). With the painstaking industry that characterises Scandinavian epidemiology, Hagnell personally interviewed over 3000 inhabitants of Lundby in South Sweden. The interviews lasted between 0.5 h and over 2 h, and the whole project took nearly 2.5 years to complete. In addition to personal interviews with the respondents, Hagnell used three key informants who had lived in the area for 25, 30, and 60 years. They had actively participated in both official and private events and were all interested in their fellow people. In some cases, their information was extremely accurate, whereas in others, they were completely unaware of psychiatric disturbance in the recent past. For instance, in one case, a depressive illness 5 years earlier, lasting 6 months, was not mentioned by the key informant. In another case, an organic confusional state lasting for 1 year was not referred to. Examples of omissions of this magnitude cast considerable doubt on the use of key informants as the sole source of data in population surveys.

Surveys can also be conducted by a two-stage process involving a self-administered screening instrument, such as the General Health Questionnaire (Goldberg & Blackwell, 1970) to identify 'cases'. However, this method is not applicable to preliterate or semiliterate societies. Another way of economising is to use trained interviewers to screen the population under study. Their aim is to identify subjects who are definitely or possibly suffering from psychiatric conditions. Those selected are then interviewed by psychiatrists, to confirm or refute their 'caseness', and to make a diagnosis. To check on the reliability of the screening interviews, it is also necessary for the psychiatrists to see a random sample of those judged initially to be normal. A selection of one in ten normal subjects is probably sufficient to assess the judgement of the screening interviewers, and does not add a great deal to the work required of the psychiatrist. The success of this strategy rests on the effectiveness of the training for the screening interviewers. Recent experience (Sturt *et al*, 1981) has shown that some people without any psychiatric background can pick up the interviewing and rating techniques easily and rapidly, whereas others fail to grasp the issues involved. This underlines the importance of careful monitoring and selection of interviewers during the training period. With this proviso, the use of lay interviewers to screen the population, backed up by psychiatrists to do second interviews, is probably the most efficient and economical method of conducting surveys of psychiatric morbidity. The majority of the studies that have been conducted have been carried out in Western countries, but there are now more than 20 published studies from developing countries. Of those reviewed here, five relate to African countries, nine were conducted in India and Sri Lanka, three in Taiwan, two in Japan, and one in China. This chapter discusses those from Asia.[1]

The earliest study in this group is that by Lin (1953). He surveyed the Chinese population of three areas: a small village; a provincial town; and a seaport on the island of Taiwan off the South China coast. The Chinese arrived on the island in the 17th century and gradually displaced the aborigines, Malayo-Polynesians, who became confined to the mountains in the interior. The method of the survey consisted firstly of a preliminary stage of gathering information from elders, officials, policemen, physicians, and

---

[1] For ease of comparison, rates from all the surveys discussed are presented in Table XII pp. 110–111.

school teachers. From these key informants, it was possible to identify a considerable number of psychiatrically ill people. This stage of the inquiry was followed by a house-to-house survey conducted by teams of doctors and medical students, accompanied by the elder or official of the village. The team interviewed each member of every family for about 5 min. If psychiatric abnormality was suspected, or the respondent had already been mentioned by a key informant, he or she was interviewed in greater detail. The final diagnosis was made by Lin, who reviewed every case and interviewed all those in whom the presence of abnormality was equivocal. The interviews were not standardised, but as one psychiatrist made all the diagnoses, we can assume that the application of diagnostic criteria was reasonably consistent. An astonishing number of subjects, 19 931 in all, were interviewed in the course of 16 months. A total of 214 cases in the three areas were diagnosed as having psychiatric disorders, and included both active cases who showed current abnormalities and inactive cases who had been psychiatrically ill at some previous time. A count of the active cases would give an estimate of the point prevalence (see Fig. 7, p. 86).

Some authorities would also include inactive cases of schizophrenia in the point-prevalence figures, maintaining that 'once a schizophrenic, always a schizophrenic'. There is room for disagreement here, since a proportion of people suffering from a first episode of typical schizophrenia will never experience a second attack in thier lifetime, and will appear completely normal once the episode is over. Regardless of diagnosis, the inclusion in the figures of people who have ever had an attack of psychiatric illness during their life changes the point prevalence to a lifetime prevalence. The distinction between these different ways of presenting data must be carefully noted if valid comparisons are to be made between studies.

Lin found no significant differences in the overall rate of psychiatric disorders between the three areas surveyed. The lifetime prevalence of schizophrenia was calculated as 2.1 per 1000, of manic–depressive psychosis as 0.7 per 1000, and of neuroses as 1.2 per 1000. It is important to note that the average age of the population studied was much lower than that of a Western country. Over half the population was aged under 20 years and only 5.5% were over 60. This is characteristic of the age structure found in developing countries, resulting from a high birth rate and a relatively low life expectancy. It has a crucial effect on the rate of psychiatric disorders, since both psychotic and neurotic conditions have their peak incidence in adult life, and psychoses are extremely rare under the age of 15 years. It is obvious from this that rates of disorder for the total population cannot be directly compared between Western and non-Western countries, since the proportion of the population at risk for psychiatric disorders is substantially smaller in the latter than in the former. It is necessary to express the rates of psychiatric disorder in terms of specific age groups, a procedure known as age stratification. A comparatively simple way of dealing with this problem is to calculate the rates for the population over the age of 15 years. Lin's figures quoted above are expressed in terms of the total population, although he also gives the age distribution of the psychiatric disorders he found, so that it is possible to recalculate his rates for the population over the age of 15 years. This results in an increase of 72% in the above figures.

It is very surprising that he found neuroses to be less common than schizophrenia, but the author comments that there was "difficulty in identifying all cases of neurosis in the communities". The reasons for this were discussed in Part I. Of the 24 cases identified, nine were suffering from a condition called *Hsieh-Ping*, which is Chinese for devil's sickness. It is characterised by a trance state in which the subject identifies with a dead person for a period of from 0.5 h to many hours. The subject talks in a strange tone of voice, the content being mostly of a religious nature related to ancestor worship. The subject imitates the manner of the dead person and makes demands for him. It is clear from this description given by Lin that *Hsieh-Ping* is identical to possession states found in virtually every traditional culture throughout the world. It was argued in Chapter 2 that possession states should not be considered as illnesses at all, so that Lin's prevalence rate for neuroses becomes even lower.

This survey of the Chinese population of Taiwan was followed by a study of the aboriginal Malayo-Polynesians on the island using the same techniques (Rin & Lin, 1962). At the time, the total population of aboriginals was 200 000. The people were semiliterate and lived in agricultural, traditional communities. It is noteworthy that their life expectancy was only 40–45 years, representing a substantial reduction in the period at risk for psychiatric disorders. As with the Chinese, the study began with the establishment of a liaison with community leaders. By this means, 70% of cases diagnosed as psychiatrically ill were identified before the household surveys. The language of communication was Japanese, which was understood by the majority of the population between the ages of 20 and 45. The discussion of the language of emotion in Chapter 4 suggests considerable difficulties in the identification of neurotic conditions for subjects who are not interviewed in their mother tongue. In all, the team interviewed 11 442 people, representing 5% of the aboriginal population.

Altogether, 154 cases of psychiatric disorder were identified, yielding a prevalence of 13.5 per 1000. Of these, 45 were suffering from a psychosis, classified as either active or inactive as in the earlier study. A substantial proportion of inactive cases, 12 out of the 25, were classified as 'malarial psychosis'. This refers to people who were discovered to be suffering from malaria during the period of psychotic behaviour. The problem of the relationship between acute infectious fevers and psychosis in tropical countries is discussed in Part IV, but note that some cases of schizophrenia may well be included under the rubric of 'malarial psychosis'. Hence, the number of cases of schizophrenia identified in this survey, amounting to ten, is probably an underestimate of the true number. The prevalence arrived at by expressing this figure as a rate for the total population is 0.9 per 1000.

Unfortunately, the age distribution of the population was not available, so this figure cannot be corrected for the skew towards the younger age groups and the relatively low life expectancy. These factors, as well as cases of schizophrenia camouflaged as 'malarial psychosis', if taken into account, would increase the prevalence rate considerably. The number of cases of manic–depressive disorder found was also ten, yielding the same uncorrected prevalence of 0.9 per 1000. Only nine cases of neurosis were identified, corresponding to a prevalence of 0.8 per 1000, but this is certainly a gross underestimate, for the reasons already given.

These two large-scale population surveys in Taiwan, conducted by the same researchers, represent important pioneering ventures. The rates for psychoses can be compared between the two studies, but the lack of standardised techniques for clinical examination and diagnosis render comparisons with other studies dubious. Furthermore, the use of 'malarial psychosis' as a classification, and the failure to standardise by age in the aboriginal survey, undermine the value of the prevalence rates derived.

Fifteen years after the original survey of the Chinese population, Lin *et al* (1969) returned to the same three areas and repeated the study using the same techniques. In the period between the two surveys the total number of Chinese inhabitants in the three communities rose from 20 000 to 29 000, an increase of 46%. The age distribution changed in the direction of a higher proportion of the population in the older age groups. The percentage of the illiterate fell from 37 to 20% and there was a significant shift in occupation from farmers and fishermen to labourers. From the first to the second survey there was no significant change in the prevalence of psychoses as a total group, although schizophrenia showed a significant drop from 2.1 per 1000 to 1.4 per 1000. During the same period, the prevalence of neuroses showed a huge increase from 1.2 per 1000 to 7.8 per 1000. This increase was greatest in the upper social class, least in the middle class, and intermediate in the lower class. It was particularly marked in people with no formal education. One can speculate that it might be due to the change in age structure of the population, to increasing industrialisation, or to greater literacy leading to more psychological expression of emotional distress (see Chapter 4). It is not possible to determine the relative importance of these factors on the basis of the data presented by Lin and his colleagues.

A population survey has also been repeated after an interval of some years in Japan (Kato, 1969). The Japanese Ministry of Health and Welfare carried out two nationwide prevalence surveys of psychiatric disorders in 1954 and 1963. A random sample of households was selected from 100 national census areas in 1954, and 203 census areas in the second survey. Surveys of 4895 households containing 23 993 persons were conducted on the first occasion and of 11 853 households containing 44 902 persons on the second. Each district was investigated by a team of one or two psychiatrists, a public-health nurse and/or a psychiatric social worker, and a public-health statistician. The supervisors carefully selected 100 psychiatrists in 1954, and

203 in 1963, who were in close agreement on diagnostic standards. A 1-day point-prevalence rate was determined in each survey. The investigators were concerned only with active cases, defined as persons who had shown psychiatric symptoms in the previous year, with the exception of manic-depressive symptoms, where the time span was limited to 6 months. It should be noted that this is a more restricted survey than those of Lin and his colleagues, who were interested in both active and inactive cases. Nevertheless, the prevalence rate for schizophrenia, which was identical in both Japanese surveys at 2.3 per 1000, was very close to that found by Lin in 1953 for the Chinese on Taiwan, namely 2.1 per 1000. The prevalence rate for manic–depressive psychosis represents a 6-month prevalence in the Japanese surveys, and was 0.2 per 1000 on both occasions. The 1-year prevalence of neurotic disorders was found to be 3.0 per 1000 in the first survey and 2.8 in the second.

More population surveys for psychiatric illness have been conducted in India than in any other developing country. Sethi *et al* (1967, 1972, 1974) have carried out three surveys employing the same techniques. In the first two, they studied 300 urban families and 500 rural families, whereas in the most recent they interviewed a random sample of 2000 families from the North Indian city of Lucknow. In their 1974 paper, they reported the data obtained from the first 850 families investigated. Each family was interviewed by a research team comprising a psychiatrist, a clinical psychologist, and a social worker. The personnel had experience conducting field interviews, as the same team had been employed in the two earlier surveys. Family members were interviewed with a questionnaire consisting of a list of psychological and somatic symptoms usually observed in psychiatric disorders. It operated as a screening device, so that if the responses suggested the presence of any psychiatric problem, the person was immediately given a full psychiatric assessment. A detailed case history, and a clinical evaluation, were recorded for every suspected case, and the completed questionnaires were checked by a senior psychiatrist for confirmation of the diagnosis.

A total of 4481 people were screened, and of these, 300 were designated as psychiatric cases. The authors give period prevalence rates for various diagnostic categories, but regrettably fail to specify the period concerned. Hence, we do not know whether they considered inactive as well as active cases, and it is not possible to compare their figures directly with any other survey. The period prevalence rates they give are 2.5 per 1000 for schizophrenia, 1.1 per 1000 for manic–depressive disorders, and 27.1 per 1000 for neuroses. Their rates for the psychoses are very close to those in the studies we have already considered, whereas their rate for neurotic disorders is strikingly higher. This might be attributable to different diagnostic criteria, or to the fact that this is the first study considered so far in which a standardised screening instrument was used.

One of the most extensive Indian surveys was executed by Dube (1970). He organised a field survey of the area around the North Indian city of Agra, including urban, semirural, and rural populations. The technique was very similar to that used by Sethi, including the application of a standardised screening schedule and thorough examination of suspected cases by a psychiatrist. The cases underwent a second interview by another psychiatrist to ensure a correct diagnosis. Active cases were defined as suffering from a psychiatric condition during the 18 months preceding the survey, whereas inactive cases had suffered from such a condition at any time prior to 18 months, but had experienced no active symptoms since then. The total population of the area under study was 29 468, but only 16 725, or 57% were aged over 15 years. This is very similar to the age structure of the Chinese population of Taiwan studied by Lin. Prevalence rates are given by Dube for active cases alone, and for active and inactive cases combined. He also gives age-specific prevalence rates for a number of age groups. It is thus simple to calculate his rates for the population over the age of 15 years. In terms of the total population, he found the prevalence of active cases of schizophrenia to be 1.49 per 1000, while for all cases it was 2.17 per 1000. The latter figure is very close to the lifetime prevalence rates determined in the other studies discussed above. His figures for manic–depressive psychosis were 0.51 per 1000 for active cases and 1.26 per 1000 for all cases. The corresponding rates for neuroses were 9.4 per 1000 and 12.6 per 1000. When these figures are expressed in terms of the population over the age of 15 years, they are increased by 76%. The resulting age-corrected lifetime prevalence for schizophrenia then becomes almost identical to the corresponding figure derived from Lin's (1953) survey of the Taiwan Chinese.

An innovation in methodology was introduced by Elnagar *et al* (1971) in their study of a small village community in West Bengal. The team conducted a house-to-house survey of all 184 families in a circumscribed area. The survey included a thorough clinical examination of all individuals by a health physician in conjunction with a health assistant, to eliminate the possibility of any psychiatric disorder associated with physical illness. A schedule was used to screen for psychiatric symptoms and detailed case histories were obtained of suspected cases. The final diagnosis was made by a non-Indian psychiatrist, which casts some doubt on the reliability of ascertainment of neurotic disorders. The authors included both active and inactive cases, and their prevalence rates were 4.3 per 1000 for schizophrenia and 1.5 per 1000 for neuroses. They do not give a rate for manic–depressive conditions. They divide the population into those aged 15 and over and those under 15, so that it is possible to correct the prevalence rates for age. This increases the figure for schizophrenia to 8.0 per 1000, the highest corrected prevalence rate we have encountered so far. However, it must be emphasised that the total population surveyed was relatively small, yielding only six cases of schizophrenia, so that the prevalence rate cannot be accepted with total confidence.

The city of Lucknow, first surveyed by Sethi *et al* (1974) was also the site of a survey by Thacore *et al* (1975). Whereas Sethi had randomly sampled the general population, Thacore concentrated on families registered at an urban health centre established in 1965. The 500 families registered at the centre represented a cross-section of the resident population, and formed the sample for the study. Family members were screened during house-to-house visits by a team using a health questionnaire designed to elicit information on the mental and physical health of the respondents. Individuals suspected of suffering from psychiatric disorders were then examined by a psychiatrist either at their homes or at the centre. The authors do not state whether they counted both active and inactive cases, but refer to their rates as representing a 1-year prevalence. The rates for the total population of 2696 surveyed were 1.9 per 1000 both for schizophrenia and for manic–depressive psychosis, and 20.4 per 1000 for neurotic disorders. These rates, when expressed in terms of the population aged over 15 years, increase to 3.3 per 1000 and 36.5 per 1000, respectively.

The last two Indian studies discussed here were both initiated by Nandi *et al* (1975, 1980). In the first, they surveyed a village near Calcutta which had no electricity, virtually no latrines, and in which all but one family were cultivators. The team of interviewers used a psychiatric questionnaire and a case-record schedule to screen the total population of the village, which amounted to 1060 people. They used a definition of caseness formulated by the World Health Organization. All cases identified were examined both physically and psychiatrically by two senior psychiatrists. Any differences of opinion were discussed and resolved by re-examining the case. The prevalence rates determined in this study were 2.8 per 1000 for schizophrenia and 67.0 for neurotic disorders, by far the highest figure yet encountered. In evaluating this result, it should be noted that Nandi's study employed the most rigorous technique of all the Asian surveys, including a standardised psychiatric screening instrument, an internationally recognised definition of caseness, and physical examination of all patients.

In the second study, Nandi *et al* (1980) interviewed 4053 people living in 28 villages in two different districts of West Bengal, an area in which the small-scale survey of Elnagar *et al* (1971) was conducted. The same techniques as in Nandi's earlier study were used, and the prevalence rates found were 2.2 per 1000 for schizophrenia and 16.8 per 1000 for neurotic disorders. The latter figure is several times smaller than the corresponding rate from Nandi's first survey. However, it conceals a wide variation in rates shown by the different castes studied. The prevalence of neurosis among tribal people and lower castes was as low as 5.5 per 1000, while among Brahmins it reached 43.2 per 1000, a rate comparable with that from the first study. The prevalence of schizophrenia was also higher among the Brahmins, 7.2 per 1000 compared with less than 2.0 per 1000 for the other centres, but these rates were based on four cases and five cases respectively, so can be accorded little weight.

Next a survey from Sri Lanka carried out by Wijesinghe *et al* (1978) is considered. This was a well-designed and carefully conducted study, equal to the best of the Indian surveys. A screening interview was constructed by a clinical team on the basis of the case records of 100 patients attending a psychiatric clinic of a general hospital. The interview consisted of a general health inquiry followed by psychiatric items, and was administered by social workers. They screened 7653 people in a semi-urban area. Criteria for caseness were laid down, and anyone satisfying them was referred for a psychiatric examination. Prevalence was calculated for the 6-month period of the survey, and only cases active during that time were included in the figures. This would seem to be a relatively restricted period compared with other surveys considered, but the majority of cases detected were chronic, so would also have been included in an annual prevalence or even a life-time prevalence. Of all the cases found, 69% were over 2 years in duration. Furthermore, every case of schizophrenia had lasted more than 2 years, and 62% for at least 10 years. The period prevalence rates derived from the cases were 3.8 per 1000 for schizophrenia and 25.2 per 1000 for neuroses. As a check on the effectiveness of the social workers' screening procedure, a random sample of respondents who were not referred to the psychiatrists was given a psychiatric interview. A substantial number of these was found to be suffering from an active psychiatric condition, in almost every case a neurosis. An estimated prevalence rate, based on these extra cases, comes to about 60 per 1000. This is close to the highest figure found in all these Asian surveys, by Nandi *et al* (1975), and indicates that increasing scrupulousness in case finding hardly alters the prevalence of schizophrenia, but makes an enormous difference to the prevalence of neurotic conditions.

Wijesinghe *et al* (1978) also give the age distribution of their screened population so that it is possible to correct their prevalence figures for age. The rates per 1000 population aged 15 and over come out as 5.6 for schizophrenia and 89.0 for neuroses. We can infer from this methodologically sophisticated study that the very highest rates found in the Asian surveys are likely to represent the most realistic estimates of the true prevalence of neuroses.

Finally, a prevalence study conducted in China was reported by Lin *et al* (1980) who had access to a mimeographed report, by Xia *et al*. An area of Shanghai containing 4 000 000 inhabitants was surveyed during the period 1972–1978. Key informants were used to identify possible cases. The informants consisted of 'barefoot doctors', nurses, health workers in factories, and lay people serving on regional committees, all of whom had received short courses of psychiatric training by local psychiatrists. The diagnosis of the identified cases was then ascertained by psychiatrists through home visits. The figures produced were an overall prevalence rate of mental disorder of 7.3 per 1000, and a prevalence rate for schizophrenia of 4.2 per 1000. These data are not age-corrected, and the overall prevalence rate is not very informative in the absence of a more detailed diagnostic breakdown. Nevertheless the rate for schizophrenia is of considerable interest since epidemiological data from China are rare.

9 Knocking on doors in Africa

Far fewer psychiatric surveys have been carried out in Africa than in Asia. The earliest was of the Yoruba people of Nigeria by Leighton *et al* (1963), and involved the introduction of major innovations in methodology. The most important was the use of instruments and techniques that had already been employed in a population survey in a Western country. Until recently, this was the only study in a developing country, the results of which could be directly compared with data from a developed country. The publication of Orley & Wing (1979), which is discussed below, adds a second study of this kind.

Leighton's (1959) second innovation was the development of a method for identifying cases. He produced this in the context of the Stirling County Study, a psychiatric population survey of a rural area in northeast America. The essence of his approach is the avoidance of diagnostic categories where possible, and their replacement with assessments of the degree of psychiatric disturbance and impairment of function. This departure from traditional psychiatric practice was prompted by Leighton's concern over the unreliability of psychiatric diagnoses. Whatever its advantages in avoiding this problem, his method has the distinct disadvantage that the resultant data do not yield prevalence rates for specific conditions.

The psychiatric questionnaire used in the Nigerian survey was a somewhat modified and expanded version of the one employed in the Stirling County Study. The new version was dubbed the Cornell-Aro Psychiatric Questionnaire and included additional questions considered to be appropriate to the Yoruba, such as: "Do you ever have creeping feelings in the skin?" and "Are you troubled by having a feeling of expanded head and goose flesh?" The questionnaire was translated into the Yoruba language and was administered by psychiatrists. There were six in all, two of whom were Nigerian and interviewed respondents in Yoruba. The other four used interpreters to conduct interviews, a procedure that introduces an additional source of potential unreliability.

101

The survey was conducted in 15 villages, ranging in size from 37 inhabitants to 2130, in each of which a random sample was drawn, and in eight sections of the city of Abeokuta, with a random sample drawn from each section. The Yoruba villages were rural farming settlements, while the city was the main commercial and governmental centre for the area. The data were compared with those from the Stirling County Study, in which a random sample of 1010 adults was interviewed. The age structure of the Yoruba respondents was very similar to that of the Stirling County sample. A total of 262 villagers and 64 townspeople constituted the Nigerian sample. This was a small-scale survey compared with most of the Asian studies reviewed, the size of the sample being limited by the use of psychiatrists to conduct every interview. If the Asian figures are applicable to Nigeria, not more than one or two schizophrenic people would be expected to appear in a survey population of 362 adults. In fact, three cases were detected, but it would be misleading to express such a small number as a prevalence rate, since one case more or less would alter it drastically.

There is another problem in accepting the number of schizophrenic people detected at face value and this is highlighted by a study done by Harding (1973). He carried out a point-prevalence study of a psychosis severe enough to remove the patient from the family home. He surveyed the rural district of Ibarapa, 40–60 miles north of the area covered by Leighton's study, identified all traditional healers in the area who treated psychiatrically ill patients, and arranged for groups of medical students to visit them on a given day and count the number of psychotic patients under treatment. In addition, the number of vagrant psychotic people was ascertained by information from the police and local authority. It was found that 43 patients from Ibarapa with a psychotic condition were living with traditional healers, with an additional eight vagrant psychotics. The population of Ibarapa was 140 000, so that the prevalence rate of psychotic people living away from their homes was 0.36 per 1000. By no means all of these were suffering from schizophrenia, but none of them would have been identified by the usual technique of random selection of households.

In the absence of derived prevalence rates, the material is presented using Leighton's (1959) categorisation, as it is at least comparable with his data from Stirling County. He uses four ratings for the degree of psychiatric disturbance: A represents the evaluator's certainty that he or she is dealing with a case of psychiatric disorder, B is accorded to a probable case, C is for doubtful cases, and D is given to respondents who are free from significant symptoms. A rating of A was given to 23% of the Yoruba respondents, compared with 31% of the Stirling County sample. It will be noted that these represent very high proportions of cases in a general population sample, suggesting that the threshold for pathology applied by Leighton and his colleagues was relatively low. When men and women were considered separately, it emerged that the proportion of men given an A rating in the Yoruba villages (22%) was almost identical to the figure for Stirling County men (21%), while the village women (20%) appeared to be psychiatrically much healthier than the Stirling County women (40%). B ratings were given to 17% of the Yoruba sample compared with 26% of the Stirling County respondents. It is also worth noting that depressive symptoms were found much more commonly among Yoruba villagers (30%) than among the people of Stirling County.

Gillis *et al* (1968) published the second African survey, which was conducted among the coloured people of the Cape Peninsula. These people have evolved over 300 years as a distinct ethnic group, and at the time of the survey numbered 200 365. A random sample of 500 of this population was interviewed by a team of three psychiatrists and 14 specially trained social workers. Interviews were also held with reliable people who knew each respondent. A questionnaire was constructed, consisting of 600 items, including some from the Cornell-Aro instrument described above. The exact wording to be used by the social-worker interviewers was laid down, but they could ask additional unspecified questions. The responses were evaluated by the psychiatrists using the methods developed by Leighton, and already described. Of the total coloured population interviewed, 12% were given an A rating and another 12% a B rating. It appears from these figures that the Cape coloured people are considerably healthier from a psychiatric point of view than either the Yoruba or the Stirling County folk. However, as the authors point out, they were only concerned with psychiatric disturbance at the time of the survey, whereas Leighton *et al* were covering the whole of the respondents' past life. Prevalence rates in these accounts are sorely missed as it is very difficult to interpret these global judgements of caseness that eschew diagnostic categories. Fortunately, Gillis *et al* record that they identified 27 cases of psychoneurosis. This would give a prevalence rate for neurosis of 54 per 1000, which is close to the highest rate recorded in the Asian surveys. When one considers that this represents a point-prevalence rate rather than a lifetime prevalence, it becomes apparent that the Cape coloured people do not have a special claim to psychiatric health in the developing world.

Giel & Van Luijk (1969*a,b*) also utilised Leighton's form of classification in two population surveys they conducted in Ethiopia, one in a rural village, the other in a small town. For the town survey, they randomly sampled 100 households and interviewed whoever was present and sufficiently informed to give reliable information. In the majority of cases, this resulted in an interview with the head of the household or his wife, as others were unwilling to discuss the inmates of the house. The authors, a psychiatrist and a sociologist, were accompanied by an interpreter and a community nurse from the town's health centre. The interview centred round a checklist of symptoms and disease entities, including some of the more familiar behavioural and psychological disturbances. If considered necessary, a short physical examination was also conducted. Giel & Van Luijk were well aware of the shortcomings of having to rely on an interpreter: "Interpreters, especially if they are trained in medicine, tend to be very selective in their translations. They look for what they consider to be medically relevant and leave out all the rest of a patient's statements. They feel embarrassed or they become ironical when a patient tries to express himself in his own words and uses his own familiar images.''

Having collected all the information, the authors rated the degree of certainty that the individual was a psychiatric case using Leighton's method. Of the 384 people covered by the household survey, 6% were appraised as certain cases of psychiatric disorder and 3% as probable cases. These figures are even lower than those of Gillis *et al* for the Cape coloured. Only a single case of schizophrenia was encountered among the Ethiopian townspeople, but 16 cases of psychoneurosis were detected. This gives a prevalence rate of 41.7 per 1000, or 63.5 per 1000 of the population aged 15 or more.

The second Ethiopian survey was of a rural village, a 5-h mule ride from the nearest roadside town. Giel & Van Luijk (1969*b*) studied the village of Muti, whose inhabitants, the Kafa, speak their own language, Kafinya. The village was ill defined so that it was not possible to select a random sample of households. Instead, the authors started with the houses around the market place and on the mission compound, working away from these two centres until they had visited 100 houses. The technique of interviewing was exactly as in the town survey, and as before they relied on an interpreter. Of the 370 people covered by the survey, 6% were judged to be certain cases of psychiatric disorder and 3% probable cases, exactly the same proportions as in the town survey. Altogether, 19 cases were diagnosed as neurosis, yielding a prevalence of 51.4 per 1000 or 93.1 per 1000 of the population aged 15 years or more. This is the highest age-corrected rate we have yet come across in these population surveys.

Another African psychiatric survey was by Orley & Wing (1979). Orley was trained both as a psychiatrist and an anthropologist, and before he attempted the survey, he carried out anthropological and ethnopsychiatric fieldwork in Uganda over a period of 5 years. He surveyed the total population of two villages in a rural area of Uganda. The instrument used for detecting psychiatric symptoms was the PSE (Wing *et al*, 1974), which had already proved to be applicable in a variety of cultures, including a number of traditional ones (World Health Organization, 1973). Orley had learned the local language, Luganda, and translated the PSE into it. Some problems were encountered with the translation, particularly the items referring to unpleasant emotional states, but were not found to be insuperable. The interviews were conducted jointly by Orley and a research assistant, who was from the area. The survey took 8 weeks in the first village, and 14 weeks in the second village. Of the 221 subjects aged 18 years or more, all but 15 were successfully interviewed.

A novel technique was used to determine the number of cases in the sample. Wing *et al* (1974) had already developed the Catego program for standardising diagnosis on the basis of PSE symptoms (see p. 36). Catego is only applicable to subjects exhibiting a certain level of pathology, of the kind usually encountered among hospital in-patients and out-patients. To determine the level of caseness reached by subjects in a population survey, it was considered necessary to develop another program. This is known as the Index of Definition (Wing *et al*, 1978) and assigns subjects to one of eight levels of definition of psychiatric disorder. Levels one to four lie below the threshold for a case, level five is considered to be the borderline, and levels six to eight constitute definite cases. The level a subject reaches is determined partly by the number of symptoms and partly by their type. Thus, single 'key symptoms', such as depressed mood, autonomic anxiety, or hypomanic affect, can push a subject up to a relatively high level even if there are few other symptoms present. In this way, the same hierarchical approach that characterises Catego is also built into the Index of Definition. The two programs can be used in conjunction, so that any disorder above the threshold point is classified by Catego, producing the equivalent of a clinical diagnosis. This technique standardises the process of judging caseness, which in all the other surveys discussed has depended on the assessment by individuals, which may well vary from case to case. One might equate the definite and threshold levels of the Index of Definition with the certain and probable categories of Leighton, but the degree of correspondence between these two systems of determining caseness has not been investigated.

Using the Index of Definition, Orley found that 11 respondents were assigned to levels six or seven (none reached level eight) and hence were considered to constitute definite cases. A further 42 cases reached level five, and were categorised as threshold cases. Combining all cases at threshold level and above, 27% of the women and 24% of the men were considered to have a psychiatric disorder. These overall prevalence rates can be directly compared with the findings of two recent general population surveys carried out in the Camberwell district of south-east London using the same techniques. In the first survey, in which only women were interviewed, 11% reached level five or above (Wing *et al*, 1978). The second survey was carried out in the same area but included men as well as women (Bebbington *et al*, 1981*b*). The overall prevalence rates were found to be 15% for women and 6% for men. Thus, the use of a standardised interviewing technique combined with a computerised method of determining caseness has demonstrated that Ugandan villagers of both sexes show a considerably higher level of overall psychiatric morbidity than people living in an inner London suburb.

Breaking down the overall psychiatric morbidity into specific diagnostic categories is necessary to make comparisons with the other studies considered. Too few cases of psychosis were identified in any of the above surveys to calculate reliable prevalence rates. For neurosis, Orley & Wing found a prevalence of 269 per 1000 population between the ages of 18 and 65 years for women and 174 per 1000, for men. These are far and away the highest prevalence figures for neurosis found in any population survey in a developing country. However, they are matched, at least for the women, by figures from a carefully conducted survey of an urban population in the Argentine. Tarnopolsky *et al* (1977) found the total prevalence of neurosis per 1000 population aged 15 and above to be 287 for women and 94 for men. A study in Athens, using an identical definition of cases to Orley & Wing's, produced prevalence rates for neurosis of 222 per 1000 for women and 82 per 1000 for men (Mavreas *et al*, 1986). The figures for Londoners between the ages of 18 and 65 were 106 per 1000 for women in the first Camberwell survey, and in the second survey 135 per 1000 for women and 58 per 1000 for men.

Instead of looking at the prevalence of caseness, one can examine the distribution of depressive symptoms, regardless of the level reached by the subjects on the Index of Definition. The syndrome of depression, compounded of a small number of symptoms and signs from the PSE, was found in 20% of Ugandan women and 23% of Ugandan men. The corresponding figure for the Camberwell survey was 10% of the total population (Bebbington *et al*, 1981*b*). This echoes the finding of Leighton *et al* (1963) that depressive symptoms were found much more commonly among Yoruba villagers than among their American respondents.

The Camberwell surveys we have considered were too small to yield useful prevalence figures for psychotic conditions. Larger-scale surveys have been conducted in the Scandinavian countries and the USA, but the data are presented in such a way that it is very difficult to extract prevalence rates for schizophrenia and manic–depressive psychosis. One study that does give lifetime prevalence rates is that by Helgason (1964), who conducted an epidemiological survey of 5395 people in Iceland. The rates he gives for schizophrenia are 4.3 per 1000 for males and 7.6 per 1000 for females.

An alternative approach is to derive such rates, not from population surveys, but from case registers. A case register is a continuously updated record of all contacts made with a particular kind of health service by people from a defined catchment area. The Camberwell Register (Wing & Hailey, 1972) records all contacts with psychiatric services by residents of the London borough of Camberwell. It is relatively simple to extract from the register an annual prevalence rate for any psychiatric illness. This figure includes all inhabitants of the borough who have been either in-patients or out-patients of the psychiatric services during a specific year, and who have been given the relevant diagnosis. The figure does not include patients who were in contact with the services prior to the year under scrutiny, but who have subsequently lost contact. Thus, it is not a total prevalence rate, but it is possible to make an adjustment for these lost cases as we shall see. The prevalence rate for schizophrenia for the year 1977 derived from the Camberwell Register is 3.1 per 1000 total population. When this is adjusted for the population aged 15 years and over, the rate increases to 3.9 per 1000. A study was conducted by Leff & Vaughn (1972) of Camberwell patients with functional psychoses who had been in contact with the psychiatric services up to 31 December 1969, and who had then been out of contact for at least 1 year. They identified 27 patients with schizophrenia who satisfied these criteria. It cannot be assumed that the pool of Camberwell schizophrenic patients out of contact with the services increases by an additional 27 patients every year, because some of those who lost contact previously re-establish contact when they fall ill again, or for other reasons. Thus, it is not possible to use this figure to calculate the total number of Camberwell schizophrenic people out of contact with the services at any one time. However, it does provide an idea of the scale of the adjustment required. These 27 cases represent an additional prevalence rate of 0.2 per 1000 population over the age of 15 years. The total age-adjusted prevalence rate for schizophrenia is thus likely to lie between 4 and 5 per 1000 for the population of Camberwell.

Comparable figures can be derived from the Salford Case Register, which was established in 1968 to cover the residents of a county borough in the English Midlands. The point prevalence rate for schizophrenia per 1000 population age 15 and above was 4.39 in 1968 and 6.00 in 1978 (Wooff *et al*, 1983). This rise over 10 years is probably accounted for by a considerable fall in the population of Salford, the more able-bodied, healthy people moving to live elsewhere. An identical figure to the 1978 rate for Salford was arrived at by Tsuang *et al* (1982) in a study of relatives of controls for genetic research in schizophrenia in Iowa.

One case-register study in the West which is not in accord with these figures was conducted in Ireland (Walsh, 1985). Data on in-patients in Ireland have existed since the late 1850s and have shown that the Irish psychiatric hospital-stay rate was the highest known. One reason for establishing case registers was to investigate this alarming finding. There are two registers in Ireland, the St Loman's Register and the Three Counties Register, the latter covering a mainly rural population. The point prevalence rate for schizophrenia derived from the St Loman's Register is 3 per 1000 population age 15 and over, similar to the figures from Camberwell and Salford. However the comparable prevalence rate from the Three Counties Register is 8 per 1000. This high figure cannot be ascribed to a difference in diagnostic habits, as it has been checked in a research project in which the PSE was administered to every register patient given a diagnosis of schizophrenia. Study of the Irish register data has revealed that rates of contact of persons beginning new episodes of care for any psychiatric condition are significantly lower than in other register areas. However, the prevalence rates are much higher, indicating that Irish patients contact psychiatric services less frequently, but once they enter the psychiatric network they are less likely to leave. This might be the explanation for the high prevalence of schizophrenia in the Three Counties area.

In addition to the population surveys reviewed, a handful of studies have concentrated on estimating the prevalence of schizophrenia in developing countries. One of them used a survey technique, while the others relied on hospital admission rates, a much less reliable method. Ben-Tovim & Cushnie (1986) surveyed six villages in a remote rural area of Botswana over a period of 1 year from June 1981 to June 1982. The local village health workers acted as key informants, as did tribal authorities, community workers, traditional healers, religious healers, and schoolteachers. This study is unusual in that the researchers were also providing a clinical service to the villages, and therefore visited them at regular intervals over the course of a year. This form of scrutiny is more likely to detect transient illnesses than a point-prevalence survey. Patients identified by the key informants were given diagnostic interviews by the research psychiatrists, who used a semi-structured interview. These data were supplemented by a 1-day census of all patients under treatment in the only mental hospital in Botswana, and the monitoring of all psychiatric patients admitted during the year of the study. A government census of the country had been carried out just prior to the beginning of the study, so the population of the six villages was known accurately. The number of those age 15 or over was found to be 1133. Both authors agreed on the diagnosis of schizophrenia in six individuals. All satisfied the criteria of ICD–9, but one was above the upper age limit for a DSM–III diagnosis of schizophrenia. This means that all six patients must have been ill for more than 6 months, and that no acute transient psychoses were included. Furthermore, no patients from the study area were found in the mental hospital or were admitted to hospital during the study year. The only omission from this comprehensive case-finding technique is a survey of patients resident with traditional healers, of the kind Harding (1973) conducted. However, since Ben-Tovim & Cushnie used traditional healers as key informants, they probably covered this possible source of cases. The prevalence figure from their data based on an ICD–9 diagnosis is 5.3 per 1000.

Lastly, two estimates of prevalence, from developing countries outside Africa, are provided by Murphy & Taumoepeau (1980) in Tonga, and Torrey *et al* (1974) in Papua New Guinea. In the Tongan study, the records of the psychiatric hospital were used to calculate a first-admission rate, but no diagnostic breakdown was possible, as there was no psychiatrist. To gain a better idea of the rates, Murphy & Taumoepeau used key informants on the island of Eua to determine whether psychotic people were kept at home, since the mental hospital was heavily stigmatised. They found three chronically ill schizophrenic and two chronically ill manic–depressive people who had probably never been to hospital. The population of the island aged over 15 was 2250, giving a very low prevalence rate for schizophrenia. However the case-finding technique was not as thorough as in the Botswana study, so that the reliability of this figure is not as sturdy. The study in Papua New Guinea was considerably less satisfactory, since Torrey *et al* (1974) relied entirely on mental-hospital admission rates. The reasons why this source of data inevitably underestimates the true incidence and prevalence of schizophrenia in a developing country was discussed above. Consequently, the figures produced by Torrey *et al* are not comparable with the prevalence data generated by the other studies reviewed here.

It is evident from Table XII that the prevalence rate for schizophrenia from a variety of population surveys in developing countries varies within relatively narrow limits. The rate uncorrected for the age structure of the population ranges between 0.9 and 4.3 with an average of 2.6 per 1000. This compares with the uncorrected figure from the Camberwell Register of 3.1 per 1000. However, because of the very different age distributions of the populations of developing and developed countries, it is more valid to compare the age-corrected figures. The range for developing countries is 1.3 to 8.0 with a mean of 4.4 per 1000. This is not as representative a figure as we would like, since it is possible to produce age-corrected data for only seven of the 15 studies included. We have estimated the true age-corrected rate for Camberwell to lie between 4 and 5 per 1000, while the current figure from Salford and from Iowa is 6 per 1000. The highest register figure we have encountered is 8 per 1000 from Ireland, but this is equalled by the age-corrected rate for West Bengal (Elnagar *et al*, 1971). The lowest rates from developing countries were found among Taiwan aborigines (0.9 uncorrected) and Tongans (1.3 age-corrected). These are matched by the prevalence rates found by Eaton & Weil (1955) in a study of American Hutterite communities: 1.1 uncorrected and 2.1 age-corrected per 1000. It is evident that variations in the prevalence of schizophrenia from place to place are not attributable to the developed/developing dichotomy. Differences in prevalence may of course reflect variations in incidence or in long-term outcome. It is possible, for example, for a high incidence to be associated with a good outcome, so that relatively few chronic cases would contribute to the prevalence. It is clear that careful and thorough incidence studies are required in developing countries. One international study of this kind, recently completed (Sartorius *et al*, 1986) is discussed below.

The rate for manic–depressive disorders in seven population surveys ranges from 0.7 to 1.9 with an average of 1.2 per 1000. These are uncorrected figures, and exclude the results of Kato's (1969) surveys, which covered a period of only 6 months. The mean of the age-corrected figures is 1.9 per 1000. For the neuroses, a dramatic contrast to the psychoses is found, in the range of figures encompassed. Table XII shows that the prevalence of neuroses ranges from 0.8 per 1000 in Taiwan aborigines (Rin & Lin, 1962) to 269.0 per 1000 in Ugandan women (Orley & Wing, 1979). As previously anticipated (end of Part I), difficulties were encountered in comparing the frequency of neurotic conditions across cultures, borne out by the enormous variation in prevalence rates. The latter reflects three major problems. First, cultural influences on the form of neurotic disorders leading to somatic presentations in developing countries, which are difficult to disentangle from physical illnesses. Second, variations in interviewing techniques undoubtedly contribute to the wide range of figures. Higher prevalence rates usually result from surveys in which every subject is interviewed with a standard clinical

TABLE XII

Prevalence rates per 1000 from population surveys

Population surveyed	Schizophrenia	Manic–depressive illness	Neuroses	Study
Taiwan Chinese	2.1	0.7	1.2	Lin (1953)
corrected for age over 15	3.7	1.1	2.1	Rin & Lin (1962)
Taiwan aborigines	0.9	0.9	0.8	Lin et al (1969)
Taiwan Chinese	1.4	—	7.8	Lin et al (1969)
Japanese	2.3	0.2[1]	3.0	Kato (1969)
N. Indians – Lucknow	2.5	1.1	27.1	Sethi et al (1974)
N. Indians – Agra	2.2	1.3	12.6	Dube (1970)
corrected for age over 15	3.8	2.2	22.2	
W. Bengal	4.3	—	1.5	Elnagar et al (1971)
corrected for age over 15	8.0	—	2.7	
N. Indians – Lucknow	1.9	1.9	20.4	Thacore et al (1975)
corrected for age over 16	3.3	3.3	36.5	
W. Bengal	2.8	—	67.0	Nandi et al (1975)
W. Bengal	2.2	1.5	16.8	Nandi et al (1980)
Sri Lanka	3.8	—	25.2 (60.0)[2]	Wijesinghe et al (1978)
corrected for age over 15	5.6	—	89.0+	
Chinese – Shanghai	4.2	—	—	Xia et al (Lin et al, 1980)
Botswana		—	—	Ben-Tovim & Cushnie (1986)
corrected for age over 15	5.3	—	—	

Group				Reference
Tonga	1.3	0.9	—	Murphy & Taumoepeau (1980)
corrected for age over 15	—	—	54.0	
S. African Cape coloured	—	—	41.7	Gillis et al (1968)
Ethiopian town	—	—	63.5	Giel & Van Luijk (1969a)
corrected for age over 15	—	—	51.4	
Ethiopian village	—	—	93.1	Giel & Van Luijk (1969b)
corrected for age over 15	—	—	287.0	
Buenos Aires women (15)[2]	—	—	94.0	Tarnopolsky et al (1977)
Buenos Aires men (15)[2]	—	—	222.0	
Athens women (18–74)	—	—	82.0	Mavreas et al (1986)
Athens men (18–74)	—	—	269.0	
Ugandan women (18–65)	—	—	174.0	Orley & Wing (1979)
Ugandan men (18–65)	—	—	106.0	
Camberwell women (18–65)	—	—	135.0	Wing et al (1978)
Camberwell women (19–65)	—	—	58.0	Bebbington et al (1981b)
Camberwell men (18–65)	—	—		

[1] Rate for 6 months only.
[2] Corrected for cases not interviewed.

schedule, rather than relying on key informants and unstandardised clinical impressions. The third problem concerns the definition of a case of neurosis. This problem hardly affects the definition of schizophrenia, since the key symptoms just do not occur in normal people. By contrast, minor neurotic symptoms are distributed throughout the general population. As we have seen, depressive symptoms were found by Leighton *et al* (1963) in 30% of Yoruba villagers, and by Orley & Wing (1979) in over 20% of Ugandan villagers. Whereas schizophrenia is a discrete condition, the neuroses lie on a continuum with normality, and the judgement as to where to interrupt this continuum in order to separate cases from non-cases is inescapably arbitrary. However, where the same judgement is made across several studies, the prevalence of neuroses can be directly compared. This is the case with no more than two sets of studies dealing with Western and non-Western countries; those by Leighton *et al* comparing rates in North America and Nigeria, and by Orley & Wing (1979) comparing villages in Uganda with a district in London. The study by Orley & Wing is the more advanced of the two methodologically, since it incorporates a computerised judgement of caseness, which is not subject to variation in the way human judgements invariably are. The studies by Leighton *et al* revealed little difference in the prevalence of neuroses between Stirling County and Abeokuta, whereas Orley & Wing found a considerably higher prevalence in the Ugandan villages than in south-east London.

The findings of these carefully conducted surveys clearly overrule the earlier clinical impressions of Western psychiatrists working in developing countries that neurotic conditions were uncommon. We need to pay particular attention to the study by Orley & Wing, since they employed the most sophisticated techniques available. However, their finding of a greater prevalence of neuroses in Uganda compared with London is difficult to interpret in the absence of incidence rates. It is likely that some of the excess is accounted for by the lack of available treatment for neuroses in developing countries. Nandi *et al* (1976) carried out a trial of antidepressant drugs in previously untreated people identified as suffering from depression in a community survey they conducted in West Bengal. They found that the depressed people in the community, who had never sought treatment, responded just as well to antidepressant drugs as patients attending a psychiatric clinic. This finding suggests that if appropriate treatment was as available in a developing country as it is in the West, the duration of neurotic conditions in the former could be curtailed, thus decreasing the prevalence rate.

Once more we are faced with too many possible interpretations of the data because of the lack of information about incidence. The determination of incidence rates for psychotic and neurotic conditions in developing countries is obviously of high priority. These endeavours need to utilise the latest advances in standardisation of psychiatric interviewing and of processing the data collected. Without these, a great deal of effort is likely to be expended with very little return, and the question that prompted this part of the book will be no nearer to being answered.

Fortunately, a WHO study of the incidence of schizophrenia in a variety of cultures has now been published (Sartorius *et al*, 1986). This was designed as the successor to the IPSS (World Health Organization, 1973), but in contradistinction to it was epidemiologically based. Twelve centres participated, comprising four in developing countries – Agra, Cali, Chandigarh, and Ibadan, and the remainder in developed countries – Aarhus, Dublin, Honolulu, Moscow, Nagasaki, Nottingham, Prague, and Rochester. The aim was to identify every resident of each catchment area, within the age range 15–54, who had made a first contact in the previous 3 months with a helping agency for a possible psychotic illness. The term 'helping agency' was intended to cover a wide range of facilities, from local psychiatric services to traditional or religious healers. In some centres, in addition to mental-health professionals and GPs, police stations and prisons were included in the case-finding network. Thus, the study attempted to cover all the possible sources of cases shown in Table XI (p. 89) for a developing country, except vagrants and persons in the general population who had not sought help for their problems. Case-finding continued over 2 years or more, to even out any seasonal fluctuations. Checks were carried out in each centre to determine whether any possible cases were slipping through the net. The results of this precautionary measure suggested that the coverage was incomplete in five centres – Agra, Cali, Ibadan, Prague, and Rochester, which were consequently omitted from the analysis of incidence rates. This is particularly unfortunate, since three of them are in developing countries.

Patients passing the screening criteria were assessed with the PSE, and other standardised instruments to collect data on history and social performance. The PSE data were processed with the Catego program (described on p. 36) (Wing *et al*, 1974). Patients ascribed to one of the Catego classes S, P, and O, and/or receiving a clinical diagnosis of schizophrenia according to the International Classification of Diseases (ICD) were retained in the sample for analysis. The total study population consisted of 1379 patients, of whom 745 were men and 634 women. The great majority of subjects were urban residents, except in the Agra centre and in the rural area of Chandigarh.

An almost identical proportion of patients in developed and developing countries had a duration of illness before contact of less than 6 months. However, while half the patients in developing countries had an acute onset, defined as the development of a florid psychotic state within a week, this was true of only one-quarter of those in developed countries. This difference provides ammunition for critics of the study, considered below.

It is important to present the degree of concordance between the Catego classification and clinical diagnosis. The two systems were in agreement in 1036 (75%) of the study population. There were 79 (6%) patients with a Catego S, P, or O class and a non-schizophrenic ICD diagnosis, and

263 (19%) patients with an ICD diagnosis of schizophrenia who were assigned to other Catego classes. Thus the Catego classification of schizophrenia proved to be narrower than the clinical diagnosis, as in the IPSS. It is worth noting at this point that patients ascribed to Catego class S + (exhibiting at least one of Schneider's first-rank symptoms) had a generally more florid clinical picture, with many other delusions and hallucinations, than patients allocated to classes S, P, and O.

The incidence rates for the seven centres with reliable data were calculated per 10 000 population aged between 15 and 54, since this was the age range of patients accepted into the study. The patients from the Chandigarh centre were separated into those with urban and with rural domicile, because of a marked contrast between these two locations in socio-cultural features. The incidence rates are displayed in Table XIII. Figures have been calculated for the broadest diagnosis of schizophrenia – Catego S, P, or O and/or ICD schizophrenia, and for the narrowest – Catego S + .

The incidence rate for the broadest category of schizophrenia ranges from 1.5 per 10 000 in Aarhus to 4.2 in rural Chandigarh. This variation in rates is statistically significant. By contrast, the range for S + cases is 0.7 to 1.4, a non-significant variation. The reason for this difference in range between the broad and narrow categories of schizophrenia becomes clear when the proportion of S + cases in each centre is examined. Whereas nearly two-thirds of the Nottingham cases of broad schizophrenia were classified by Catego as S + , only one-quarter of the Chandigarh cases were. As a consequence, the rates for Chandigarh urban and rural areas dropped from the highest to almost the lowest when the narrow definition was applied. These cross-cultural differences in the relative frequency of Schneider's first-rank symptoms have been recorded before. For example in the London centre of the IPSS, first-rank symptoms were detected in 68% of schizophrenic

TABLE XIII
Annual incidence rates of schizophrenia per 10 000 population aged 15–54

Centre	Broad group[1]	Catego S +	Broad group – Catego S +	S + as percentage of broad group
Aarhus	1.5	0.7	0.8	47
Chandigarh urban	3.5	0.9	2.6	26
Chandigarh rural	4.2	1.1	3.1	26
Dublin	2.2	0.9	1.3	41
Honolulu	1.6	0.9	0.7	56
Moscow	2.8	1.2	1.6	43
Nagasaki	2.0	1.0	1.0	50
Nottingham	2.2	1.4	0.8	64

[1] Catego S, P or O and/or ICD schizophrenia.
From Sartorius *et al* (1986).

patients, closely similar to the proportion among Nottingham patients in Table XIII. In a study of schizophrenic patients in Sri Lanka, however, Chandrasena & Rodrigo (1979) found them to be present in only 25%, almost identical to the proportion in Chandigarh patients in Table XIII.

The purpose of conducting studies of the incidence of diseases is to throw light on their aetiology. The important findings of the WHO study indicate that the broad category of schizophrenia almost certainly subsumes more than one disease. Schizophrenia defined narrowly by the presence of Schneider's first-rank symptoms has a similar incidence across a variety of cultures, suggesting that the aetiological factor(s) are common to all the cultures studied. This does not mean that the aetiology of S + schizophrenia is exclusively biological. There could still be a contribution from environmental factors that operate across a range of cultures. For example, the recent WHO study of life events in schizophrenia provides evidence that they play a similar role in precipitating episodes of illness regardless of the cultural setting (Day *et al*, 1987). Once S + schizophrenia has been removed from the broad category, the rates for the remainder vary more than fourfold from 0.7 per 10 000 in Honolulu to 3.1 in rural Chandigarh. We can deduce from this that non-S + schizophrenia is a clinical grouping in which environmental factors probably play an important aetiological role. It is of great interest that S + schizophrenia comprises an identically small proportion of the broad category in both rural and urban Chandigarh. This should stimulate a search for the common factors in these two environments, which are so different in many respects. The similar finding in Sri Lanka provides another clue that needs following up.

The WHO incidence study has been criticised by Torrey (1987) for not including centres in countries with a reportedly high incidence, such as Sweden, and a reportedly low incidence, as in some tropical areas. Of course this would be ideal, but is very difficult to achieve for remote places in the Third World. The centres in developing countries were chosen by WHO because they had sufficient personnel to conduct the research, and in most cases had already gained experience in international collaborative studies. Great perseverance and a meticulous approach to technique is essential for the conduct of incidence studies. In the WHO study, even centres with considerable resources and past experience of research, such as Prague and Rochester, were unable to maintain the standards necessary. It is almost inconceivable that such a study could be successfully carried out in Papua New Guinea or Tonga, using local personnel belonging to the relevant culture.

A different criticism has been levelled at the study by Stevens & Wyatt (1987). They draw attention to the much higher proportion of cases with an acute onset in the developing countries compared with the developed countries. They point out that these would be designated as acute reactive, brief, or schizophreniform psychosis by DSM–III criteria, and question their inclusion under the rubric 'schizophrenia'. They also suggest that this type of disorder will introduce a bias towards a more favourable course for schizophrenia in developing countries. These salient issues will be discussed later when we come to consider variations in the outcome of schizophrenia across cultures.

III. Are psychiatric conditions treated differently in different cultures?

10 Extraction and exorcism

The answer to this section title appears to be self-evident: on the one hand there are the pre-scientific methods of treatment used in traditional societies; and on the other there are the scientific remedies developed in the West and exported to the rest of the world. But are the scientific and traditional methods as different as they seem to be at first glance? This part of the book reviews the methods of treatment of psychiatric conditions employed by traditional healers and by ordinary people as part of the practice of folk medicine. The concepts of psychiatric illness formulated in traditional cultures are examined, since particular treatments often stem directly from these. Throughout this section traditional and scientific methods of treatment are compared, to highlight similarities and differences between them.

The scientific view of illness of any kind is firmly based on the concept of a disturbance of normal bodily function. The causes of the disturbance may include external agents, such as excessive intake of alcohol or intolerable psychological pressures, but these are considered to operate on the internal milieu to produce the illness. In many traditional cultures, illness is conceptualised in a concrete way as an external object which has intruded into the body. Such alien objects do not merely cause the illness, they *are* the illness. Thus the healing procedure consists of removal of the offending substance, which may be either inanimate or animate, from the sufferer's body. Allen (1976) records that, among the Nepalese, the medium extracts the illness from the patient either by sucking or with the aid of a wand. He produces a piece of grit or some unidentifiable fragment of animal or vegetable origin, and hands it around on a brass plate amid applause, as a proof of his success.

Ngubane (1976), in discussing Zulu traditional medicine, notes that certain types of disease can be taken out of a patient and discarded as a material object. Once discarded in this manner, diseases may hover around in the atmosphere, which is considered polluted and dangerous. The danger arises from the unattached disease, which can enter someone who unwittingly comes into contact with it. This concept is, of course, close to the scientific view of infectious diseases, except that it is applied generally to all illnesses, including psychiatric conditions, many of which carry no risk of contagion. The idea of illness as a material object that can be transferred from one individual to another is illustrated by a cure for fever recommended in the *Talmud*, the Rabbinical commentaries on the *Old Testament*. "Let him sit at the cross-roads, and when he sees a large ant carrying a load, let him take it, throw it in a copper tube, stop it up with lead and seal it with sixty seals. Then let him shake it and carry it to and fro, exclaiming 'Thy load be upon me and my load (viz. the fever) be upon thee' ''. Another commentator objected that it might happen that the ant chosen may have already had someone's fever unloaded on to him. In this case, the second invalid would merely be exchanging one fever for another! To counter this objection, he was recommended to say, "My burden *and* thine own burden be upon thee". (Cohen, 1968).

Onyango (1976) interviewed a Kenyan traditional healer to gather information about his healing techniques. The healer categorised psychiatric patients into various types, one of which seems to correspond closely to manic–depressive disorders. According to the healer, patients suffering from this type of disorder had worms in their heads. "The worms have hairy bodies and these interfere with brain function. When the worms are awake in the head, the patient becomes very excited, talkative, his voice changes and the eyes become red. But when the worms are sleeping, the patient becomes too sad, never talks, refuses food and he may become very violent as he is constantly irritated in the brain by the hair of the worms". The treatment was to remove the worms from the brain by giving the patient medicine to make him sneeze. When the patient was very ill, the healer employed a fumigation method, involving the burning of herbs in a room in which the patient was locked naked for 1 h. The smoke caused the patient to perspire and sneeze, and the healer claimed that he often saw worms on the floor after this treatment. Giel *et al* (1968) described the place of worship of a healer-priest in Ethiopia and wrote, "insects and other vermin vomited in the process of healing adorn the walls and attest to the cures that took place".

The extraction of objects from the body to cure disease is, of course, the basis of modern surgery. It is not unknown for patients to keep their extracted gallstones or kidney stones on the mantelpiece, confirming the powerful psychological effect of viewing the material 'cause' of your illness demonstrably outside your body. It will be objected that it is spurious to draw a parallel between magical object extraction and modern surgery, since the latter is based on scientific knowledge of disease processes occurring in the body. However, we have only to reflect on the number of normal appendixes removed, and on the operation for removing much of the large bowel to prevent 'self-poisoning', which was fashionable in the earlier part of this century, to see the comparison as more than fanciful. If traces of magical procedures are still detectable in the practice of modern surgery, influences in the reverse direction can also be identified. These are shown most clearly by the 'psychic surgeons' of the Philippines. These native healers carry out 'operations' on their clients without using any instruments. With their bare hands they knead the abdomen of patients and materialise tissues which have the appearance of blood, mesentery, and internal organs. Indeed, that is just what they are, but analysis of the 'extracted' tissues prove them to belong to animals. The same sleight of hand that enables healers to produce objects from patients' bodies is here being used to mimic the dramatic procedures of modern surgery. Links with older techniques are revealed by the Philippino 'surgeons'' removal of beans from under patients' eyelids to cure eye disease.

The techniques described above exemplify the most concrete form of extraction of illness. The next step in abstraction involves the transfer of an invisible illness principle from the subject to an external inanimate object. In these cases, the illness is ascribed to harmful spirits who have to be lured from the sufferer's body. In Thailand, the spirits are induced to leave by placing a sticky ball of rice on various parts of the patient's body, starting from the tips of the toes and working upwards to the top of the head (Suwanlert, 1976). The names of spirits are called out during this procedure and the patient is asked to pray with the healer. The rice ball is then thrown away, indicating that the spirits have departed. Among the Eskimos of Alaska, insanity and episodic hysteria are usually ascribed to the intrusion of spirits. The healer has the patient lie down near an inanimate object, such as a log of wood or a saw, and then, with sweeping motions, he brushes the sickness from the patient on to the object. When the transfer has been accomplished, the object is broken to pieces (Murphy, 1964).

A further degree of abstraction is involved in the replacement of the inanimate recipient of the illness with an animate being, invariably an animal of some kind. Examples of this procedure abound in the literature; some are reviewed in detail to identify the common elements. One of the earliest accounts of modern times is that by Borelli (1890), who studied healing techniques in Ethiopia. He wrote, "the most efficacious remedy then consists in taking a hen and swinging it round the head of the possessed, subsequently throwing it upon the ground. If the hen dies at once or soon afterwards it is a good omen; the Zarr or Buddha has passed into the body of the fowl and caused it to perish". A very similar ritual is described by Hes (1964) among the Yemenite Jews. These people formed a community in Yemen, surrounded by their Arab neighbours, from well before 400 BC. They emigrated *en masse* to Israel in 1949 to 1950, and were then studied by Hes. They represent an isolated, encapsulated group, whose traditions have probably changed less over the centuries than those of Jews in any other country. The Yemenites believe that some mental illnesses are caused by *shedim*, or spirits possessing the patient. These can be exorcised only by the most powerful and high-ranking healers, who are called *ba'alei hefetz* (masters of the will). One method used by the native healer, or *mori*, to exorcise spirits is to take a sheep, dove, or chicken and revolve it three times around the patient. The *mori* then whispers to the spirits, "Masters, please have mercy upon the patient and take the sheep instead". Immediately afterwards, the sheep is slaughtered.

A similar, but more complex procedure, is found among the Shona of southern Africa (Gelfand, 1964). One cause of madness they identify is angered ancestral spirits, or *ngozi*. The healer, or *nganga*, takes the patient and a black hen to a pool. He orders the patient to sit under a particular tree growing near the water's edge. He cuts off the hen's smallest toe and then makes small incisions on the front and back of the patient's neck. He dips the hen's toe into some powder and rubs the mixture of powder and blood into the cut he has just made. He then dips the hen into the water, rotates the patient's head, and says, "Ngozi, leave the patient alone and come to the hen". The patient is instructed to step into the pool and wade to the other side without looking back. The hen is left at a crossroads and disappears into the woods, where it is soon lost, and with it the spirit transferred from the patient. This technique involves the introduction of a number of additional elements – the use of water, the specification of crossroads, and the prohibition on looking backwards. The last-named injunction is also encountered in the Biblical story of Lot's wife and in the Greek myth of Orpheus and Eurydice, where it apparently serves the same purpose as in the Shona ritual, namely to prevent evil from attaching itself to the individual. We have already discovered the use of crossroads in the Talmudic cure for fever, which advises the sufferer to wait at the crossroads until an ant comes into view. In southern Italy the following incantation is used against skin diseases: "Wicked damned wind. Go drown thyself in the sea. There thou hast nothing to do with this blessed flesh". Having said this, the patient must put his clothes down at a crossroads and the first person who passes by will pick up the illness (Risso & Böker, 1968). This element also appears in the European myths about vampires. When a vampire has been killed by driving a wooden stake through its heart, it is recommended that it be buried at a crossroads. The most likely explanation of this strategy is that if the evil spirit wanders abroad it will be confused by the choice of four possible directions and will be unable to find its way back to the original sufferer.

Water as a cleansing agent is, of course, a component of many rituals, but has a special place in the transfer of spirits causing illness. A ceremony marking the recovery from psychosis is performed by the native healers of the Yoruba in Nigeria (Prince, 1964). The patient is dressed in a new, white cloth, and has her head shaved while standing waist-deep in a swiftly flowing river. Three doves are used as living sponges to wash away the evil from the patient. They are then either drowned or decapitated and their bodies flung downstream. The patient takes off her white wrapper, which also floats away. The evil is borne away by the river on the bodies of the doves and on the white cloth, and anyone touching them will contract the illness.

Plowden (1868) gives an early account of spirit expulsion in Abyssinia: "The favourite remedies are amulets and severe tomtoming, and screeching without cessation, till the possessed, doubtless distracted with the noise, rushes violently out of the house, pelted and beaten, and driven to the nearest brook, where the Zar quits him, and he becomes well". A river also features in another exorcism ritual described by Gelfand (1967) among the Shona. The native healer, or *nganga*, treats a possessed woman by standing her next to a sheep or hen in the forest. He says to the sheep, "I am giving away this spirit", and the sufferer then prays to her dead mother, telling her that today she has thrown out this bad spirit, and asking her not to allow it to return to her, but to allow it to enter someone else. After this the *nganga* takes a few grains of each crop that is grown and puts them into a black cloth. He then stands on the bank of a river and throws the bundle into the water.

The elements common to all these procedures of transferring spirits from humans to animals can now be summarised. The native healer commands or beseeches the spirit causing the madness to leave the patient and enter into an animal. The patient's head is commonly the focus of activities aimed at extracting the spirit. When this has been achieved, the animal is either killed, presumably putting an end to the spirit, or driven off with precautions ensuring that it will not return. An additional feature is the use of water to cleanse the patient of evil, and sometimes the introduction of flowing water to carry the spirits away forever, since rivers never run backwards! Having identified these common elements in exorcism rituals, we can turn to one of the oldest accounts of such healing techniques, which is found in the *New Testament*.

It is evident from the Gospels that a substantial part of Christ's healing mission concerned the mentally ill: "And Jesus went about all Galilee, teaching in their synagogues, and preaching the Gospel of the Kingdom, and healing all manner of sickness and all manner of disease among the people. And his fame went throughout all Syria: and they brought unto him all sick people that were taken with divers diseases and torments, and those which were possessed with devils, and those which were lunatick, and those that had the palsy; and he healed them" (Matthew 4: 23–24).[1] "When the even was come, they brought unto him many that were possessed with devils: and he cast out the spirits with his word and healed all that were sick" (Matthew 8: 16). "As they went out, behold, they brought to him a dumb man possessed with a devil. And when the devil was cast out, the dumb spake" (Matthew 9: 32–33). "Then was brought unto him one possessed with a devil, blind and dumb: and he healed him, insomuch that the blind and dumb both spake and saw" (Matthew 12: 22).

It is hardly surprising that such dramatic cures attracted people who had been through the hands of the medical establishment and had suffered as much from the remedies as from the disease. "And a certain woman, which

---

[1] All quotations from the *New Testament* are from the Authorised Version.

had an issue of blood twelve years, and had suffered many things of many physicians, and had spent all that she had, and was nothing bettered, but rather grew worse. When she had heard of Jesus, came in the press behind, and touched his garment. For she said, If I may touch but his clothes, I shall be whole. And straightway the fountain of her blood was dried up; and she felt in her body that she was healed of that plague'' (Mark 5: 25–29).

It is likely that many of these patients were suffering from hysterical disorders, but one case history in the Gospels concerns a man who was almost certainly psychotic. The most circumstantial account is given by Mark. ''And when he was come out of the ship, immediately there met him out of the tombs a man with an unclean spirit, who had his dwelling among the tombs; and no man could bind him, no, not with chains; because that he had been often bound with fetters and chains, and the chains had been plucked asunder by him, and the fetters broke in pieces: neither could any man tame him. And always, night and day, he was in the mountains, and in the tombs, crying and cutting himself with stones.'' (Mark 5: 1–5).

It is evident from the above that the patient was wandering about without a fixed home, but usually returned to the cemetery, where presumably he found some shelter from the elements. He was clearly violent and attempts had been made to subdue him by putting him in chains. This is a common method of dealing with violent psychiatric patients in countries without sophisticated medical facilities. Native healers often have one or more psychiatric patients restrained with shackles within their compounds. However, this particular man is credited with the unusual strength often ascribed by folklore to the madman, as he was able to break out of any restraint. He is also described by Mark as shouting; we may surmise that this was in response to auditory hallucinations. His habit of cutting himself with stones may have been either self-mutilation or attempted suicide.

Luke gives a similar description of the man, but adds two items of information, namely that he was naked and that his illness was chronic. ''And when he went forth to land, there met him out of the city a certain man, which had devils long time, and ware no clothes, neither abode in any house, but in the tombs. For he had commanded the unclean spirit to come out of the man. For oftentimes it had caught him: and he was kept bound with chains and in fetters; and he brake the bands and was driven of the devil into the wilderness'' (Luke 8: 27–29).

There is therefore strong evidence that the man was suffering from a chronic psychotic condition. How did Jesus deal with this? ''But when he saw Jesus afar off, he ran and worshipped him, and cried with a loud voice, and said, What have I to do with thee, Jesus, thou Son of the most high God? I adjure thee by God, that thou torment me not. For he said unto him, Come out of the man, thou unclean spirit. And he asked him, What is thy name? and he answered, saying, My name is Legion, for we are so many. And he besought him much that he would not send them away out of the country. Now there was nigh unto the mountains a great herd of swine feeding. And all the devils besought him, saying; Send us into the swine, that we may enter into them. And forthwith Jesus gave them leave. And the unclean spirits went out, and entered the swine: and the herd ran violently down a steep place into the sea (there were about two thousand) and were choked in the sea'' (Mark 5: 2–13).

In Jesus' healing technique we find all the elements that are common to the exorcism procedures used by native healers throughout the world when dealing with mental illness. He commands the devils to leave the possessed sufferer, he transfers them into the bodies of animals and the animals are subsequently killed. There is the additional element of water to wash away the spirits, which entered into some of the rituals considered above.

Thus, we have evidence of a form of ritual for exorcism persisting unchanged over several thousand years. Its endurance over time and its widespread distribution throughout a variety of cultures argue for an important psychological effect on the participants. In the case of the psychotic man exorcised by Jesus, the procedure was reported as successful. ''And they came to Jesus, and see him that was possessed with the devil and had the legion sitting, and clothed, and in his right mind'' (Mark 5: 15).

In general, we would not expect a ritual of any kind to have more than a temporary effect in chronic psychotic conditions, although Farmer & Falkowski (1985) describe the case of a psychotic Tongoese woman whose illness of 4 months' duration completely resolved during a traditional healing ceremony. However, it is likely that a substantial proportion of patients suffering from neuroses would respond, particularly if the ritual were an integral part of their culture. It is also conceivable that this form of treatment might shorten the duration of an acute episode of psychosis. There is a substantial body of evidence concerning the powerful therapeutic effect of placebo procedures on both neurotic and psychotic conditions. It is somewhat ironic that our knowledge of placebo effects is derived largely from drug trials, in the context of which they are regarded as a nuisance that has to be controlled for. Their therapeutic potential has hardly been deliberately exploited by modern psychiatrists who, in turning their backs on the 'magical' procedures of the traditional healers, may be depriving themselves of a potent therapeutic tool. It might be argued that the public in Western nations is too sophisticated to respond to the dramatic appeal of exorcism ceremonies, but this is not so. Exorcism is still carried out within the Catholic and Anglican Churches, albeit somewhat infrequently. However, the demand far outstrips the supply. One team of religious exorcists claimed that in 4 years they dealt with 7000 people who were convinced they were possessed. Only 58 of these were considered to be genuinely in need of exorcism and took part in the appropriate ritual (*Evening News*, London,

14 April 1975). Evidently, there is still a clientele for exorcism procedures in the West, who are not bringing their problems to doctors, since they know they will not receive the kind of treatment they crave. Further consideration of the use of alternatives to modern medicine by the public in Western countries is given later.

11 Possession and divination

Throughout recorded history, man has maintained an ambivalent attitude to the powers of evil. On the one hand, they are feared as the cause of misfortune and illness; on the other hand, there is the attractive possibility that they might be harnessed and their power used to further the aims of anyone who is bold enough to make the attempt. There are numerous examples of the second attitude in world literature, including Faust, Frankenstein, and the story of the Golem, most of which end disastrously for the would-be controller. This ambivalence is represented by the dichotomy between exorcism and possession states. Whereas exorcism is a means of expelling spirits that cause disease, states of possession are often deliberately sought in order to make use of spiritual powers hovering in that shadowy world surrounding us. Chapter 2 showed that possession states occur in nearly all traditional cultures and that they are to be distinguished from psychiatric conditions. Indeed, one of their most frequent uses is in the treatment of illness, both physical and psychiatric. First, the methods used to induce states of possession are considered.

The two most common components are rhythmic sound and rhythmic movement. The sound is often produced by repetitive drumming and chanting, while the movement may take the form of dancing in which many people take part. Dancing or other repetitive movements continue for long periods, leading to physical exhaustion, which probably also plays a role in altering the subject's state of mind. Another important, if not essential, ingredient is overbreathing. The subject breathes faster and more shallowly than normal with the result that the level of carbon dioxide in the blood is lowered. This in turn gives rise to a feeling of lightheadedness, due to a lowering of the level of consciousness. An additional feature sometimes included in the ritual is the inhalation of fumes from herbs or of incense. Finally, and perhaps of most importance, is the social expectation of the onlookers. The ceremony is put on in order that one or more subjects will go into a trance, and all who attend expect that they will either experience this themselves or will see others overtaken by it. This aspect, combined with the dramatic nature of the ritual, can be referred to as suggestion, which is believed to play an important part in hypnosis. Indeed, there are close parallels between the hypnotic state and possession states, in that both types of phenomena are characterised by a lowered level of consciousness, by altered behaviour that does not appear to be under the subject's control, and by amnesia for the period during which the subject is in the state. Unfortunately, we understand almost as little about hypnotism (Barber, 1969) as we do about possession states, so that their similarity throws no light on the cerebral mechanisms involved. It is usual to invoke the term *dissociation*, but this is no more than a cloak for ignorance. Sargant (1957) indulges in the interesting speculation that the altered state of consciousness found in these trances is induced by the particular periodicity of the rhythmic movement and sound. He notes that "certain rates of rhythm can build up recordable abnormalities of brain function".

Whatever the physiological mechanism responsible, there is a further similarity between possession states and hypnosis, namely an insensitivity to pain. Hypnosis can abolish the subject's response to painful stimuli and has even been employed to produce anaesthesia in dentistry and surgery. During possession states, subjects quite frequently expose themselves deliberately to pain or injury as a demonstration of the 'magical' quality of their experience. Among the Fukienese on Taiwan, the traditional healer, after going into a trance, practises self-mutilation – cutting the tongue or back with swords, piercing the cheeks with iron rods, flailing the back with a nail-studded ball (Li, 1976). The whirling dervishes also pierce the tongue and cheeks with metal skewers. In a number of cultures, subjects in a possession trance will walk barefoot across glowing coals to demonstrate their invulnerability, while in possession ceremonies in Sri Lanka, the dancers run flaming torches along their bare arms.

Possession states fulfil a variety of functions in different cultures, some religious and some secular. Their appearance may mark a change in role or status for the subject. Thus, the Gnau of New Guinea recognise a condition known as *bengbeng*. Affected people breathe in a rapid and uneven manner, while rapid cries are seemingly jerked out of them and their bodies convulse in time with the cries. They stride around chanting incomprehensibly, speak messages from spirits, or utter warnings. Their cries or jerks may crescendo to the point of collapse, or else fade away into stillness or silence. The Gnau believe *bengbeng* is due to possession by a spirit, and that the behaviour is not due to illness, nor that it is itself an illness. Possession may, however, reveal illness and after it had occurred some women were regarded as ill and behaved in the appropriate withdrawn manner (Lewis, 1976). Instead of heralding illness, the appearance of possession states may mark out the subject as a healer. Among the Navajo, hysterical seizures may take the form of hand-trembling, which is regarded as a sign that the sufferer may become a diagnostician or shaman (Neutra *et al*, 1977). In Sri Lanka, the multitude of spirits are organised in a hierarchy. Possession by lesser spirits is of little import, but a subject may be possessed serially by spirits of increasingly high status. When possessed by a god, it is clear to everyone that the subject has reached the status of a healer (Wijesinghe *et al*, 1976). In Taiwan each temple usually has one healer who serves for life (Tseng, 1972). When he becomes too old to perform, the elders of the temple will announce that they are seeking a successor. They beat the golden drum in the temple every night, attracting young people in the neighbourhood. Some onlookers carry a sedan chair on their shoulders, and sway in time to the beating of the drum. After a while, one of the sedan-chair carriers or some other bystander will suddenly fall unconscious. This man is believed to have been possessed by a god and selected for the role of healer. If several men happen to fall into this state at the same time, the one who remains comatose the longest is considered to be the chosen one. Possession has also been regarded in Christianity as a sign of the divine spirit entering the subject, although such exuberant manifestations have met with increasing disapproval from the clerical establishment from St Paul onwards (see Chapter 1).

Possession states are commonly entered into by the traditional healer as a technique either to determine the causes of illness or else to heal the sick. The diagnostic powers of the possessed healer are presumably strengthened by the spirit that has entered him or her. Frequently, the healer's behaviour changes as he or she becomes possessed and appears to be under the control of a greater force than his or her own will. A dramatic manifestation of this is a change in the quality of the voice, and often in the content of speech, which sounds like some strange tongue. Healers who 'speak in tongues' in this way usually have a trained interpreter standing by to convey the meaning of their utterances to the audience. Among the Fukienese, the healer is known as *dang-ki*, which means "youth into whom a spirit descends". The *dang-ki* will usually speak a kind of language that is unintelligible to all but the interpreter, who acts as an assistant. In almost every Taoist or folk temple in Taiwanese villages, there is a *dang-ki* for the worshippers to consult (Li, 1976). The same situation is found in Zambia, where some of the healers, or *ng'angas*, go into a trance during which spirits speak through them. An assistant listens, interprets where necessary, and relays the information to those consulting the healer (Frankenberg & Leeson, 1976).

Practitioners of the ancient Hindu system of medicine, the *Ayurveda*, also use the possession states for diagnosis, but speak intelligibly to the client. A *patri* acts as the medium for a spirit or *bhuta*. After drum-beating and the burning of incense, the *patri* goes into a trance, possessed by his master *bhuta*. The spirit possessing the client is then asked to show itself and the client breaks into a weird dance. The spirit speaking through the healer then engages the spirit possessing the client in a dialogue. There is an established hierarchy of spirits, as in neighbouring Sri Lanka, and if the healer's spirit is more powerful, it orders the other to leave the body of the client. If the latter has the ascendancy, the healer's spirit pleads, asking the other to state its conditions for releasing the client. The client's spirit declares its conditions, which may be an animal sacrifice, a ritual feast, or a 'house' for its use. After this, both the healer and the client throw a final fit, foam at the mouth, and pass into unconsciousness. Neither of them remembers what transpired during the ceremony, but the audience does (Carstairs & Kapur, 1976). This dialogue between the spirit causing illness and the healing spirit exemplifies the dual attitudes towards the spirit world that often exist in a traditional culture. Mary Douglas (1973) highlights this point in her discussion of the Nuer and Dinka, two neighbouring Nilotic tribes: "The Nuer attitude to possession is that it is dangerous in the first phase (the patient), and produces an abnormal specialised role in the second phase (the healer, usually a close relative of the patient); a role whose specialised task is to counteract the dangers of first phase possession." She contrasts this duality with the attitude of the Dinka "that trance is the primary manifestation of unspecialised benign power. It is not restricted to a specialised role in the sense of calling for special initiation, by affliction, asceticism or training, but is open to all adult males of a clan, and normally experienced by them all."

Where possession is not universal, as it is in the Dinka, but restricted to a chosen few, as in the Nuer, it may increase the subject's social status. Wijesinghe *et al* (1976) conducted a population survey in Sri Lanka to determine the prevalence of possession states. They found 40 subjects who had experienced possession states out of a population of 7653, representing a prevalence of only 0.5% in a semi-urban neighbourhood. One subject regularly became possessed with one of three gods. He considered himself very fortunate in being a favourite of the gods and in having received this dispensation. He was treated with a certain amount of respect by his family as well as by the neighbours, on account of his extraordinary powers. Carstairs & Kapur (1976) conducted a similar survey in a South Indian village, and found that 5% of women and 2% of men had experienced possession states. They noted that people capable of voluntary possession gained a great deal in terms of status.

Bourguignon (1976) points out that a possession trance involves role playing, taking roles not otherwise available to the actor, and demonstrating one's performance of these roles to others. Lebra (1976) adds the observation that people are able to express themselves more freely by taking a supernatural role than by representing themselves. The spirit-possessed Japanese can play informant roles that allow them to make a statement to others that would be too embarrassing or audacious to make outside that role. These remarks lead to another function of possession states, namely the provision of opportunities for behaviour which would normally be socially unacceptable.

This is clearly illustrated by the zar cult, which probably originated in Ethiopia, but is now found the length of the Nile, from Alexandria in Egypt to Khartoum in the Sudan (Kennedy, 1967). Zar ceremonies are designed to placate evil spirits who have possessed people and thereby caused illness.

The zar is primarily a female activity, and it is generally felt that men should not attend women's ceremonies, although males may play the principal roles of leader and musicians. If the leader is a male, he is called the *sheikh*, if a woman, the *sheikha*. The *sheikh* usually has available several costumes for changes during the performance according to the personalities and desires of various spirits. Songs are sung, each addressed to a different spirit. When a spirit is called that is associated with some person in the audience, she begins to shake in her seat. She moves toward the central dancing area, sometimes dancing and shaking until she falls exhausted to the floor. Before the spirit consents to leave, it usually demands special favours such as jewelry, new clothing, or expensive foods. The wish-fulfilment aspects of this behaviour are transparent; however, Kennedy points out that in some cases where material items are demanded, they are given for a temporary pacifying of the spirit and returned after the ceremony. The response of the audience is an affirmation of social support and a temporary indulgence of normally unattainable desires. It is important to recognise that women are of low status relative to men in the cultures in which the zar flourishes, which accounts for another aspect of these ceremonies, the possession of women by a male spirit. In these circumstances, the spirit may call for whisky and cigarettes, which are then partaken of by the whole audience. The male-possessed woman may also shout and swear and issue commands, which have to be obeyed. This behaviour by women is either forbidden or greatly disapproved of in the culture at large. Okasha (1966) studied the participants in zar ceremonies and found that 63 of 100 women interviewed were married. The majority of the married women had an unhappy marital life because of infidelity of their husbands, sexual dissatisfactions, or marital disharmony. He considered zar ceremonies to be a means for women to abreact their frustrated desires. Wijesinghe *et al* (1976), from their experience in Sri Lanka, hold a similar view, that possession states can act as socially sanctioned modes of exhibiting aggression, particularly for women.

A similar ritual is incorporated in spiritism in Puerto Rico (Harwood, 1977). A form of this cult with African origins is known as Santeria, in which 15 saints figure prominently. A celebrant possessed by a saint exorcises everyone present at the *séance* and behaves in the manner dictated by the personality of the particular saint. For instance, St Barbara is extremely aggressive and energetic, so that a devotee possessed by her becomes imperious and commanding in manner. Another example of the compensation function of possession states is provided by the Teke Tsaayi of the Congo (Dupré, 1976). In this culture, women are excluded from decision-making and from owning objects. A woman who becomes possessed by the *mukisi* spirit, which lives under water, experiences trance states in which she speaks in tongues and dreams of coveted possessions. During this period, the possessed woman gains men's privileges; she is given objects, she does no work, she eats the choicest foods, and drinks palm wine. The period ends with the fetching of a board carved with symbolic designs, and then a ritual bath in a stream, in which all the remains of her food are thrown. The spirit possessing her is believed to return to the stream during this ceremony. The woman then takes several months to relearn her language, and to accustom herself to cooking food and doing work. She goes from village to village and receives various gifts from the villagers, which will cover part of the expenses of treatment.

A further use that is made of trance states is encountered among the Masai of Kenya. This does not involve the notion of possession by a spirit, but is worth mentioning here because of its psychiatric implications. For a young male Masai, the most important achievement is to attain the status of *moran* or warrior. This can only be reached by killing a man belonging to another clan. The Kenyan government has attempted to prohibit this homicide, but it is very difficult to suppress it completely. At certain times in the year, the various clans meet together. During these meetings, a state of truce prevails; nevertheless, confrontations between young men of different clans are extremely tense. In these situations, one of the protagonists will start to overbreathe, and will go on to jerking of the limbs so that he has to be held tightly by other males of his clan until he loses consciousness. Mechanisms to induce trance states are clearly being used here to check and discharge aggressive impulses that are normally encouraged, except in the special circumstances of the meetings of the rival clans.

In reviewing possession states, we have seen that the mechanisms for producing the desired psychological effects are remarkably similar throughout the world; however, the uses to which they are put show considerable diversity from culture to culture, satisfying a variety of local needs. One of the functions we touched on was divination while in a trance state; but divination can also occur in clear consciousness and this area of healing requires detailed consideration.

Divination, like other aspects of traditional healing, has a very long history. The oracle at Delphi was a woman who received direct inspiration from Apollo, the god of divination. After entering a trance state, she would be asked questions and would give the god's response in unintelligible speech. This would be interpreted by an assistant, who would write it down in hexameter verse and hand it to the questioner. The equivocal nature of the replies has become famous in history, and indeed one surname of Apollo was *Loxias*, meaning the Oblique One. This ambiguity is returned to later, but for the present, it is sufficient to note that the priestess spoke with the voice of the god on only 9 days of the year. Because of this restricted period, only a very small proportion of those who wished to consult the divine oracle was privileged with an answer. Most of the pilgrims' questions were answered in a different manner, namely by drawing lots. This kind of divination took place every day of the year in public view, and was the most common method as regards simple questions that could be answered yes or no (Andronicos *et al*, 1974). This ancient form of divination by drawing lots inaugurates the following survey of similar methods in contemporary traditional societies.

Two techniques for divination have been elaborated by the Azande of the Sudan. One involves the use of two sticks – one sweet, the other sour – which are inserted together into a termite hill. According to which one is nibbled by the termites, the answer is given. The second method is known as the *benga* oracle. A strychnine-like poison is fed to a chick, and the answer to the question posed is yes or no, depending on whether the chick lives or dies. The Dogon, who border on the Sahara, make patterns in the sand representing people, places, and propositions. Grain is scattered over the patterns to attract the white desert fox. The animal comes at night and eats the grain, making tracks that obscure some of the sand-drawn symbols and leave others untouched. Interpretations are made of the intact patterns. In the Ayurvedic system, the traditional healer screens for the cause of problems by picking out a handful of shells or rice grains from a heap in front of him. If the number selected is even, a spirit is said to be the source of the trouble (Carstairs & Kapur, 1976). The Kenyan diviner studied by Onyango (1976) threw irregularly shaped beads to make a diagnosis. If the pointed ends of the beads faced the wall inside the house, this was taken to indicate that the evil spirit was within the patient's family. However, if the pointed ends faced the door, then the evil spirit was being sent from outside by an enemy.

In ancient China, the diviner would burn a cow's shoulder blade or a tortoise shell while a question was being asked. The pattern of cracks produced by the heat would be interpreted by the diviner as providing an answer (Hsu, 1976). Another Chinese method of divination that has survived to the present day is drawing *ch'ien* (Tseng, 1976). In Chinese temples, a bamboo pipe is placed near the altar. It contains a set of 100 bamboo sticks, each inscribed with a number. A *ch'ien* client, after worshipping the god at the altar and presenting the problem, selects a stick at random. The client tells the number to an old man sitting at a desk in the temple and receives the corresponding *ch'ien* paper. On each paper a poem is written, which is of obscure meaning and has to be interpreted for the client by the old man. The emphasis of the interpretation is not on the supernatural and the esoteric, but on behaviour and social adjustment. The ways of coping with problems suggested by the *ch'ien* interpreter always tend to be conservative. People are advised to make peace and not fight with others, and litigation is discouraged.

Maclean (1971) studied the method of divination among the Yoruba. The *babalawo*, or father of mysteries, casts 16 kola nuts 16 times. The outcome of each set of four throws is recorded as marks upon a wooden *ifa* tray covered in sand. The patterns of marks relate to specific verses within the *odu*, or corpus of sayings relating to *ifa*. There are a total of 256 verses corresponding to all the possible combinations of the 16 throws. The diviner interprets the contents of the oracle for his clients. The remedies prescribed after divination are concerned with the reordering of the client's relationships with the spiritual world or with members of society. An emphasis is placed on the need to restore good feelings between relatives.

From this brief view of methods of divination, it is apparent that the simplest form is some chance procedure that gives yes-or-no answers to direct questions. Simons (1957) comments on this type as follows: "Divination, like science, stems from mankind's stubborn refusal to submit passively to disease, death, and other adversity. Both are designed to cope with and control nature. Both provide evidence of an enquiring mind, and involve trial and error". The next stage of sophistication is the linking of the random procedure with a verse or saying that is obscure or ambiguous in meaning. The ambiguity ensures that whatever comes to pass has been foretold, thus reinforcing the omniscience of the deity inspiring the diviner. This was certainly the case with Apollo Loxias and the Delphic oracle. However, in many cultures, a new dimension has been added to divination by having a human intermediary interpret the god-given messages. In this way the inflexibility of the god is replaced by human wisdom and experience. An informative account of the way a diviner elucidates a client's problem is given by Harwood (1977) in his description of Puerto Rican spiritism. During communication with the spirit realm, the medium makes statements about the client with which he must indicate agreement or disagreement. He is constrained by the ideology of the cult to exercise this corrective function in order to prevent malevolent or capricious spirits from clouding the medium's clear view of the client's condition. The medium starts with general statements and gradually focuses down. In the course of this procedure, the client's social relationships are assessed. The medium spends some time on the psychological state of the client, then moves to an exploration of his family, job, and love life. The final diagnosis names a spiritual cause which relates to the social circumstances revealed during the dialogue. The qualities of this kind of diviner are summarised by Harvey (1976) in describing the Korean *mudang* as "keenly intuitive and perceptive persons who make good use of their knowledge of people and human problems in helping their clients make the best of their situations. They give conservative advice, provide clients with outlets for potentially disruptive emotions, and get substantial help from the passage of time in solving clients' problems." No Western psychotherapist would feel slighted at being characterised in this way.

We have seen that the Chinese interpreter of *ch'ien*, the Nigerian *babalawo*, and the Korean *mudang* all attempt to regularise the client's social relationships within the structure of the client's own culture. In this respect, they act as agents of social control. However, this view glosses over the subtlety and sophistication of their methods of interpreting the given statements or verses. We need to examine one procedure of this kind in great detail in order to appreciate its quality. An excellent account of one such divination is given by Werbner (1973), and we will draw extensively on it in the following pages.

Werbner studied domestic divination among the Kalanga of Botswana. He refers to domestic *séances*, by which he means gatherings at a client's home, in which all of the small congregation, including the local diviner, live nearby or are close relatives. One consequence of the local nature of the ritual is that the diviner has "extensive, intimate, and up-to-date information about the personal and family histories of each member of the congregation". Among the Kalanga, domestic diviners are exclusively men and are usually over 40. This contrasts with the Zulu, whose diviners are usually women. Zulu men can become diviners, but since this is considered to be a woman's job, such men become transvestites for the remainder of their lives as diviners (Ngubane, 1976).

The Kalanga domestic diviners are not believed to be assisted by ancestral spirits, and they do not undergo possession. The chance element is represented in their ritual by the throwing of four clearly distinguishable pieces of ivory. Each piece has two surfaces, one marked, the other unmarked, so that there are 16 permutations. The ivories are also classified according to age and sex, so that there are old female, young female, old male, and young male pieces. The client throws down the pieces and the permutation is noted, each one bearing a name which is best understood as a metaphor relating to the age and sex terms of the throw. Each permutation is linked with its opposite through the obverse surface of the ivories. Thus *endurance* is the complementary permutation to *fatigue*. Each cast of the ivories has a number of stock verses associated with it, but the individual diviner varies as to his repertoire of verses.

Werbner describes a divination ceremony that was held for a patient suffering a painful pregnancy. At the *séance*, the illness was attributed to affliction by demons, although there was also concern about the possibility of someone affecting her by sorcery. Werbner analyses in detail the fifth cast of a series of seven, in which all four pieces of ivory fell marked-side upwards, the name for this being the *tower*. After the *séance*, the diviner stressed that all the pieces showed colour; that is, they were marked. He said, "It astonishes you, so what is said about it must dazzle, just as the Tower of all dazzles". At the time, he recited, "The shadows have turned. Where is the guinea fowl? Where is its brood? The shadows would belong to them". This refers to a bird and its brood exhibiting dazzling colours when they preen themselves and, by analogy, to women who are possessed by demons, which makes them behave in a very colourful way. The implication was that a woman initiated into the cult of possession, termed a host, and her daughter (the guinea fowl and its brood) should perform a ritual. Specifically, he was referring to the pregnant patient and her mother.

He then recited, "Of lads, of turtle-doves, people towering to see". He later explained this as follows: "Just as the Tower is above all and its prominence is in a gathering of many together (a reference to all the marked pieces), so too a head of grain stands above others, with many together". His interpretation was that turtle-doves flock about and raise dust, while crops are standing, or while grain waits to be threshed. Then lads gather and shout to scare away the birds, and people gather, towering over one another, to see if beer is to be prepared from the grain as part of a feast.

Finally he recited, ''A genet is a bird, a guinea fowl is a bird; and black when it flutters away, it comes with the colours of the dead''.

First, there was a play on the word for lion, *shumba*, substituting for it the word *simba*, which means a genet or wild cat. This is a deliberate evasion, because a woman possessed by demons becomes wild like a lion, but a direct comment about a woman's status as the host for demons is forbidden in her presence at a time when she is not possessed. The reference to colours is also important in this respect, because the genet displays three colours, red, white, and black, which are also the colours of the ritual garments worn by the possessed host. In deliberately misclassifying the genet as a bird, he was drawing attention to what the genet and the guinea fowl have in common, namely spots of colour, and the capacity of this attribute to be transformed to its opposite, namely darkness. Thus, the closing phrase, ''black when it flutters away, it comes with the colours of the dead'' referred to a familiar alteration of perception: birds appear black against the sky when in flight, but are revealed in all their brilliant colours when they are close by. This familiar but arresting transformation also contained a cryptic allusion. At the onset of demonic possession, a woman rushes from the hut, disappears into the night and darkness, and then returns irridescent as a host of demons.

The condensation of language and imagery in the diviner's comments on a single throw of the ivories is astonishing. This poetic form of communication can only work if the audience shares with the diviner the full range of metaphorical meanings of the images, as well as an understanding of the specific human situation to which they are being applied. Werbner argues that the very factor that makes such allusive communication possible also renders it necessary. The domestic diviner is an integral part of his community and has to be very circumspect about what he says. After all, he is no more immune to sorcery than any of his clientele. He often makes explicit comments during the divination about equivocating: ''We speak indirectly; we speak in allusions''. This style of speech is not peculiar to Kalanga diviners. Gatere (personal communication) comments that in many African cultures the concept of *double talk* is common and forms an integral part of the culture. A similar point was made by Henry (1936) in describing *Kaingang*, a Brazilian Indian language. *Kaingang* allows construction of sentences with neither a subject nor object, making it possible to talk about things and people without mentioning them at all. This characteristic of the language enables people to talk about disagreeable things without specifying what or whom they are referring to. Henry wrote, ''They allude to subjects that are only remotely connected with the true subject, for often the true subject is too delicate or sensitive''. This problem regularly faces diviners, whose evasive tactics show a considerable similarity across cultures as the following examples demonstrate.

In Ayurvedic medicine, as practised in South India, a high level healer or *pandit* often needs to discuss symptoms stemming from a psychosocial problem which the patient cannot make explicit outside a clinical context. The *pandit* subtly discusses sensitive issues relating to family interrelationships and personal problems, by referring to humoral imbalances (Nichter, 1981*b*). *Nervios* is a term used in Costa Rica as an acceptable label for distress due to family or economic pressures. Low (1981) states that it expresses in a coded form information that would otherwise be culturally inappropriate or difficult to articulate. "Within the consultation the patient is initially hesitant to directly discuss 'private' family data, and the physician capable of misunderstanding: *nervios* provides a medium by which social and emotional issues can be explored." In Taiwan, the *dang-ki's* interpretation centres on a devil, a ghost or a god, which can serve as a symbol of a significant person in the client's life. Instead of relationships with spouse, parents, or neighbours being spoken of directly, which would be unacceptable, a deceased relative's spirit or ghost is identified as the source of the problem. In this way, the real-life drama is played out in the insubstantial world of spirits (Tseng, 1976). The same device is used by traditional healers in Tonga, where explanations about spirit interventions allow the expression of disharmony without the need for disruptive open confrontation (Parsons, 1984).

As we concluded in Chapter 6, in much of the developing world, distress resulting from problematic interpersonal relationships is presented to the doctor or healer in the veiled form of bodily complaints. The diviner is appropriately named: it is not that he is capable of seeing into the future, or discerning the intentions of the gods, but that his personal qualities and experience equip him to divine the interpersonal problems that are disguised as complaints about the client's body. However, the cultural constraints that prevent direct reference to the source of the client's distress apply equally to the diviner. Having decoded the somatic message, he then has to recode it in the form of another set of metaphors, be these humoral imbalances, discontented ghosts, or poetic imagery.

We may wonder whether the client is always able to understand the true meaning of the diviner's pronouncement. In practice, this is probably not essential, because the diviner's diagnosis is usually accompanied by a prescription that involves a reordering of the client's social relationships. Again this is achieved by subtle means, since direct interventions are likely to fail, as discovered by Racy (1980). He successfully decoded the somatic complaints of Arab women and then tried to alter the environment that was creating their distress: "I have on occasion, attempted to encourage Saudi women to assert and emancipate themselves. But I soon discovered that as a psychiatric consultant I could not be a social reformer. The patients belonged in their cultural set and distressing as it may be to them and to the observer, that reality could not be easily and safely altered". The diviner, however, is integrated in the culture and has developed strategies for achieving change that do not threaten the social structure. For example, a *pandit* studied by Nichter (1981*b*) focused the attention of the family on to the general well-being of the patient by involving family members in the preparation of time-consuming medicines and special meals. A parallel can be drawn between the metaphorical, allusive language used by the diviner and the symbolic interpretations given by the Western psychotherapist. In both cases the communication is at a high level of abstraction, but refers to a specific problem in relationships. Both the diviner and the psychotherapist direct their attention to the network of social relationships surrounding the client. Psychotherapy in the West is beginning to return to the diviner's technique of including key people in the therapeutic sessions, with the move towards family therapy and the even broader network therapy, which Speck & Reuveni (1969) have aptly named *tribe treatment*. We can now appreciate that in its most developed form, divination, far from being a random procedure, is a sophisticated form of social therapy comparable in many respects with Western psychotherapy.

12 Eclecticism and the survival of traditional healing

In the preceding two chapters, a variety of healing methods that are essentially psychological were described, where the healer attempts to alter the client's state of mind by a form of communication. They are generally also social, involving the client's relatives and neighbours in the treatment. However, these do not by any means exhaust the traditional healer's repertoire. Herbs are an important resource for psychiatric conditions as well as physical ailments. The nature and possible effectiveness of most of these herbal remedies are unknown to Western scientists. One of the outstanding exceptions is *Rauwolfia serpentina*. This is prepared from a plant, whose name reflects the snakelike configurations of the roots. *Rauwolfia serpentina* was recommended for mental disturbances in the Ayurvedic writings of India, which date back more than 2000 years. It has also been in use in African traditional medicine for an unknown period of time, as there are no written records. A hint of the antiquity of this practice in African healing is given by Prince (1960), who worked as a government psychiatrist in western Nigeria. In the course of his duties, he saw many patients who came to the clinic soon after having attended a traditional healer, and who exhibited extrapyramidal signs. These are commonly seen as side-effects of modern psychotropic drugs, and it was evident that the healers were using drugs with very potent biological activity. He spent 2 weeks at the home of a famous traditional healer with a five-generation pedigree of specialising in the treatment of mental illness. His most important medicine, which was given to almost all his patients, was identified as a preparation of *R. serpentina*. Prince's account suggests that *R. serpentina* has been used as an antipsychotic agent in African traditional medicine for at least 100 years.

Rauwolfia serpentina was first introduced into Western medicine in 1954 (Kline, 1954), but was ousted within a few years by chlorpromazine, because it was found that after an initial sedative effect, *R. serpentina* produced turbulence. Furthermore, it was noted that some patients treated with *R. serpentina* became severely depressed. Subsequently, the opinion has been growing that chlorpromazine and its derivatives also produce depression in a substantial proportion of patients, so that it is possible that *R. serpentina* was not given a fair chance to compete with the phenothiazine drugs. Be that as it may, it is a sobering thought that an effective antipsychotic agent was known to traditional healers for thousands of years before Western medicine produced an alternative. *Rauwolfia serpentina* is not the only psychotropic drug used by traditional healers. Gatere (personal communication) has seen patients in a state of acute excitement given a herbal preparation that renders them unconscious for at least 24 h. On returning to consciousness, the patients no longer show excitement. Unfortunately, some of them are brought to out-patient clinics and are found to have brain damage. Clearly, a powerful psychotropic drug, with profound effects on the brain, is being used by the traditional healers. In general, we are ignorant about most of the remedies used in traditional medicine. This is partly due to the secrecy surrounding some of the preparations, and partly to lack of interest by pharmacologists. However, in Delhi and Peking, there are institutes dedicated to the analysis and testing of traditional herbal remedies.

Apart from using herbs, some healers understand the importance of rehabilitation for psychiatric patients. The Kenyan healer interviewed by Onyango (1976) stated that in most cases the patients worked for him: "After a week some recover, then I do not let them stay idle. They cultivate, fetch water, I send them to market and to the flour mill, and they cut grass in the compound." They carry out these jobs until they are discharged home. He is reported as being quite careful in the way he allocates jobs to his patients, and he would not send a patient to cultivate or to the market unless he was sure the patient was well enough for these tasks. A similar account is given by Harding (1973) of a traditional healer in Nigeria. He found that acutely excited patients were restrained by the use of chains, but that these were used on individual patients for no more than 2 weeks. By the end of this period, their excitement was usually controlled by herbal preparations, including *R. serpentina*. During the whole period of treatment, attention was paid to the patients' psychological needs, and as they recovered, they were progressively involved in increasing amounts of work in and around the healer's compound. This study demonstrates the eclecticism of some traditional healers, who initiate an integrated programme of pharmacological, psychological, and social treatments, an approach which is widely acknowledged to characterise the best of Western psychiatry.

Not all traditional healers are as admirable as this particular man, and there are undoubtedly quacks and charlatans among their ranks whose only interest is in making money out of the sick. Like any professional group, traditional healers are a mixed bag, but in this case, the mixture contains even more extremes than usual, as there are no controls on entry into the profession. Maclean (1971) notes that Yoruba practitioners are divided into the *onishegun*, who are primarily herbalists, and the *babalawo*, who practice divination. She describes a "wild Ibadan prophet, Samson Tella, (who) has much more in common with the conventional picture of the witch doctor than have the quiet and dignified *babalawo.''* This diversity was also commented on by Frankenberg & Leeson (1976) who studied traditional healers in Zambia. They found some to be pure herbalists while others divined during possession-trances. They wrote that "ng'angas are a heterogeneous collection with no unanimity of theory or practice. There is no written body of knowledge or beliefs". Buckley (1976) remarked on the astonishing variety of radically different ideas put forward by Yoruba herbalists, who fail to agree on the nature of specific diseases, or the effective cures. Nevertheless, he postulated "an unconscious blueprint . . . by which the Yoruba have fashioned and understood their political, social, religious and economic relationships" and which underlies their theories of disease. He gives the following account of it. In Yoruba thought, the human body is formed by the coming together of sperm and menstrual blood at the time of conception. Sperm and blood are united in the womb and emerge at the time of birth, but are still concealed by the black exterior of the body.

Colour is very important to the Yoruba, but their words for colours do not readily translate into English. Yellow is often confused with red, and blue is sometimes mistaken for green or black. There are only three major distinctions of colour in the Yoruba language: *dudu* (black), *pupa* (red), and *funfun* (white). In Yoruba thought, the sky is white and the earth is red. Elements which are associated with the colour white (sperm, urine, rain) flow normally and beneficially between areas that are hidden (the belly, the earth) and areas that are exposed (the sky, the outside of the body). It is considered dangerous to expose hidden elements associated with the colour red. When there is no black soil and the red earth is exposed, the land is infertile. Menstrual blood is viewed as dangerous since it flows from a hidden inner source on to the black surface of the body, and most herbalists fear that the presence of a menstruating woman will destroy the power of their medicines. In religious symbolism, black is used to indicate secrecy, and red and white, even when used together with black, imply a dangerous revealed secret.

Buckley shows how these fundamental theories about colours underlie notions of certain diseases. Thus, various skin conditions are explained by redness becoming apparent on the black surface of the body, and are attributed to intercourse during or just after menstruation. He makes no such specific links with psychiatric conditions, but other authors have done so in writing about different cultural groups. Thus, we have already noted in Werbner's (1973) account of divination among the Kalanga, that the colours of the ritual garment worn by a possessed person are red, white, and black. Ngubane (1976) notes that there is an invariable colour sequence in medicine used by Zulu traditional healers; black being used first, followed by red, and then white.

Turner (1967) has studied the Ndembu of north-western Zambia, and reports that, like the Yoruba, they have primary terms for three colours only, white, red, and black. He writes that "white seems to be dominant and unitary, red ambivalent, for it is both fecund and 'dangerous', while black is, as it were, the silent partner, the 'shadowy third', in a sense opposed to both white and red, since it represents 'death', 'sterility', and 'impurity'. The colours are conceived as rivers of power flowing from a common source in God and permeating the whole world of sensory phenomena with their specific qualities. More than this, they are thought to tinge the moral and social life of mankind with their peculiar efficacies". Turner has found that colour symbolism underlies the treatment of all diseases and analyses the specific links in the treatment for severe headache. The condition is considered to be partly the result of witchcraft or sorcery and hence has a 'black' character. The colours white and red are used in the ritual treatment, for example, to decorate a medicine pot which is hung over the patient's doorway. The treatment is carried out at sunset and sunrise to coincide with the waning and waxing powers of the sun, a 'white' object. The medicines used all have a 'strong' aggressive character associated with redness. Hence, white and red are regarded as working in combination to rid the patient of the black disease.

Apart from the widespread significance ascribed to colours, other cosmological theories are encountered which may have a local or a general acceptance. The Rejang live in south-west Sumatra and suffer from epidemic diseases in the hot season, whereas the wet season is accompanied by colds and bronchorespiratory illness. The traditional healer or *dukuen* views heat as a greater source of danger and illness than cold, which is seen as operating through a chill wind. Wind is conceived of as a cosmic life force that actively resides in space awaiting opportunities to enter humans (Jaspan, 1976). The patient must on no account be left alone to brood in isolation or to experience bodily or psychological needs that may remain unfulfilled, as this renders him vulnerable to entry by the wind. For these reasons the *dukuen* expects the patient's relatives and friends to be in constant attendance. Heat, cold, and wind also feature in the Ayurvedic system of medicine (Carstairs & Kapur, 1976). Illness is believed to be due to an imbalance between natural elements, leading to an excess of heat, cold, bile, wind, or fluid secretions in the body. The humoral disease theory of the Greeks may have developed from the Ayurvedic concepts. In the mental sphere, it is believed that excessive heat can cause excitement, excessive cold can lead to depression, and excessive bile to hostility.

Few writers have integrated ideas about psychiatric conditions into an overall cosmology in the way Buckley has. His account is intellectually satisfying, although one may question the extent to which it actually pervades the thinking of every member of the culture. What is of great interest to us is the result of the clash between traditional concepts of psychiatric conditions and Western scientific ideas on the same subject, which are introduced along with modern medical facilities. The outcome of the confrontation has proved to be remarkably similar in a large variety of cultures. Orley & Leff (1972) examined concepts of illness held by Ugandans and found that one of the distinctions they made was between native and European illnesses. Native illnesses were characterised as being sent by others rather than occurring spontaneously, and were believed to respond to native remedies and not to European treatments. Polio was categorised as a European illness, whereas psychiatric conditions were considered to be native illnesses. Among the Maori (Ritchie, 1976), there is a common belief that sicknesses are of two kinds: one that can be cured by Western medical therapeutics; and the other, *mate maori* (Maori illness) that cannot. In Tonga the majority of the population still rely on the traditional healer to treat sickness not identified as Western in origin, *mahaki faka-palangi*. The latter include respiratory disease, severe abdominal pain, gastric ulcer, and diabetes (Parsons, 1984). The Zulu categorise illnesses either as *umkhulane*, those which come by themselves and are understood by a Western-trained doctor (for example, measles, malaria, smallpox), or as *ukufa kwabantu*, diseases of the people, which can only be understood by African people (Ngubane, 1976). By contrast, the Yoruba include smallpox with madness as diseases that do not respond to Western methods. Both are believed to emanate from the same god, *Shopanna* (Maclean, 1976). In the study by Onyango (1976), patients in the psychiatric hospital in Nairobi were asked their views on mental illness. Of the respondents, 61% thought mental illness was infectious, a killing disease, and that Europeans could not catch it. Over half the patients were discontented with Western medicine and felt that their illness could only be cured by traditional methods. One patient complained: "One has to take this medicine of yours on and on. It is not easy to swallow tablets, but I have to do this because I am a Christian and the church does not allow me to go to traditional doctors".

Simons (1957) points out that the scientific revolution has come to Africa not as the universal heritage of all men, but as 'white man's knowledge', something distinct from, and incompatible with, tribal beliefs and practices. As a consequence, Western scientific theories about disease have made few inroads on traditional theories. Healers and their clients in traditional societies have retained their theories of illness intact, at least for the time being, and have managed to do this by reclassifying certain conditions as belonging to the Western system rather than to their own. This attitude of 'rendering unto Caesar that which is Caesar's, and to the gods that which is the gods' ' , to paraphrase the Biblical quotation slightly, is applied to illnesses that Western medicine has been conspicuously successful in treating or preventing, such as the epidemic diseases. Fortes (1936), working in the Gold Coast, noted that the dispensary at Zuarungu, which had been established for more than 15 years, had completely displaced the native treatment for yaws, which was lengthy, expensive, and unreliable. Western methods of treating psychiatric illnesses in their acute stage are probably not dramatically more effective than traditional healing methods, while the idea of prevention by taking maintenance drugs for long periods of time is totally alien to patients used to traditional healers. Furthermore, it can hardly be claimed that scientific theories of the origin of psychiatric conditions are compelling in terms of the evidence that can be mustered in their support. It is not surprising, therefore, that psychiatric conditions are viewed as remaining firmly in the sphere of traditional healing practices. Clearly, this militates against psychiatrically ill people reaching the Western doctor in the first instance, although the failures of the traditional healers probably arrive at Western-type facilities in the end. As argued in Part II, this biases the view of psychiatric illness in a developing country when the focus is on the psychiatric services.

Although traditional theories of illness have survived contact with Western medicine, the more dramatic techniques and technology introduced from the West have had an influence. We have already referred to the 'psychic surgeons' of the Philippines (p. 121). Frankenberg & Leeson (1976) found that some Zambian healers used a divining apparatus seemingly operated by magnets, while others consulted the spirit via a horn transmitter–receiver connected by a cord to a shrine. Other healers often employed scarification, tattooing, and rubbing herbs into the wounds, but referred to the treatment as 'African injections'. A Buddhist healer in a meditation ceremony described deities coming to heal the patient. They 'appeared' in their traditional forms, Thep, for example, riding on a water serpent, but were described as giving injections and pills, curing cancer, and extracting diseased bones by surgery (Tambiah, 1977). Gatere (personal communication) reports that some Kenyan healers display glass paperweights and imply that their magical powers are responsible for enclosing the shrunken building within its glass case. Eclecticism of this kind indicates a degree of flexibility of traditional healers that augurs well for their survival. Indeed, we have only to glance around us in a Western country such as Britain to appreciate that traditional healing techniques flourish despite competition with scientific psychiatry for 100 years. It is worth considering in detail which of the techniques used by traditional healers in developing countries still draw a large clientele in the West.

We began this section by considering methods of extracting illness from patients, ranging from the concrete to the abstract. A healing method currently used in the West which has an affinity to these techniques is the laying on of hands. This was used by the kings of England and France throughout the 14th to 17th centuries to treat scrophula, a tuberculous infection of the skin, which was consequently known as the King's Evil. The healing power of the king's touch was believed to stem from his divinity, and as monarchs became regarded as increasingly human, this practice waned. In its heyday it was very popular and Charles II is recorded as having laid his hand on a total of 92 000 people. In his boyhood, Dr Samuel Johnson was touched by Queen Anne in an attempt to cure his scrofula. The laying on of hands is no longer a royal prerogative, although the religious context of the procedure persists and the importance of faith is emphasised. Harry Edwards, a British manual healer, claimed to have treated well over 1 million people since World War I. This technique is also used by the traditional healers, or powwow doctors, of the German community in Pennsylvania (Guthrie & Szanton, 1976). They rely on texts called the Sixth and Seventh Books of Moses, and use prayer and the laying on of hands to treat a wide variety of physical disorders and the mentally ill. The powwow doctor believes that by his physical touch he takes the illness to himself and then 'puts it off'. There is a clear link here on the one hand with the techniques for extracting and discarding illness that were described in Chapter 10, and on the other with modern spiritualism.

Skultans (1974, 1976) has made a study of spiritualism in South Wales. The spiritualist healer is believed to be an instrument of the healing act of a spirit, frequently of a deceased doctor. The healer usually becomes aware of possession by a tingling sensation in his fingertips. When this occurs, the healer places his hands on that part of the patient's body to which he is guided by the spirit. Hence, there is a diagnostic as well as a therapeutic skill being exercised. The patient feels an intense heat emanating from the healer's hands and penetrating the body. The healer usually strokes the patient's body, and sometimes shakes the hands after each stroke, symbolically discarding the sickness that has been drawn out of the patient. There is a bowl of water by the healer's side in which he washes his hands after the spiritual healing of each patient. We have already referred to the use of water in traditional exorcism rituals to wash away the evil spirits. In modern spiritualism, we can identify elements common to the traditional healing techniques described above. In particular, we note the combination of the extraction of illness by physical contact with the healer, and the use of spirit possession for diagnosis and healing. Like many traditional healers, the spiritualist aims to locate the sources of tension in a person's social relationships insofar as these might be responsible for the lack of physical well-being.

In the technique just described, the healer does not show any dramatic manifestation of possession, but in some *séances* in which the aim is to communicate with the dead, the medium enters a trance state of the kind seen in traditional societies. The medium's voice alters, as though a spirit were speaking through her, and she relays messages from the spirit world. Here there is a difference from possession states in traditional cultures, in that the utterances of the medium are usually intelligible to the audience.

Thus, we find that extraction, exorcism, which is still employed by the clergy, albeit infrequently, and possession continue to be used for the treatment of mental and physical disorders outside the confines of scientific medicine. Of the traditional techniques reviewed, divination and herbal remedies remain to be identified in a Western context. Personal consultation for divination has become a rarity in the West and is virtually confined to gypsy fortune-tellers at fairs and carnivals. However, less peripatetic diviners continue to operate in Western cities as can be seen from the following extract from a hand-out distributed recently in London: "I am descended from a long line skilled in spiritual reading. I am endowed with power far beyond that of other fortune-tellers. I have seen things that point to the future and have done things that are unsurpassed. Even if you are deformed or sick I can help you. Just as there are people with greater physical powers than others, there are those with greater mental powers than others. I have strange and mystic powers. Problems of love, marriage, quarrels, enemies, or bad luck present no problems to me. No doubt you have tried others. Maybe you have tried many others and had no luck. Then you should come to me and I will guarantee results.''

Apart from such professionals, divination undoubtedly continues in a domestic setting between friends and neighbours, taking forms such as reading tea leaves at the bottom of a cup, but it is probably not taken very seriously. However, on a public scale, divination remains an important and popular procedure, judging by the number of newspapers that carry a daily horoscope. The supposed influence of the stars and planets on human affairs has formed the basis for divination since antiquity. In Ayurvedic medicine, the *mantarwadi* is a master of the zodiac and discovers the cause of problems through the zodiac (Carstairs & Kapur, 1976). Horoscopes in daily news-papers are couched in the kind of ambiguous language that has characterised divination from the Delphic oracle onwards. It is even possible to telephone an astrologer, according to the following advertisement in the London Underground. ''Russell Grant's Zodiac line presents your personal horoscope forecast. Russell Grant bases his personal telephone horoscope forecast on your actual day, month, and year of birth, so you won't get the same forecast as the millions of other people who share your sun sign. Instead Russell will tell you what prospects he can see for you today in business, in finance, in your love-life – and, maybe a couple of other rather personal things just between you and him'. What appears to be missing in the West is the domestic diviner with an intimate knowledge of the client, who goes beyond ambiguity to prescribe therapeutic changes in the client's social relationships. However, as we have already indicated, in our opinion this role has been taken up by the psychotherapist working within the ambit of scientific medicine.

Finally, we need to consider the status of herbal treatments in the West. Herbalism is a recognised branch of knowledge, and in Britain is represented by the National Institute of Medical Herbalists, which trains and accredits herbal practitioners. Some herbal remedies, such as digitalis and quinine, have become important treatments in scientific medicine. But influences also operate in the reverse direction, as we have seen with other forms of traditional medicine. One herbal remedy for 'nerve troubles' contains several B vitamins in addition to powdered motherwort, mistletoe, wild lettuce, and other herbs. The inclusion of the B vitamins is justified in the accompanying brochure on the grounds that ''the therapeutic values of the herbal ingredients are greatly enhanced because the 'take-up' by the cells of the herbal healing substances is rendered much more efficient''.

Herbalist shops are common in Western cities, but even more common are chemists' shops in which a large variety of patent medicines are available. A booklet issued by the Office of Health Economics in London (1968) states that the total expenditure on medicines in the UK in 1966 was £267 million, of which £188 million was for medicines prescribed within the National Health Service. The other £79 million was spent by the public on medicines bought without a doctor's prescription. The booklet goes on: "Whereas it was the original concept that all sickness should come within the scope of the Health Service, it is now acknowledged that much treatment must fall outside it". An estimate is put forward that two out of every three ailments suffered by the population are probably not taken to the doctor. Instead, as we have seen, the public has recourse to a range of treatments, all of which have their equivalents among the remedies offered by traditional healers in non-Western countries.

To consider, then, the question that opened this part of the book, the traditional healing techniques applied to psychiatric conditions in developing cultures throughout the world have survived in a recognisable form in the West, where they coexist, more or less peacefully, with modern psychiatry. The practitioners of most of these techniques operate outside conventional medicine. However, the psychotherapist, whether medically qualified or not, can be seen as the direct heir of the traditional diviner. The triumphs of Western psychiatry lie in the field of pharmacology and not in the area of social management, which is well understood and practised by traditional healers. On the other hand, Western psychiatry may benefit from a closer study of the herbal remedies employed by healers to treat their psychiatrically ill clients. Alternative therapies flourish in areas in which conventional medicine is unsatisfactory. Psychiatry in the West is currently such an area, and will continue to be so in the foreseeable future, so that the survival of traditional healing techniques is assured.

IV. Do psychiatric conditions have a different course in different cultures?

13 Outlook East and West

A paradox encountered repeatedly is that the very characteristics that make developing countries so interesting from the point of view of our questions also make it difficult to provide the answers. The course of psychiatric disorders in developing countries is relatively uninfluenced by Western medicine, since aftercare facilities are virtually non-existent. Furthermore, the concept of preventive or maintenance treatment is alien to traditional healers. As a result, it is possible in developing countries to observe the natural history of psychiatric disorders. However, to make the relevant observations over extended periods of time, it is necessary to keep contact with a cohort of patients, and this is very difficult to achieve in the absence of a well-developed network of aftercare services. As with the determination of incidence and prevalence rates, the issue of the representative nature of the samples studied is crucial. Any cohort of patients forming the basis of a study of the course of a particular illness obviously needs to be representative of the illness in question. In the case of psychiatric disorders in developing countries, representative cohorts can only be drawn from the general population, because of the high degree of selection involved in attendance at the sparse psychiatric facilities. In fact, only a single study using this strategy in a developing community has been published, that by Gillis & Stone (1973).

These workers followed up subjects interviewed in their original population survey of the Cape coloured community (Gillis *et al*, 1968), which was discussed in detail in Part II of this book (p. 103). The original cohort was seen in 1963, and specific groups were reinterviewed 6 years later in 1969. All subjects initially judged as definitely or probably psychiatrically disturbed, and 10% of those assessed as normal, were followed up in the second survey. Of the 161 individuals eligible for follow-up examination, 16 had died, one refused to attend, and only seven were not traced. Over half of those showing definite psychiatric disturbance in the original survey were unchanged 6 years later. All the rest had improved, but only a small proportion had lost all their symptoms. It is of particular interest that only three of the 12 psychotic people identified initially remained ill at follow-up examination, the remainder having undergone remission after a transient illness. These figures excluded one subject who died and another who refused a second interview, so that the remission rate for psychosis was 70%. Just under half of those with probable psychiatric disturbance remained unchanged at follow-up examination, while a similar proportion improved. Twelve per cent actually got worse, whereas a higher proportion, 19%, of those originally assessed as normal, had developed a psychiatric disturbance at follow-up examination. Only about 10% of psychiatrically disturbed subjects were recognised as ill and received treatment during the 6 years of the study, so that the findings give a reasonably accurate picture of the natural history of psychiatric disorders in the community.

The outcome of psychiatric disorders in the Cape coloured community can be compared with the findings of a follow-up study of new cases of psychiatric illness identified in a survey of 46 general practices in London (Shepherd et al, 1966). The comparison is not completely valid, because in the London survey, only patients who had been identified by their GPs as suffering from a psychiatric disorder were studied. People suffering from neurosis who had not sought medical help were not included, although it has been shown that they represent a substantial group (Hurry et al, 1980). Furthermore, the patients in the London survey had all presented for the first time, whereas in the South African survey, both new and recurrent illnesses were included. The London patients were followed up 3 years after the index consultation, and as many as possible were interviewed: in the event 81% were traced, and a sample of 100 out of the original 524 cases was interviewed (Kedward, 1969). It was found that 73% of all new cases were free from psychiatric symptoms at the time of follow-up examination. The great majority of these were suffering from neuroses, as in the Cape coloured survey, so that the outcome for neurotic conditions appears to be a great deal better in London than in the Cape. This may be a consequence of two factors, namely that all the London patients were new referrals, which in itself is linked with a good prognosis, and that they all received treatment, whereas very few of the Cape coloured subjects did. It is difficult to find a study that permits a closer comparison with that of Gillis & Stone (1973), but the 10-year follow-up of psychiatric cases in a Swedish population by Hagnell (1966) yields some comparable data. He was dealing predominantly with neurotic conditions, and recorded that over the 10-year period, the duration of psychiatric illness was more than 3 years for 20% of those ill. Once more we find a better outlook for neurosis in a Western country. Before accepting this finding as conclusive, we need more follow-up studies of general population samples both in developing and Western countries.

Fortunately, there are considerably more studies on the outcome of psychoses around the world, but their interpretation is clouded by the problem of selection. As already found in Part II, population surveys have to be on a very large scale to identify reasonable numbers of psychotic patients. Consequently, research is conducted much more frequently on psychotic patients in contact with the psychiatric services, allowing large samples to be collected. However, this source of subjects may be heavily biased by the factors that prompt psychotic patients to seek treatment from the medical services. It was concluded above (p. 88) that a sample drawn from these sources is likely to be representative of psychotic patients in the community in a Western country. By contrast, such a sample in a developing country will be shaped by the selection factors determining contact with Western-style services and is likely to be grossly unrepresentative. This epidemiological consideration dominates our presentation of the available data, and will receive detailed attention in the following chapter.

One of the earliest scientific studies of the outcome of schizophrenic illnesses in a developing country was conducted in Mauritius (Murphy & Raman, 1971). Murphy chose the island of Mauritius because it represented a tropical setting where the level of psychiatric care approached Western standards, although the culture remained in many respects traditional. Furthermore, being a relatively small island, it was feasible to trace patients after a period of some years. The population at the time was 600 000, two-thirds of whom were Indian in origin, and the remainder mainly African. The lack of Westernisation is exemplified by the fact that in 1962, 45% of the adult population had never attended school. On the other hand, in 1956, there were 1.2 psychiatric beds per 1000 population, which can be compared with 2.9 per 1000 for London and 1.0 per 1000 for Aarhus (World Health Organization, 1973). These figures substantiate to some extent Murphy & Raman's claim that the culture was relatively un-Westernised, whereas the psychiatric service was well developed. Regrettably, however, they give no information about the attitudes of the public towards psychiatric disorders and their treatment, factors having a crucial effect on the referral of patients to Western-type facilities. Furthermore, they did not search for untreated schizophrenic people in the population, so that it is impossible to evaluate their statement that "the hospitalized group is as representative of the total as is true for a Euro-American population".

The study began with a review of all admissions to the only psychiatric hospital on the island during the year 1956. All first admissions with a diagnosis of schizophrenia were selected for follow-up examination. This was conducted by two experienced psychiatric nurses, one for the Indian patients, one for the others. The nurses' tasks were to trace the patients, conduct a home visit, and interview both the patients and some person close to them. The information gathered was brought back to the authors to make assessments of course and outcome. Where the current psychiatric state of the patients was unclear, means were used to bring them to the hospital for a clinical examination.

From the data collected in 1956, the authors were able to calculate age-specific first-admission rates for schizophrenia. These turned out to be very similar to the comparable incidence rates for England and Wales at the same period. The authors were very successful in tracing their cohort, although the follow-up was 12 years after the first admission, and failed in less than 2% of cases. They faced the difficult problem of how to assess outcome, which may be measured in terms of readmission, freedom from symptomatic relapse, or social performance. They rightly rejected readmission on its own, since this is dependent on many factors unconnected with the course of illness, such as availability of beds or distance from the hospital. Instead, they combined readmission with a judgement of the severity of disturbance. They compared their data with figures from a 5-year follow-up of British schizophrenic patients admitted for the first time to one of three large psychiatric institutions in 1956, the same year as the beginning of the Mauritius study (Brown *et al*, 1966). The worst prognosis was shown by patients who were either in hospital at the time of follow-up or who were in the community but showed severe disturbance. The proportion with this outcome in the British (28%) and Mauritian (24%) samples is very similar. The best outcome is represented by patients who recovered completely from the initial episode of schizophrenia and had no further episodes during the follow-up period. Here, there is a marked difference between the two cohorts, 34% of the British sample falling into this group compared with 59% of the Mauritian patients. This difference in outcome becomes even more impressive when we consider that maintenance treatment with phenothiazine drugs was employed for half the British sample, but for only a small proportion of the Mauritian group. This result could be attributed to differences in diagnostic concepts between Mauritius and Britain, of the kind revealed by the US:UK Project (p. 32). Thus, a broader concept of schizophrenia in Mauritius might include patients who would be diagnosed by British psychiatrists as manic–depressive, whose prognosis on the whole is usually better than narrowly defined schizophrenic patients. This consideration engenders some doubt about the interpretation of Murphy & Raman's findings, so that they have to be viewed in the context of other similar studies.

One was carried out in Hong Kong, where all the psychiatrists have had a British training, so that their diagnostic habits can be assumed to be very close to those of British psychiatrists. Lo & Lo (1977) screened the notes of all patients between the ages of 14 and 60 who attended the Hong Kong Psychiatric Centre for the first time in 1965 and were given a definite diagnosis of schizophrenia. Of the 133 patients in the cohort, 82 (62%) attended for a follow-up examination 10 years after their first admission. Four had died and the remaining 47 (35%) failed to attend. The fully evaluated patients were compared with those not attending, on a number of basic characteristics, and only one significant difference was found; more patients in the former group had a supportive relative. Of those fully evaluated, 21% recovered from the initial episode and had no recurrences, while an additional 44% had remissions and relapses with no or only mild personality deterioration. Thus, a total of 65% of the patients interviewed at the 10-year follow-up could be said to have had a good outcome. However, this is not as impressive a finding as Murphy & Raman's, partly because of the relatively high proportion of the cohort for whom no information was available, and partly because of the much lower percentage (21) with no further episodes over a 10-year period compared with the equivalent Mauritian figure (59%). Indeed, the outcome of the Hong Kong cohort is no better than that of the British cohort used as a comparison group by Murphy & Raman.

Another study from a developing country that conflicts with Murphy & Raman's findings is that by Kulhara & Wig (1978). These research workers from the city of Chandigarh in North India modelled their study on that by Brown *et al* (1966) referred to above. They selected patients attending the department of psychiatry who came from a catchment area defined as the city of Chandigarh and neighbouring villages within a 20-mile radius. Chandigarh is unique in India, being a Western-style city designed by the French architect Le Corbusier, and built from scratch in the 1950s. The housing units are European in proportion, limiting the size of families, so that one finds an uncharacteristically high percentage of nuclear families within the city. The surrounding villages, on the other hand, are relatively uninfluenced by the presence of the city, and families conform to the traditional Indian pattern, with large households being the norm. The cohort consisted of patients seen for the first time in the department of psychiatry between 1 January 1966 to 31 December 1967, and given a diagnosis of schizophrenia. Diagnostic practices in the department are closely modelled on British principles. The follow-up period ranged from 4.5 to more than 6 years. Of the 173 eligible patients, complete follow-up information was available for only 100 (58%), a success rate very similar to that of Lo & Lo (1977) in Hong Kong.

The clinical outcome of the patients followed up was assessed on criteria very similar to those used by Brown *et al* (1966). The worst outcome, as before, was for patients who failed to recover from the initial episode of schizophrenia. These formed 32% of the Chandigarh cohort, a very similar proportion to that found in Britain and Mauritius. The patients showing the best outcome, a complete recovery from the initial episode and no relapse, constituted 29% of the Chandigarh sample, being very similar to the British figure, and much lower than the proportion in the Mauritian cohort. This report is not explicable in terms of the unusual urban character of Chandigarh, since the outcome for patients from the villages was no better than for those from the city itself. Twenty-five per cent of the cohort received no aftercare, but their outcome was no worse than for those who attended the clinic on a regular basis. The main doubt that hangs over the findings of this study is that such a high proportion of the cohort was untraced (nearly 30%), and this might represent patients with a particularly good prognosis.

A recent study of outcome of schizophrenia from a single developing country was conducted in Sri Lanka by Waxler (1979). During the years

1970–1971, she sampled a cohort of 89 schizophrenic patients admitted for the first time to a psychiatric ward in Sri Lanka and later discharged. The diagnosis was that made by the hospital psychiatrist at discharge from the first admission. Some patients had been continuously ill for 5–10 years before being admitted for the first time. In all, 83% of the sample came from rural areas. The sample was followed up 5 years after the first admission, and all but two were traced and reinterviewed. Information on the course of illness was obtained both from hospital records and from relatives. Waxler found that 29% of the cohort remained seriously and continuously ill for the 5-year period, a figure very similar to those from the other studies reviewed. On the other hand, 40% had no further episodes after the one that led to the first hospital admission. This is somewhat better than the British figure used for comparison, but falls far short of the proportion in the best outcome group in the Mauritian cohort.

Waxler made some subsidiary inquiries, to investigate possible explanations for her finding. In particular, she postulated that the high proportion with a good outcome in her sample might be due to a pool of untreated, severely ill schizophrenic people in the community. She checked on the possible selection bias in her sample by conducting an epidemiological survey of four randomly selected villages in the catchment area of the admitting hospital. Out of 771 people surveyed, she found six who were defined by family members as having had a psychiatric illness at some time in the past. It was established that all of them had been treated at one or more government hospitals or clinics. Hence, there was no evidence of a large pool of untreated schizophrenic people in the catchment area from which her initial cohort was drawn, and it can be assumed that the cohort was a representative sample of schizophrenic people in the community.

The results of the four outcome studies in developing countries are presented together in Table XIV, with the British figures for comparison. There are undoubtedly difficulties in defining different types of outcome accurately. However, there is probably little variation in the best type of outcome, namely a complete recovery from the initial episode and no further recurrences. The worst type of outcome is more subject to individual judgement; nevertheless, there is remarkably close agreement on the proportions in this category from all the studies. The wide range in the proportions with the best outcome seems to bear some relationship to the degree of success in tracing the total cohort. Thus, the lowest figures are found in the studies from Hong Kong and Chandigarh, in which a substantial proportion of the samples were lost to follow-up examination. This raises the distinct possibility that patients who recover completely and remain well are reluctant to make any further contact with the psychiatric services, and hence fail to come to follow-up interviews. This consideration would not apply to the difference between the Sri Lankan and Mauritian studies since, in both, the researchers achieved virtually total success in reinterviewing their original samples. Waxler's is undoubtedly the more rigorous, since

TABLE XIV
Outcome of first-admission cohorts of schizophrenic patients

Location	Length of follow-up in years	Percentage with full information	Percentage with best outcome[1]	Percentage with worst outcome[2]	Study
Britain	5	100	34	28	Brown *et al* (1966)
Mauritius	12	98	59	24	Murphy & Raman (1971)
Hong Kong	10	62	21	32	Lo & Lo (1977)
N. India	5	58	29	32	Kulhara & Wig (1978)
Sri Lanka	5	98	40	29	Waxler (1979)

[1] Complete recovery from initial episode and no recurrence.
[2] Failure to recover from initial episode, or partial recovery with recurrences.

she interviewed all the patients personally, whereas Murphy & Raman relied on screening interviews by psychiatric nurses, who might conceivably have missed episodes of psychosis occurring some time in the 12 years covered by their inquiry. Furthermore, Waxler carried out an epidemiological survey in parallel with her follow-up study, showing that she was not dealing with a sample biased by selection for contact with the services. There is certainly enough evidence here to support more carefully standardised follow-up studies in a variety of cultures using comparable techniques for diagnosis and clinical assessment. Fortunately, two such studies have been carried out by the World Health Organization (1979) and Sartorius *et al* (1986).

The first was a follow-up of the original samples of patients collected in nine different countries as part of the IPSS (already described in detail in Part I, p. 33 ff.). An integral feature of the original design of this international project were follow-ups at 2 and 5 years of the patient samples. Both follow-ups have now been successfully completed, but only data from the 2-year follow-up have been published. A basic feature of the IPSS was the standardisation of clinical assessment through the use of the PSE. Further standardisation was applied to the diagnostic process by computer programs such as Catego, which revealed that in seven of the nine centres there was close agreement on the diagnosis of schizophrenia. Fortunately, those seven centres span both Western and non-Western countries, so that the outcome of clinically comparable groups of schizophrenic patients can be studied. It must be emphasised that the patients studied in each centre were not selected on any epidemiological basis, and hence there are problems of interpretation, which will be discussed when the results are presented.

We have already encountered difficulties in defining outcome in the studies considered above. In the IPSS, a number of ways of assessing outcome were employed, and attempts were made to standardise these by having the judgements made at WHO headquarters by a group of psychiatrists on the basis of data provided by the individual centres. This group of assessors achieved reasonably high levels of agreement on the various measures of outcome, with the exception of social functioning. By collapsing the levels of social functioning into a dichotomous scale, a more acceptable level of agreement between the raters was achieved. The five main measures of outcome used in this international study were: the symptomatic picture at follow-up interview, the length of the episode of inclusion, the percentage of the follow-up period spent in a psychotic episode, the pattern of course, and the degree of social impairment.

Although patients with diagnoses other than schizophrenia were included in the original IPSS samples, there were too few of them to make meaningful comparisons of outcome between centres. Therefore, we will review here the findings for the schizophrenic patients only. The overall success rate in reinterviewing patients with the PSE at the 2-year follow-up was 76%. It was over 70% in every centre except London, where shortage of research staff limited the follow-up study to patients admitted from the local catchment area, resulting in no more than 21% of the original sample being reinterviewed. Excluding London, the average percentage reinterviewed in developed and developing countries was identical at 84.

The results for the schizophrenic patients successfully followed up are presented in terms of each outcome measure in turn. The symptomatic picture at the time of the 2-year follow-up was generally undramatic. Florid symptoms were uncommon and were overshadowed by negative symptoms such as flatness of affect, lack of insight, and difficulties in co-operating. All centres showed a very similar picture in this respect, with the exception of Moscow, which, with Washington, embodied a broader definition of schizophrenia than the other centres (see p. 37).

The second measure, the length of the episode of inclusion, was derived from the follow-up psychiatric history. It was quite distinct from the length of initial hospital stay, which was influenced by local sociocultural factors and the availability of services. The mean length of the episode of inclusion varied from 3.8 months in Ibadan to 13.9 months in Aarhus. The shortest average durations were found in Ibadan (3.8 months), Moscow (6.4 months), Agra (7.1 months), and Cali (8.1 months). In these four centres, more than one-third of the patients had an episode of inclusion that lasted less than 1 month.

For the third measure of outcome, the follow-up psychiatric histories were reviewed to estimate the percentage of the follow-up period spent by the patients in a psychotic episode. The average for all centres combined on this index was 37%. The lowest means were shown by Ibadan, Agra, Moscow, and Cali, in ascending order. With the exception of Moscow, these centres had more than 20% of their patients spending less than 5% of the follow-up period in a psychotic episode.

TABLE XV
Outcome of IPSS samples of schizophrenic patients

Centre	Percentage with full information	Percentage with best outcome (group 1)	Percentage with worst outcome (group 7)
Aarhus	91	6	50
Agra	90	51	20
Cali	77	19	26
Ibadan	49	58	7
London	57	23	30
Moscow	90	7	18
Taipei	99	27	27
Washington	58	21	47
Prague	96	17	30

Adapted from World Health Organization (1979), Table 6.16.

The next measure, the pattern of course, is of particular interest to us since it provides data that can be compared with that from the earlier studies reviewed. The patients in the IPSS follow-up were assigned to one of seven groups, depending on the pattern of course they demonstrated during the interval between the initial evaluation and the 2-year assessment. It is clearest if we take the two extremes, as before, patients in group 1 showing the best outcome with a full remission after the episode of inclusion and no further episodes. The worst outcome is represented by group 7, which comprises those who were still in the episode of inclusion at the time of the 2-year follow-up. These results are presented in Table XV, but in comparing them with those in Table XIV it must be remembered that, in the latter, all patients are on first admissions, whereas in the former, the patients are a mixed group of those first admitted and those readmitted. Hence an overall worse outcome would be expected in the World Health Organization series than in the earlier studies.

It is evident that there is a great deal of variation both in the best outcome and in the worst outcome. Two centres, Agra and Ibadan, have a strikingly high proportion of patients with complete recovery from the initial episode and no recurrences. One of these centres, Agra, had a high success rate in following up patients, while in the other, Ibadan, the rate was low. The percentages with the best outcome in these two centres in developing countries come close to the figure of Murphy & Raman (1971), even though their samples were not purely first-admitted patients. The figures from the London centre are similar to those of Brown *et al* (1966), although the success rate in following up patients was much lower, and it was not a first-admission cohort.

The final outcome measure was the degree of social impairment during the follow-up period. As we have already seen, it was necessary to divide the patients into two groups, those with severe social impairment, and the rest, in order to achieve acceptable levels of interrater reliability. When all the centres were combined, the average percentage showing severe social impairment was 23. Five centres scored below this figure: Ibadan (5%); Agra (18%); Taipei (20%); Moscow (21%); and Cali (22%).

Viewing these different assessments of outcome as a whole, a clear pattern emerges of a group of centres consistently showing the best results. Agra, Cali, Ibadan, Moscow, and Taipei feature with the best outcome on at least two measures, while Agra and Ibadan come off best on every measure. The appearance of Moscow among this group of centres in what are otherwise developing countries emphasises the crucial effect of diagnostic practices on outcome. The Moscow psychiatrists were using a relatively broad concept of schizophrenia, which included a substantial proportion of patients that psychiatrists in the other centres (except Washington) would have diagnosed as affective psychosis or neurosis. These patients would be expected to have a better outcome than narrowly defined schizophrenic patients, and hence would improve the outlook of the Moscow sample when compared with the samples of schizophrenic patients from other centres. This interpretation is supported by another feature of outcome that was examined in this study, namely the diagnostic character of any subsequent episodes during the follow-up period. It emerged that Moscow was the centre with the highest proportion of patients (32%) having episodes of affective psychosis subsequent to the inclusion episode that was diagnosed by the centre psychiatrists as schizophrenia. The Moscow figure may be contrasted with the equivalent percentages for London (4%), Taipei (5%), and Prague (7%), where a narrow definition of schizophrenia is evidently in operation.

Hence, in interpreting these outcome data, we would be well advised to restrict our comparisons to centres with closely similar diagnostic practices. The use of the Catego program as a reference classification demonstrated that seven of the IPSS centres were in close agreement on a narrow definition of schizophrenia (see p. 40). These included all the centres in developing countries, and the Western centres in Aarhus, London, and Prague. This finding legitimises comparisons of outcome of schizophrenia between these centres, and gives us some confidence in regarding Agra and Ibadan as showing unusually good results. The main drawback to the Ibadan data is the low percentage of patients with full information at follow-up examination. It was argued previously that the relatively poor outcome shown by patients from Hong Kong and Chandigarh could be due to the patients with a full recovery being lost to follow-up study. It would indeed be capricious to argue exactly the opposite in the case of the Ibadan sample. Nevertheless, there should be more confidence in the Agra findings, as these derive from a 90% successful follow-up. The outcome of the Agra schizophrenic patients is so conspicuously superior to that of similarly diagnosed patients from Aarhus, London, and Prague that further careful studies of this phenomenon are obligatory.

First, possible explanations for the findings must be considered. The simplest concerns an issue we have raised several times, namely the selection of patients for treatment by the psychiatric services. Where these are scarce, as in many developing countries, a particular kind of patient tends to be referred for treatment. It is characteristic of these patients that they cause considerable disturbance in their community. Gatere (1980) sampled attitudes to psychiatric illness among the general public and deliverers of health care in Kenya. The latter included doctors, pharmacists, clinical officers, and traditional healers. The respondents were asked, "What four things make you know that a given person is mad?" The types of behaviour on which they all agreed, listed in order of priority, were: aggression (particularly attacking people); making a noise; walking naked; and talking to oneself. Gatere comments that if a psychiatrically ill person does not conform to this stereotype the chances of being treated early are small.

A similar picture emerges from the study by Westermeyer & Kroll (1978) of the use of the term *baa* by villagers in Laos. The English equivalents are insane, crazy, or psychotic. They studied 35 people labelled as *baa* and found that over half of them had assaulted others, while one-quarter had destroyed property. Only seven of the group showed no violence towards others, themselves, or property at any time during their *baa* condition. However, six of these subjects exhibited considerable hostile verbal expression, cursing people and yelling insults or threats at both strangers and acquaintances.

The popular stereotype of 'madness' that emerges from both these studies is of a person creating a public disturbance by violence to people or property, or by offences to public morality. When schizophrenia is viewed as a whole, patients showing these symptoms are generally in the minority and represent the most emotionally excited and physically overactive group. It is conceivable that patients with these characteristics might have a better prognosis than the others, as well as being more likely to receive treatment, and hence would bias a sample in contact with the services towards a better outcome. Evidence against this explanation is forthcoming both from Murphy & Raman's study and from the IPSS follow-up. In neither study was physical overactivity or emotional excitement associated with a good prognosis. Further contrary evidence comes from Waxler's demonstration that there was no pool of untreated, severely ill schizophrenic people in the area of Sri Lanka she studied.

The most convincing rebuttal of the selective-referral explanation is provided by the second WHO follow-up study of schizophrenia (Sartorius *et al*, 1986). This international collaborative venture, described on p. 113, was an epidemiologically based study of patients making their first contact with a psychiatric facility. Great care was taken to ensure that all patients presenting with schizophrenia in each catchment area were included. Hence a selective bias was avoided. A 2-year follow-up was conducted, and data on pattern of course were obtained in 76% of the original cohort of patients from developed countries, and in 71% of those from developing countries.

In this preliminary communication, a full breakdown of the patterns of course is not given. Instead, patterns 1 and 2 have been amalgamated and include patients with one relatively brief episode followed by a remission with or without some residual symptoms. This 'mild' pattern is thus not entirely comparable with the data from the IPSS in Table XV. Nevertheless the results are unequivocal, since 56% of patients in developing countries showed this pattern of course, compared with 39% of patients in developed countries, a significant difference ($P < 0.001$). In presenting the above study (see p. 113) attention was drawn to the significantly higher proportion of patients with an acute onset in developing countries compared with the developed countries. We also noted the caution expressed by Stevens & Wyatt (1987) that this feature might well bias comparisons of outcome. In fact, Sartorius *et al* (1986) have taken this into account in their analyses. They found, as expected, that patients with an acute onset were significantly more likely to have a more favourable outcome. However this relationship did not fully account for the better prognosis of cases in developing countries, since over 40% of those with a gradual onset had a 'mild' pattern of course compared with less than 30% in developed countries.

The findings of this epidemiological study rule out selective referral to psychiatric facilities as an explanation of the better outcome for schizophrenic patients in developing countries. They also suggest that the greater frequency of acute, rapidly resolving psychoses in developing countries may not fully explain this phenomenon. The possibility that these conditions may only mimic schizophrenia and should not be included under the same rubric deserves due consideration. An alternative explanation is based on the assumption that schizophrenia in developing countries is the same illness as in the West, but has a better prognosis. This would then be ascribed to more favourable social conditions in developing countries, including more tolerant attitudes and better opportunities for re-employment. The two arguments are examined in the next chapter.

14 Illuminating the twilight states

"The African is evidently prone to develop a type of twilight or confusional state – sometimes brief (a matter of hours), sometimes more prolonged (a matter of weeks) – but always tending to spontaneous recovery within a limited time." So wrote Carothers in 1951, encapsulating the problem in a nutshell. The dilemma he raised remains unresolved, namely whether these transient psychotic states are really confusional in nature. As we saw from the hierarchical pyramid of psychological symptoms (Fig. 2, p. 36), patients with organic brain disease exhibit symptoms from every level of the hierarchy, including those specific to schizophrenia. On the other hand, patients with schizophrenia are excluded from showing symptoms of organic brain disease. Thus, if these transient psychotic states are characterised by symptoms of organic cerebral dysfunction, they should not be included with cases of schizophrenia in international comparisons of course. It follows that it is of vital importance to determine whether or not these patients show confusion and other organic cerebral symptoms.

The problem is confounded by widespread laxity among psychiatric professionals in the use of the term *confusion*. For instance, Simpson (1984) examined the way doctors and nurses use the word 'confused', and found that one-third of the psychiatrists participating in his study considered that hallucinations and/or delusions supported or implied a description of 'confused'. A lay person may describe as confused anyone who appears to be out of touch with reality, which would include patients suffering from functional as well as organic psychoses. However, the technical use of the term in psychiatry is properly confined to patients whose consciousness is clouded, or who are disoriented in time, place, or person, all of which are indications of organic cerebral dysfunction. Clouding of consciousness is manifested by reduced wakefulness and a disturbance of awareness. Excessive sleepiness during the day is not seen in patients with functional psychoses, unless they are treated with high doses of tranquillisers. However, awareness *is* disturbed in the functional psychoses, particularly in mania and schizophrenia. Manic patients show a heightening of awareness, resulting in an inability to shut out irrelevant stimuli. As a consequence, they are easily distracted from the business of the interview by extraneous happenings such as noises outside the room, or by features that capture their interest, such as the colour of the interviewer's tie. Whereas the manic patient shows a widening of his or her span of attention, in schizophrenia this is often narrowed. The schizophrenic patient may be so absorbed in the psychotic experience that the interviewer has to struggle continually to gain the patient's attention. Auditory hallucinations can be so frequent and insistent that the patient is unable to listen for more than a few moments to the speech of any real person. This phenomenon is usually clear to an observer.

Occasionally, the psychotic process appears to invade the patient's total experience of the world. Everything that surrounds the patient and everything that happens in the patient's environment appears changed and unfamiliar. All the usual reference points have vanished unaccountably, leaving the patient bemused and bewildered. On recovery, patients often describe the experience as similar to a dream, and these states have been labelled as *oneiroid* (dreamlike). Patients in an oneiroid state speak very little, and may completely fail to respond to questions. It seems as though they are living in a purely personal time and space, lacking any point of contact with the real world. It will be appreciated that it is very difficult to apply the usual tests of orientation to such a patient to determine whether an organic cerebral condition is present. However, on recovery, such patients often provide evidence demonstrating that, despite living in their own dream world, they were perfectly aware of the real world running its course in parallel with their psychotic experience. This ability to keep track of public space and time alongside their private, psychotic equivalents has been termed *double book-keeping*, and distinguishes the disturbances of awareness sometimes seen in functional psychoses from those that characterise organic cerebral states. The latter are correctly ascribed the technical term *confusion*; the former are not.

In attempting to dispel the confusion surrounding the use of the term *confusion*, it is recognised that the distinctions involved rest heavily on the interviewer's ability to question the patient closely. Unfortunately, many of the patients in whom the distinction is most vital are likely to be inaccessible to questions. One is then left only with observations of the patient's behaviour, which are of limited value in this dilemma. In patients suffering from organic cerebral states, the disturbance of awareness tends to fluctuate in intensity. At times, patients become quite lucid and ask what has been happening to them and where they are, but after a short time slip back into confusion and become inaccessible once more. By contrast, oneiroid states tend not to fluctuate in this way while they last. However, this is rather an insubstantial feature on which to base a diagnostic decision of great importance, and it is evident that clinical examination of patients must be supplemented by laboratory investigations. This point is discussed later, but first, the observations made by clinicians on these transient psychotic states are reviewed in the light of the above discussion.

One of the earliest relevant studies is that by Tooth (1950), which has justifiably become a classic, because of his careful clinical observations. The major part of his publication is concerned with the psychiatric complications of sleeping sickness. He describes the various stages of the infection, the first being characterised by fever, headache, pains in the muscles and joints, and sometimes irritation of the skin. These signs of infection with the trypanosome are frequently overlooked, since malaria and yaws are also endemic in the same area, so that almost everyone experiences fever with joint pains at some time or another. The second stage of the illness corresponds to invasion of the central nervous system, resulting in a mild meningeal reaction, but rarely anything as dramatic as meningismus or signs of increased intracranial pressure. It is not until the third stage, when the brain substance is involved, that the characteristic symptom of sleeping during the day appears. Tooth states that if pathological sleeping is absent there is little to distinguish trypanosomiasis from schizophrenia. Delusions of all sorts may be present and are commonly related to hallucinatory experiences. In organic psychoses, hallucinations usually predominate in the visual modality, but in the case of sleeping sickness, they are most often auditory, as in schizophrenia. One distinction between the two conditions is that fixed delusions are uncommon in trypanosomiasis, probably because even in the face of bizarre psychotic experiences, insight is seldom entirely lost.

The most difficult presentation to distinguish from schizophrenia is excitement with florid symptoms. In these states, incongruity of affect is nearly always present, and patients can hardly ever explain their attacks of weeping alternating with noisy euphoria. Many patients show the moist, cold extremities and the expressionless face considered to be characteristic of schizophrenia.

It might be thought that accompanying neurological abnormalities would alert the clinician to an organic cerebral condition. However, Tooth found them to be present in no more than half of his series. He makes a general statement that "with the exception of the acute toxic–confusional states, it is by no means easy to distinguish a psychosis due primarily to organic factors from the so-called endogenous group without facilities for thorough physical examination and laboratory tests". We would strongly concur with that opinion, but unfortunately he also states that the recognition of trypanosomes in the body fluids requires skill, practice, and good eyesight. In a number of the cases he describes in detail, it was not possible to find trypanosomes, and the diagnosis had to be made on clinical grounds alone.

It is evident that in some cases even the combination of a good history, a careful physical examination, and laboratory tests may not be sufficient to distinguish the psychiatric symptoms of trypanosomiasis from schizophrenia.

It is a possibility that the distinction might be easier with electroencephalography or brain scans, but these sophisticated investigations are rarely available in a developing country.

A year after Tooth's monograph, Carothers (1951) published an extensive paper on psychiatric conditions he had encountered in his practice in Africa. In the course of this he expounded a theory of brain function in Africans which is derogatory in the extreme. However, if one can ignore his outrageous theorising, his paper contains worthwhile clinical observations. He writes that: "In general, well developed and classical examples of the non-organic psychoses are relatively uncommon in the African; and even when one has classified abortive forms of these disorders as exhaustively as possible there still remains a number of frankly undiagnosable cases. Such cases are commonly confused, excited, incoherent and emotionally labile." Here we see a clear example of the incorrect use of the term *confused* to describe the behaviour of patients he considers to be suffering from non-organic psychosis. However his description fits the acute psychotic states with which we are concerned. He goes on to note that there is marked difficulty in making a differential diagnosis between various types of psychosis, since some of the more characteristic symptoms, particularly the delusional systems and sustained mood changes, are absent or unobtrusive.

We might be tempted to ascribe these diagnostic difficulties to the language barrier between Carothers and his patients, but his view is endorsed by an indigenous African psychiatrist. Lambo (1960) wrote about short-lived periodic psychoses in Africans characterised by nocturnal agitation and excitement. He agreed that many such cases were obscure and unclassifiable, since the attacks were often transient and the symptoms vague and ill defined. He designated them "periodic or transient psychoses" and distinguished them from schizophrenia on the grounds that they were much more subject to spontaneous recovery. This begs the question of whether they might be a form of schizophrenia with an unusually good prognosis. He goes on to give his opinion that the syndrome is an organic one, without providing evidence to back this up, and raises the possibility that it is a variant of epilepsy or migraine.

The circularity of using outcome to determine diagnostic distinctions is nowhere more clearly displayed than in Smartt's (1964) account of transient psychoses in Rhodesia. He studied 328 first admissions to the psychiatric ward at Harare Hospital in Salisbury, Rhodesia, during 1 year, who responded to short-term treatment and were discharged within 10 days. He classified 52% of these as acute confusional states, 38 cases being diagnosed as "simple confusion". The clinical description he gives of these cases includes classical symptoms of organic cerebral dysfunction such as disorientation, impairment of recent memory, and confabulation. On this basis, the term *confusion* is being used in its strict technical sense. However, he categorised 67 cases as "confusional states with schizophrenic features", and for these it is worth quoting his description in detail. "It usually begins with an attack of excitement, with anti-social behaviour, such as assault, damaging property, predatory wandering, singing, shouting, dancing, and going naked in public. It is only in hospital that the true picture emerges. The clinical picture is one of stupor with periodic attacks of excitement, often of savage intensity. During the first few days in hospital, the patient may adopt strange postures with stereotyped movements. Echo actions and ceaseless repetition of a phrase or a snatch of a tribal song are common. Many patients show cataplexy and automatic obedience, but negativism, curiously enough, is rare''. The reader will find these symptoms enumerated on p. 12 as characteristic of the picture of catatonic schizophrenia. However, Smartt writes: ''In spite of the catatonic picture, these patients are not suffering from schizophrenia. They are basically confusional states and they respond to short-term treatment''. Yet, he describes none of the symptoms of organic brain dysfunction to be found in his account of what he calls ''simple confusion''. His assertion that these are not schizophrenic illnesses appears to be based solely on their rapid resolution. Indeed, he states later: ''The true diagnosis often rests on the response to treatment, for in confusional states the patient responds rapidly''.

The fallacy in this approach can best be demonstrated by considering a disease of the kidneys, acute nephritis. This acute inflammation of the kidneys generally affects children and young adults and is believed to represent an allergic response to infection with a bacterium, the streptococcus. Most sufferers recover rapidly and completely, but in some the condition lingers on and enters a different stage, known as nephrotic syndrome, while others eventually develop chronic nephritis after many years. Occasionally the acute illness passes rapidly and irreversibly into the condition of chronic nephritis. Thus, a variety of outcomes are possible for the sufferer from acute nephritis. Not only is it impossible to predict a particular outcome from the clinical picture in the acute phase, but no additional information is gained from the microscopic examination of biopsy specimens of the kidneys at that time. The different outcomes of the disease have not encouraged nephrologists to distinguish a variety of types of acute nephritis as distinct diagnostic entities. To do so would be tantamount to declaring that the prognosis lay within the nature of the disease, and not in the patient's response to it. We are not in possession of the evidence that would allow us to make such a declaration in respect to schizophrenia. Yet, as we have noted above, the current American classificatory system, DSM–III, separates from schizophrenia, conditions with identical symptoms but a duration of illness of less than 6 months before referral to the services. Given the current state of knowledge about schizophrenia, this appears to be a premature decision.

Another fallacy connected with transient psychotic states is illustrated by Rin & Lin's (1962) survey of the Malayo-Polynesians on Taiwan, reviewed on p. 95. When they encountered subjects who were discovered to be suffering from malaria during a period of psychotic behaviour, they categorised the psychiatric illness as "malarial psychosis", and separated it off from schizophrenia in their calculations of prevalence. Now the coincidental occurrence of malaria, or for that matter any physical illness, and schizophrenic symptoms may be explained in at least three different ways (Asuni, 1967). First, the infection with malaria parasites may directly affect the brain, producing an organic psychosis with schizophrenic symptoms. Second, the patient's knowledge that he or she has contracted malaria may act as a psychological stress, which then precipitates a schizophrenic episode. Last, in an area in which malaria is common, it is likely to occur by chance in a proportion of patients developing schizophrenia, their concurrence in the same person being truly coincidental. Only the first of these possibilities could justifiably be labelled as 'malarial psychosis' and distinguished from schizophrenia. In this case it would be necessary to establish by clinical and laboratory tests that the malaria parasites or the associated fever were interfering with cerebral function.

A partial attempt at this approach was made by Nadeem & Younis (1977), working in the only psychiatric hospital in Sudan. They reviewed the medical records of patients admitted during a 2-year period for a psychiatric illness in which an associated acute physical illness was found. They made a clinical distinction between patients who showed varying degrees of clouding of consciousness and those whose consciousness was clear. Of the 39 patients in the sample, 20 fell into the former group, and 19 into the latter. The most common associated physical illness was malaria, and of the 17 patients with this infestation, eight showed clouded consciousness and nine were in clear consciousness. In the eight patients with clouded consciousness and malarial infestation, one can confidently ascribe their psychological symptoms to an organic cerebral dysfunction caused by malaria. It remains a possibility that laboratory tests such as brain imaging might provide evidence of cerebral involvement by malaria in the patients whose consciousness was clear on clinical examination. However, in the absence of such evidence, one cannot assume a direct causal link between the malaria and the psychological symptoms. It is relevant to the theme of this chapter that in Nadeem & Younis's sample there were 12 patients with schizophrenic symptoms, of whom eight showed clouded, and four clear consciousness.

Before summarising the present state of knowledge concerning acute transient psychoses, reference should be made to the French literature, in which the earliest accounts of these states are to be found. There is a good review of the relevant French work (in English) by Jilek & Jilek-Aall (1970). The term *bouffée délirante* was coined by Magnan in 1886 (quoted by Ey *et al*, 1960) to refer to a picture of oneiroid delusions and lowered levels of consciousness, developing over a period of some hours to several weeks, and as a rule remitting spontaneously. Collomb (1965), from his experience in Senegal, regarded *bouffée délirante* as a characteristic African psychopathological reaction. He described it as a transient and brief delusional attack of sudden onset, which is not a confusional state in the classical sense. He considered the typical modification of wakefulness to be like a twilight state. On the one hand he distinguishes the condition from organic cerebral states, on the other he considers it to be radically different from a schizophrenic process.

It is clear from reviewing the literature on this topic that there are more opinions than facts, and that the opinions are often based on fallacious reasoning. There is no doubt that organic cerebral conditions presenting with schizophrenic symptoms occur in Africa and the rest of the developing world, just as they do in the West. The causes are different from those in the West, reflecting the ubiquitousness of conditions such as malaria and trypanosomiasis in tropical countries. In this group of patients, symptoms of schizophrenia coexist with signs of true confusion, in a technical sense, and there should be no difficulty in making a diagnosis of an organic cerebral condition. Two other groups of patients with acute transient psychoses give rise to diagnostic dilemmas. One group consists of patients in whom an acute episode of schizophrenic symptoms with no signs of confusion coexists with a physical illness that is known to affect the brain at times. The possible associations between the psychiatric and physical symptoms were discussed above in connection with 'malarial psychosis'. The complexity of the problem is illustrated by Tooth's (1959) observations that trypanosomiasis may give rise to psychiatric symptoms even in the absence of clinical and laboratory evidence of cerebral involvement by the parasites.

The second group of patients that puzzle the psychiatrist are those who exhibit marked degrees of excitement, overactivity, and distractibility. Our experience of trying to interview such patients in India has convinced us that it is impossible to carry out a complete examination of their mental state. They often fail to answer questions, seemingly preoccupied with their own mental experiences, or else break off in the middle of a reply when their attention is captured by something extraneous to the interview. Some patients are so physically active that they cannot remain still long enough to participate in an interview. This form of presentation is rarely seen in the West, although it has been observed among West Indian immigrants to the UK (Littlewood & Lipsedge, 1978; 1981*b*). It can be viewed as the manifestation of psychotic experiences in a non-verbal form. The same can be said of catatonia, and indeed Smartt (1964) observed a high proportion of patients with catatonic symptoms among a sample of acute transient psychoses. We have explored in Chapter 6 the possible reasons why both neurotic and psychotic conditions should take a somatic rather than a psychological form in developing countries. Whatever the explanation, patients who are inaccessible to questioning pose considerable diagnostic problems, since it is virtually impossible to establish the degree of their orientation or the nature of their psychotic experiences. Hence, distinctions cannot be made between functional and organic psychoses, and between the various types of functional psychosis. The obvious strategy is to reinterview the patient when the acute phase of the illness has passed and reasonable communication can be established. This is often possible after a few days, but may not illuminate the problem as patients are rarely able to reconstruct their mental state during the period of disturbance. A recent study in Swaziland has provided data that advance our understanding of these acute transient states. Guinness (unpublished) worked as a government psychiatrist in Swaziland, and collected 156 cases of brief reactive psychosis according to the DSM–III definition, namely, having a clear relation to stress and a duration of 2 weeks in the initial psychotic episode. The patients, most of whom were admitted to the only psychiatric hospital in the country, were seen over the course of 2 years, and were followed up prospectively. Guinness compared them with past admissions given a diagnosis of schizophrenia and divided them into those with an initial episode of less than 6 months, and those with episodes lasting more than 6 months, categorised by DSM–III as schizophreniform psychosis and schizophrenia respectively. Patients were excluded from the samples if there was a history of alcohol or cannabis abuse, or any obvious current organic factors.

Guinness describes brief reactive psychoses in much the same terms as other authors. She notes physical overactivity, publicly offensive behaviour such as stripping naked or smearing faeces, pressure of speech, and fleeting experiences of changeable visual and auditory hallucinations. She records that the patient is often inaccessible, but that consciousness has more of a trance-like quality than the typical fluctuating level of awareness of acute organic confusion. She is reluctant to classify any abnormal beliefs expressed as delusions, since "the strong cultural and magico-religious content is often understandable in terms of the situation precipitating the psychosis". Instead, she employs the phrase "overvalued cultural ideas". Duration of the psychosis was several days or less in half the patients.

Two aspects of her data are of particular interest to us; a phenomenological comparison of the three diagnostic samples, and a follow-up study. The former showed that characteristic schizophrenic symptoms, including delusions of influence and formal thought disorder, were relatively common among the schizophrenic patients, affecting between 30 and 60%, were less frequent in the schizophreniform patients, shown by between 20 and 30%, and were virtually absent among those with brief transient psychoses. This could be interpreted as indicating that brief transient psychoses have little in common with classical schizophrenia. However, the follow-up study, which Guinness cautions was incomplete and retrospective, revealed that the course of brief reactive psychosis was not always benign. Some patients showed a pattern of recurrent relapses, taking the same clinical form, in response to stress. A small number, 25 cases, representing 15% of the sample, relapsed with a picture more typical of schizophrenia, with catatonic and hebephrenic features, sustained and unequivocal delusions, and thought disorder. In view of the incomplete follow-up, this probably underestimates the proportion of brief reactive psychoses that go on to develop into clear-cut schizophrenia. There is a firm message, however, that this category is clinically heterogeneous.

Guinness considers that some patients' clinical states would be best described as dissociative, with some resembling mania, while a few patients presented with a very fleeting classical psychotic depression. Although the clinical assessments in this study were unstandardised and conducted through interpreters, this sample represents the largest body of clinical data concerning acute transient psychoses collected to date. Guinness was not able to employ laboratory investigations for the presence of toxic agents, infections, nutritional deficiencies, and cerebral dysfunction, so that a study of that nature remains to be done. Nevertheless, her follow-up indicates that a proportion of these puzzling conditions develop into schizophrenia, while others resolve rapidly without leaving a trace. The constituents of what is looking increasingly like a diagnostic ragbag, probably vary in proportion from country to country. Even if we eventually discover that the majority of these patients can be assigned to Western diagnostic categories on the basis of the psychiatric phenomena, the acute onset and rapid resolution demands an explanation.

We initially embarked on this inquiry to determine whether the better outcome of patients diagnosed as schizophrenic in developing countries might be due to the mistaken inclusion under this rubric of patients suffering from organic cerebral psychoses with an inherently good prognosis. The available evidence does not point towards any conclusion, so that we are obliged to leave this question open and pass on to a consideration of the third alternative explanation proposed at the end of the last chapter.

This concerns the effects of social factors on the course of schizophrenia and involves the possibility of a more favourable situation in non-Western than in Western countries. There are two main classes of factors that are likely to be influential: the attitude of the patient's family towards the illness, and the relative ease with which patients handicapped by symptoms can be reintegrated into society. The influence of family factors on the course of schizophrenia has been established by a series of studies carried out in London (Brown *et al*, 1962, 1972; Vaughn & Leff, 1976). These workers have shown that relapse rates are higher for patients who return home to live with relatives who are either very critical of them or else emotionally overinvolved, than for patients living with less emotional relatives. Furthermore, patients who live with the former type of relatives can protect themselves from relapse by reducing their exposure to their relatives. Family life in developing countries has a different quality from that in the West. Whereas the typical Western family is nuclear, with high social contact between the members and highly charged emotional relationships, the traditional family in a developing country is characteristically extended, with several generations sharing the same household. In such a family, with a large number of members, individuals are likely to spend less time with one particular person than in a nuclear family, and emotional relationships tend to be diluted. It is possible that the lower levels of emotion and of social contact in extended families are beneficial to patients suffering from schizophrenia.

The technique of measuring relatives' emotional attitudes towards patients, which generates an index termed expressed emotion (EE), has now been applied in a variety of cultural settings. A relative is assigned to the high-EE category if he or she makes six or more critical comments in the course of the interview, shows any degree of hostility, or scores 3 or more on a scale of emotional overinvolvement (Leff & Vaughn, 1985). The presence of one high-EE relative in a household is sufficient for the household to be categorised as high EE. The proportion of high-EE households in samples of schizophrenic patients from a number of cultures is shown in Table XVI.

There is evidently a gradient which follows the degree of industrialisation and Westernisation of the cultures concerned. At one extreme, only one-third of the anglophone Los Angeles families showed low-EE attitudes, while the Mexican-American families in the same city contained 60% low-EE households. At the other extreme, less than one-third of Chandigarh urban households were characterised as high EE, while these attitudes were virtually non-existent among the peasant farmers in the same area. We can only speculate about the cultural influences that operate to produce these striking differences in attitude towards schizophrenic patients. One factor may be the degree to which the patient is held responsible for his symptoms and behaviour. Leff & Vaughn (1985) investigated this by an analysis of the content of critical remarks made by London relatives. They found that only 30% of criticisms were directed at behaviour stemming from florid symptoms such as delusions and hallucinations. The remaining 70% concerned the negative symptoms of schizophrenia, such as apathy, inertia, and lack of emotion. The relatives considered the patient to be in control of these aspects of behaviour, did not appreciate that they are an integral part of the illness, and therefore blamed the patient for them. Relatives in the Mexican–American sample were much more tolerant for negative symptoms: one mother viewed her son's habit of sleeping until early afternoon as potentially beneficial. She believed that sleep was crucial to his recovery and that he should sleep whenever he was so inclined or able (Jenkins *et al*, 1986). It is quite possible that the relatives in Chandigarh viewed the cause of schizophrenia as being outside the patient, since, in developing countries, psychiatric illnesses are often conceptualised as being sent by malevolent forces (see p. 143). Furthermore, the notion of *karma*, or fate, is prevalent in India, and also absolves individuals of responsibility for their misfortunes. Further study of the way in which relatives' attitudes to psychiatric ill health are formed in a variety of cultures would be very informative. At present, we cannot favour one explanation over another, but we can enquire whether the greater tolerance of Chandigarh relatives has an effect on the outcome of schizophrenia.

An attempt to answer this question was made as part of the World Health Organization study of the incidence of schizophrenia reviewed above (see p. 113). The first step was to determine whether the technique of rating

TABLE XVI
Proportion of high-EE households in various cultural groups

Centre study	Los Angeles (Vaughn et al, 1984)	London (Vaughn & Leff, 1976)	Aarhus (Wig et al, 1987)	Los Angeles (Karno et al, 1987)	Chandigarh (Wig et al, 1987)	
					Urban	Rural
Ethnic group or or locality	Anglo-Americans	British	Danes	Mexican-Americans	Urban	Rural
Proportion of high-EE households	67%	52%	54%	41%	30%	8%

EE could be transferred satisfactorily from English to Hindi, the predominant language in Chandigarh. This was checked by using a bilingual rater who was trained in English and then required to rate audio-tapes of interviews in Hindi without any field experience (Wig *et al*, 1987). It was found that, of the crucial EE scales, criticism and hostility could be transferred across languages without distortion. However it became evident that the field workers were underrating overinvolvement, not because of a linguistic or cultural problem, but through drift away from the original rating conventions.

Of the 209 patients from the Chandigarh centre who constituted the sample for the WHO incidence study, 78 were included in the sub-study of relatives' EE. In the households of these patients, 104 relatives were interviewed and rated on the EE scales. The rural relatives were rated significantly lower than the urban relatives on critical comments, hostility, warmth and positive remarks (Wig *et al*, 1987). Emotional overinvolvement was detected in only four relatives, one of whom lived in the countryside. Thus, the rural relatives expressed less emotion than the urban relatives in the interview with respect to both positive and negative components of the scale. We have to consider the possibility that the rural relatives felt more inhibited from expressing themselves to a stranger than their urban counterparts, who were better educated and more Westernised. If this were the case, it would invalidate the ratings made of the rural relatives, and no relationship with the outcome of schizophrenia could be expected.

In fact the EE status of relatives was found to be significantly linked with the 1-year outcome of schizophrenia, regardless of the urban or rural domicile of the patients. Five of the 16 patients living in high-EE homes relapsed over 1 year, giving a rate of 31%, which was significantly higher than the rate of 9% in low-EE homes, in which five out of 56 patients relapsed (Leff *et al*, 1987). The overall 1-year relapse rate among these Chandigarh first-contact patients was only 14%, which is half the rate for a comparable sample of London first-admitted patients, 29% of whom relapsed. Furthermore the proportion of high-EE households in the Chandigarh sample, 23%, was also half that in the London sample, 47%. These findings provide evidence that the better outcome for patients in developing countries may be partly attributable to the greater tolerance their relatives show for the symptoms and disabilities produced by schizophrenia. They support Waxler's (1979) findings that families in Sri Lanka have considerable tolerance for the deviant behaviour that often accompanies schizophrenia. In her study, families were aware that they were putting up with problematic behaviour: 28% reported that others in the family had to do extra work because of the patient's illness, and 44% wished that the patient could contribute more to the household. The burden carried by families in developing countries who care for severely mentally ill people was assessed by Westermeyer (1984) in Laos. He found that the average subject in his study caused a considerable drain on the financial resources of the family, kin, and in some cases, neighbours and the community. The greatest cost by far was represented by the loss of the ill person's productivity.

In view of this financial burden, it is logical to suppose that an extended family, with a number of adult working members, would find it easier to support an incapacitated relative than a nuclear family. There is some suggestion from a study by El-Islam (1982) that this is the case. He investigated the patterns of care by extended and nuclear families for 540 schizophrenic out-patients in the Arab state of Qatar. The majority of patients, 388, lived in extended families. He found that relatives in extended families behaved differently towards the patients in a number of respects. They were more likely than relatives in nuclear families to tolerate minor behavioural abnormalities, allow the patients temporary withdrawal, help them to assimilate their symptoms into culturally shared belief systems, occupy their leisure time, and have no expectations of feedback from them. These attitudes are typical of low-EE relatives so that one would expect that schizophrenic patients living in extended families would have a more favourable course than those in nuclear families. Surprisingly, analysis of the data from the Chandigarh study failed to show this. However, an earlier study by El-Islam (1979), involving the follow-up of male schizophrenic patients for between 1 and 7 years, demonstrated that fewer patients living in extended families developed long-standing negative symptoms than those in nuclear families. The possible link between favourable outcome and the support of an extended family clearly requires further research.

One other social factor needs to be considered, namely the ease of rehabilitating handicapped patients. With industrialisation, jobs have become increasingly technical, requiring skilled workers to carry them out. Agriculture, too, has become mechanised and the availability of jobs for unskilled workers has diminished considerably. Furthermore, the chronically high level of unemployment in the West has sharpened competition in the labour market, so that any person with an obvious handicap, such as residual psychiatric symptoms, does not stand a chance. By contrast, in an agrarian economy untouched by industrialisation, a wide range of tasks exists, from which even the most handicapped person can be found a suitable occupation. For example, the job of sitting in a field and keeping cattle away from the crops can be adequately performed by all but the most disturbed patients. Furthermore, issues such as arriving on time and doing a full day's work do not arise in a rural setting. As a consequence of the much greater flexibility of occupational roles in an agrarian economy, the majority of schizophrenic patients can be re-employed after their acute illness has subsided, even if they do not become completely free of symptoms. The possible effect this has on their morale and their feeling of integration into society may have a beneficial influence on the course of their illness (Warner, 1985).

This area has not been studied extensively in developing countries, but some light has been thrown on it by the 2-year follow-up of the IPSS (World Health Organization, 1979). In addition to the individual criteria for outcome described in the previous chapter, a composite measure was used defined by: (a) the proportion of the follow-up period during which patients were in psychotic episodes; (b) presence or absence of social impairment on follow-up; and (c) occurrence or nonoccurrence of full remissions during the 2-year period. One of the five best sociodemographic predictors of outcome for schizophrenia defined in this composite way was unemployment, which was linked with a poor outcome. However, when predictors of outcome were identified within individual centres, this factor failed to emerge as important. Furthermore, unemployment did not predict outcome within either of the groups of developed or developing countries. In view of these findings, it seems unlikely that the better outcome of schizophrenic patients in developing countries can be explained by the greater ease of their maintaining an occupational role, although this may exert a beneficial effect by moderating relatives' attitudes.

We can say very little about the outcome of neurotic conditions in various cultures since so few studies have been conducted. By contrast, schizophrenia has been the focus of a considerable number of outcome studies around the world. The WHO international collaborative studies in particular have provided comparable data on samples of schizophrenia in developed and developing countries. These have clearly indicated a better prognosis in developing countries, which the recent incidence study has shown not to be due to a selective bias in referral. The greater tolerance of families in developing countries is one factor that has been identified as contributing to a better outcome. The predominance of acute transient psychoses may be another. Makanjuola & Adedapo (1987) recently compared Nigerian patients fulfilling DSM–III criteria for schizophrenia (at least 6 months' duration of illness) with those labelled schizophreniform, having a shorter duration. The latter group had experienced symptoms for a mean of 1.7 months before referral. The two groups of patients shared a similar pattern of symptoms, including the frequency of Schneider's first-rank symptoms. However the schizophreniform patients had a significantly better outcome than the others, for both clinical and social measures. As Makanjuola & Adedapo argue, this finding may indicate merely than an acute onset in schizophrenia predicts a good outcome, rather than providing a rationale for dividing the condition into distinct entities on the basis of the nature of onset. The question remains as to why a higher proportion of schizophrenic patients have acute-onset illnesses in developing countries than in the West. A striking illustration of this difference is provided by the WHO incidence study (Sartorius *et al*, 1986) in which 52% of patients from developing countries had an onset of psychotic symptoms lasting less than a week compared with only 29% in developed countries. The proportions with an insidious onset were precisely reversed: 29% and 52% respectively. This intriguing contrast demands further research, as does the relative ease of employing patients disabled by symptoms in the Third World. Both issues are of paramount importance for the management of schizophrenia throughout the world.

V. What is the effect of migration?

15 Norwegians in the USA and West Indians in the UK

It has been shown that information of great value and interest can be obtained by comparing the type and frequency of psychiatric conditions in different cultures. Unfortunately, the practical difficulties that stand in the way of such a venture are so daunting that only a handful of studies exist that have generated truly comparable data. At first sight, it might seem that immigrants provide the perfect solution to this problem. They bring with them to the host country many aspects of their cultures, and live in close physical proximity to their new neighbours. Many of the difficulties posed by cross-cultural comparisons are obviated by this situation of close proximity. However, immigration is not a straightforward matter of transplanting representatives of a particular culture from one location to another. As we shall see, it is not possible to assume that immigrants are indeed representative of their culture of origin. A little thought is sufficient to appreciate the selective nature of migration, and furthermore to realise that different migrations in time and place involve varied selective factors. Let us take as an example the Jews, whose migration from Egypt as recorded in Exodus is one of the earliest documented. If we take the Biblical account literally, then no selection was involved in this migration, since the Jews left Egypt *en masse*. After this, the next large-scale movement of the Jews was the exile to Babylon, which was followed by the Roman wars. In AD 70, following the destruction of the temple by the Romans, most of them were forced to leave their homeland and begin their wanderings, which took them to many parts of the world. However, a small minority remained in Israel and formed a community which endured until the present. We can only speculate about the personal characteristics of the few who opted to remain under the oppressive Roman rule compared with those who were dispersed.

In recent times, the world has witnessed a mass migration of Jews from Eastern Europe to Britain and America in the late 19th century. Why certain Jews chose to migrate in order to escape pogroms and conscription and what determined their choice of Britain rather than America are crucial, but unanswerable, questions. A new migration of Jews from Europe to Palestine gathered momentum in the early part of this century, and was accelerated not so much by persecution as by nationalistic and idealistic motives. These migrants must have differed in many important ways from the Jews who remained in Europe, believing themselves assimilated, most of whom perished in the Holocaust. But there were survivors who migrated to Israel, as it became, after the war and constitute yet another highly selected group.

It is evident that individual characteristics are an important determinant of the response to a large variety of pressures that might lead to migration, and that they are further involved in the choice of a host country. It is likely that such personal qualities are also related to the liability to develop psychiatric symptoms, but as we shall see, this link remains a speculative one. There exists an extensive literature on migration and psychiatric illness, and only a small selection of the experimental work is presented here. Two groups of migrants are dealt with in depth, the West Indians and the Asians in the UK, but before doing so we will present one of the earliest studies in this field, which is a model of methodological sophistication, rarely matched by later work.

Ödegaard (1932) chose to study his compatriot Norwegians who had emigrated to the USA. This migration was not fuelled by persecution, but by the promise of economic betterment. He compared psychiatric illness rates in migrant Norwegians with those in the American-born, but also included a comparison group of Norwegians in their home country. This is an important source of additional data as any difference in psychiatric illness rates between a migrant group and its hosts can be explained in three major ways. First, it may be due to the migratory experience itself; second, it may be a consequence of selective migration of people with particular personality characteristics; and third, it may reflect a genuine difference in constitutional susceptibility to psychiatric illnesses. This last possibility can be investigated only by the inclusion of a group of non-migrants in the migrants' home country. Other than a recent study of Portuguese migrants to Switzerland (Simões & Binder, 1980), this precaution has been omitted from studies in the area of migration, probably because of difficulties in spanning both the host country and the homeland.

At the time of Ödegaard's study, the population of Norway was 2.5 million, while the Norwegian-born in America numbered 400 000. He chose an area of dense Norwegian settlement in Minnesota, and studied all Norwegian-born first admissions to Rochester State Hospital during the 40 years from 1889 to 1928. The hospital had a defined catchment area, so that true epidemiological rates could be calculated. The control material from Norway was derived from the records of Gaustad Asylum, near Oslo, and covered the same 40 years. Ödegaard randomly selected about 50 first admissions from each year, half being men and half women. This resulted in a total of 1995 cases, which were compared with 1067 Norwegian-born in the American sample.

He points out that there are very few children among newly arrived immigrant groups, most of whom are adults between 20 and 35 years of age. As a consequence, only 5–6% of the foreign-born of Minnesota were below 20 years of age, compared with 45–50% of native Americans. Since psychiatric conditions rarely present before the age of 15, the foreign-born are at a disadvantage because of their skewed age distribution, resulting in a much greater proportion of the population being at risk. This issue was encountered in Chapter 8 and it was seen that the problem can be solved by introducing a correction for the age distribution of the population. Ödegaard employed this technique, and found that age correction reduced the incidence of psychiatric disorders for the Norwegian immigrants by between 50 and 60%. Even so, they still showed a 30–50% higher incidence of psychiatric morbidity than the native Americans.

When he compared the Norwegian immigrants with the sample of non-migrants from Gaustad Asylum, he found a higher incidence in the former for each decade of life. The Norwegian non-migrants had a lower incidence of psychiatric morbidity than the native Minnesotans, so that the Norwegian migrants differed more from their sedentary compatriots than from the American-born in Minnesota. By using this three-cornered comparison, Ödegaard was able to show conclusively that the high rate of psychiatric morbidity in Norwegian migrants was not due to an increased constitutional susceptibility in Norwegians. However, a choice of explanations still remained between the stress of moving to another country and selective migration of the illness prone. In an attempt to narrow down this choice, Ödegaard made a detailed study of the case records of his subjects. He found that the recording of information was generally very good both at Rochester State Hospital and Gaustad Asylum, and he was able to make a firm diagnosis in all but 11 of his 3073 cases.

Comparison of the age-corrected figures derived from his samples for individual diagnostic categories revealed that the most striking difference involved the incidence of schizophrenia. This condition accounted for nearly half of the first admissions of the Norwegian migrants, and was twice as common among them as in the sedentary Norwegians. On the other hand, mania was 50% more common in the non-migrants than in the migrants. From his detailed study of the case records, Ödegaard came to the conclusion that "a schizoid character or an incipient schizophrenia is frequently important as an underlying or contributive cause of emigration". He opted for selective migration as the most likely explanation for the high incidence of schizophrenia in Norwegian migrants to the USA, arguing that schizoid individuals, who are particularly prone to develop schizophrenia, were overrepresented among the migrants. In this respect, however, his study is methodologically weak. Case records written at the time a subject fell ill, which might be many years after migration, do not constitute a reliable estimate of personality characteristics at the time of migration. Furthermore, there are no comparable data on the migrants and non-migrants who did *not* fall ill. To provide a sound answer to this question the personality characteristics of migrants and non-migrants at, or just prior to, migration must be compared. As this has never been attempted, the hypothesis regarding selective migration remains speculative, albeit plausible.

Ödegaard also made some attempt to explore the alternative explanation concerning the stress of migration. He examined the length of time migrants had lived in America before their first admission for schizophrenia, and found that only 11% of patients presented within the first 2 years, while one-half presented after 10 years or more. Furthermore, there was no difference in the age of onset of schizophrenia between the migrants and their sedentary compatriots. This certainly does not argue for a causative effect of the migratory journey itself or the immediate period of adjustment to a foreign country. However, it does not exclude the stressful effects of living among strangers, which Ödegaard describes so graphically that he is worth quoting verbatim.

"Everywhere you are surrounded by people with strange and unfamiliar ways and customs, and you can hardly understand anything of what they say, at any rate when they talk to each other. They do not seem to be as friendly and helpful as the people at home, and many of them do their best to profit by your lack of experience. Even if you have not had any disagreeable experience yourself, your imagination is stirred by all the stories you have heard about how crooked and dangerous they may be. You notice that your own appearance, clothing and language points you out to everybody as a greenhorn, and a big Swede at that, and you are frequently met by a mixture of mirth and contempt. You have no friends, no one to associate with and no money for expensive entertainments – frequently you live under the strain of imminent unemployment. You are forced to live among the least attractive types of Americans, because it is cheap in those sections, and this frequently means a considerable lowering of your previous standard of life. There are hundreds of similar things which tend to make you suspicious and bewildered, anxious, and lonely. Sexual adjustment also is more difficult than at home, because of the lack of social connections, and owing to financial difficulties, and the scarcity of women in the immigrant population".

The methodological innovations of this classical study, a control group of non-migrants, age stratification, and an attempt at personality assessment, are not to be found together in any later study of migrants. However, a sufficiently large body of work has been built up on West Indian migrants to the UK to make an interesting, if incomplete, story. West Indians began to migrate in large numbers to the UK after World War II, partly in response to a recruiting campaign conducted in the West Indies by London Transport. The tide of immigration was stemmed by the Commonwealth Immigration Act of 1962, with the result that the influx of West Indians reached a peak in 1964, and dropped sharply after 1965 because very few work vouchers were issued to them. This deceleration is reflected in the rate of growth of the West Indian population of the UK. Census figures are available for

Camberwell, an inner-city area of London to which immigrants tend to gravitate. The proportion of the Camberwell population made up by West Indian immigrants was 2.5% in 1961, 4.7% in 1966, and 4.9% in 1971. These figures show that the West Indian population of Camberwell stabilised between 1966 and 1971. This will need to be kept in mind in evaluating the data from the various relevant studies.

The psychiatric morbidity of West Indian immigrants to the UK has been studied at the level of the psychiatric hospital, in general practice, and in the general population. The studies are presented here in that order, with the anticipation derived from material presented in Part II that the picture is likely to be different at each level. Hemsi (1967) studied hospital admissions from the London boroughs of Camberwell and Lambeth during the single year 1961. He chose this date because it was the year of a total census, in which information concerning country of birth was collected. We have come to expect from Ödegaard's study that the age distribution of an immigrant population will differ markedly from that of the host population. This was indeed the case with the West Indians, since Hemsi found that 91% of this group in the London boroughs he studied were between the ages of 15 and 54, which contrasts with only 53% of the native-born. To take this markedly skewed distribution into account and prevent it biasing his comparisons, Hemsi chose to confine his study to patients between the ages of 15 and 54. He screened the case records of all seven psychiatric hospitals serving the two boroughs for first admissions during the year 1961. The total annual incidence for psychiatric disorders was found to be 31.1 per 10 000 population aged 15 to 54 for West Indians compared with 10.9 for the native-born. Thus, even when the figures are standardised for age, the immigrants show nearly a threefold excess over the native Londoners.

A difference in global psychiatric morbidity may conceal considerable variations in diagnostic distribution. Hemsi made his own diagnoses from the material contained in the case records. He found that he could assign the great bulk of patients to one of three categories: schizophrenia; an affective disorder; or a personality disorder. For each of these, the West Indians showed a considerably higher incidence than the natives. Schizophrenia in West Indian men showed the greatest difference from the corresponding native rate, the figures being 13.1 and 2.7 per 10 000, respectively. Could such a great excess in West Indians be produced by diagnostic errors? The occurrence, in West Indian immigrants, of acute transient psychoses of the kind discussed in the preceding chapter (p. 169) has already been noted. These would not be expected to be due to infections or infestations in people living in London, but the abuse of drugs such as cannabis might play a part. Hemsi recognised a number of patients with "atypical psychoses" but felt able to assign them to one or other of the standard diagnostic categories.

He put forward the usual explanations for high rates of psychiatric disorder in immigrants and, following Ödegaard, investigated the possible role of the stress of migration by calculating the duration of time in the UK before the onset of symptoms. This was found to be more than 2 years in 47% of the patients, suggesting a negligible influence in at least half his sample. Hemsi drew attention to the lack of data on the incidence of psychiatric disorder in the West Indies, but quoted one source (Royes, 1961) as giving a mean annual incidence for psychoses, calculated over a 12-year period, of 3.8 per 10 000. If this figure can be relied on, it certainly does not suggest a particular constitutional susceptibility to psychosis in West Indians. One is left with selective migration and the stress of living for some years in a foreign country as equally likely explanations.

Another study of psychiatric hospital admissions was carried out by Cochrane (1977). Like Hemsi, he studied a period of 1 year, but a decade later, 1971. Instead of concentrating on a small geographical area, he examined admission statistics for the whole of England and Wales. This had the advantage of producing much larger, and hence epidemiologically more reliable, figures, but the disadvantage that he had to accept the diagnoses recorded in the Mental Health Enquiry. This involved filling in a standard card for each patient admitted to a psychiatric hospital or unit and returning it to the Department of Health and Social Security. The diagnosis was usually recorded by a clerk from information available in the case record and tended to be the diagnosis made close to admission rather than at discharge, with all the inaccuracies that entailed. The other disadvantage of Cochrane's study is that he used figures for prevalence rather than incidence. As seen in Part II, differences between groups in the prevalence of psychiatric disorders can result from variations in incidence or from a differential response to treatment. For example, if West Indian patients were less likely than the native-born to attend for follow-up examination and to receive maintenance treatment, they would have a higher relapse and readmission rate, which would increase the prevalence.

Like Hemsi, Cochrane found the age distribution of West Indian immigrants to be skewed. Whereas 38% of the native population of England and Wales was over 45 years of age, only 18% of the West Indians were. He made adjustments for these differences in age distribution when working out his total prevalence figures. He found the overall prevalence of psychiatric hospital admission to be much the same in West Indian and native men, 449 and 434 per 100 000, respectively. However, West Indian women showed a considerably higher prevalence at 621 per 100 000, than native women, at 551. When Cochrane looked at individual diagnoses, he did not standardise the figures for age and found that West Indian men had lower prevalence rates than native men except for schizophrenia, where they showed a greater than threefold excess, 290 as opposed to 87, per 100 000. A very similar picture prevailed for the West Indian women, with a prevalence of 323 per 100 000 for schizophrenia compared with the native women's rate of 87. Thus, despite important differences in method, Cochrane's findings agree closely with Hemsi's on schizophrenia, although this is not true of the other psychiatric diagnoses.

Cochrane & Bal (1987) returned to this area of research 10 years later, utilising the census of 1981 instead of that conducted in 1971. The second piece of work was an advance on the first, in that incidence rates were calculated in addition to prevalence. Furthermore, these workers standardised for age within each main diagnostic category. The first-admission rate for schizophrenia per 100 000 population aged 16 years and over was 33 for West Indian women compared with 12 for women born in England and Wales. The difference was even greater for West Indian men; 39 compared with 12. Once again a threefold, or greater, rate emerged. The consistency of these findings is such that they cannot be undermined by doubts about the assignment of place of birth, and the accuracy of ascertainment of first admission. Surprisingly, Cochrane & Bal considered diagnostic inaccuracy to be the most likely explanation for the very high incidence of schizophrenia in West Indian immigrants. The reasons why this is most improbable are discussed below.

Two other hospital-admission studies have confirmed the findings regarding schizophrenia among West Indians. Carpenter & Brockington (1980) analysed the figures for first admissions to the three main hospitals serving the Manchester area between the years 1973 and 1975. They used the hospital diagnosis and confined their sample to patients aged 15–64 years. The immigrant status of the patients was derived from the case-notes and was classified as African, West Indian, or Asian. Incidence rates were calculated by relating the number of cases to population figures derived from the 1971 census. Unfortunately from our point of view, Carpenter & Brockington amalgamated the Africans and West Indians, as there were relatively few of the former. They took the measure of stratifying their sample by age, and found that the overall first-admission rate for all immigrants was twice that of the British. Among West Indians (plus Africans) the rate for schizophrenia was 11.1 per 10 000 per annum, nearly six times the British native rate of 2.0. This was not due to the different age structure of the immigrant population. For no other diagnostic group did the West Indian immigrants have a higher first-admission rate than the native British. They compared the symptoms of the immigrant group as a whole with those of the natives and found higher levels in the immigrants of only one psychotic symptom, delusions of persecution.

Another study of first admissions to hospitals was carried out by Dean *et al* (1981) for the year 1976. Their method was more rigorous than that of Carpenter & Brockington, in that the collection of cases was prospective, and a special effort was made to ensure that place of birth and other data for each first admission were accurately recorded by hospital staff. Their effort was worthwhile, as birthplace was recorded in 91% of all first admissions during 1976. They collected data from psychiatric hospitals in south-east England and analysed them by age, sex, and place of birth. The first-admission rate for schizophrenia for West Indian men was found to be 5.5 per 10 000 per annum, five times the expected British rate of 1.1.

West Indian women also showed a fivefold increased rate of 5.3 compared with 1.0 for British women. Age stratification did not eliminate this difference. It is noteworthy that the West Indian women immigrants differed from the British in their first-admission rate for one additional psychotic diagnosis, 'other psychoses'. For this miscellaneous group, the rate was twice that of the British, a result which has some bearing on the findings of the following studies.

It has been suggested by Littlewood & Lipsedge (1981 *a,b*) that the high admission rates for schizophrenia of West Indians and West Africans is largely due to misdiagnosis by British psychiatrists, faced with the problem of classifying behaviour and ideas that are not encountered in their own culture. These authors, the first of whom is trained in anthropology as well as psychiatry, examined the case-notes of 250 patients aged between 15 and 45 who were admitted consecutively to a psychiatric unit serving the London Borough of Hackney, in which 18% of this age group were born in the New Commonwealth. They included in their sample patients who were given diagnoses of schizophrenia, affective psychosis, paranoid and other psychoses, and schizoid and paranoid personality. In addition they studied those defined as "not mentally ill" and "not yet diagnosed". They judged whether the patient's mental state had a "religious flavour" on admission and furthermore, they categorised each patient as "paranoid' or "non-paranoid". They derived place of birth from the admission sheets, but ascribed to individuals under 25 years of age the birthplace of their parents if they were the offspring of immigrants. The number of people in each ethnic group in the local population was derived from the 1971 census, and the rates determined were corrected for the age distribution of the populations.

The largest group of foreign-born patients was found to be the West Indian, comprising 37 individuals. Calculated from this figure, the first-admission rate for schizophrenia was 47 per 100 000 population aged 15–45. The comparable British rate was 19. Littlewood & Lipsedge found that West Indian patients were twice as likely to have had their diagnosis changed as the British, but this change was not in any particular direction. Change of diagnosis was more common for patients with religious interests and among Pentecostals. A religious colouring to the symptoms was noted in 40% of West Indian patients compared with only 14% of the British ($P < 0.001$), but this was largely independent of religious membership. This suggested to Littlewood & Lipsedge the possibility that if religious experiences are not contained within an institutional context, they might become uncontrollable and lead to frank mental illness. An alternative possibility is that the patients had unusual religious ideas before they became ill, which did not fit easily into any existing sect. These authors found that even when the religious schizophrenic patients were excluded, there were still more West Indians diagnosed. They concluded from this that there was a genuine increase in classical schizophrenia among West Indians, which was attributable to migration.

In their second study, Littlewood & Lipsedge (1981*b*) personally interviewed 36 patients, admitted to the same psychiatric unit, who had a religious flavour to their illness. The patients were examined with the PSE on admission when possible. However, some patients were so disturbed initially that only the behaviour section of the PSE could be rated at the time. If a full PSE was then administered satisfactorily within a week, the case was termed "PSE initially impossible". This form of presentation has been discussed above in connection with acute transient psychoses (see p. 169). Of the 36 patients, 20 were West Indian, four West African, eight British, and eight from Europe. Women comprised 70% of the West Indian and West African patients, but only one-third of the other groups. Twenty-two patients were given a diagnosis of schizophrenia, of whom 12 had at least one first-rank symptom. The absence of first-rank symptoms in West Indian and West African patients was associated with an "initially impossible" PSE, a precipitating event, a religious background, a change of diagnosis in the past, and a religious experience more than 5 years before the first diagnosis. In 12 of the West Indian patients, the PSE was initially unrateable, and none of these had any first-rank symptoms when rated within a week of admission. On the initial behaviour ratings of the PSE, they all scored on gross excitement and violence, agitation, hostile irritability, and suspicion. Labile affect was rated in nine of the twelve. Orientation was good, and no patient demonstrated clouding of consciousness. Littlewood & Lipsedge observed that when the acute florid stage of these illnesses subsided, depressive features were revealed. They concluded that "It would be unwise to classify the reactions as depressive, but it might be fruitful to consider them in some way as equivalents or alternatives to depression, particularly in view of the fact that over time they become less frequent and tend to be 'replaced' by more typical reactive depression".

This interpretation ignores the well-established fact that depressive symptoms are common in classical schizophrenia, occurring in about half the patients and usually following the same course as the psychotic symptoms (Leff *et al*, 1988). It is likely that the depressive symptoms noted by Littlewood & Lipsedge in their patients were also present on admission, but could not be elicited at that time because of the difficulty in conducting a full examination of the mental state.

These authors have described a condition in West Indian and West African immigrants that is identical to the acute transient psychoses seen commonly in developing countries. Their careful observations of the mental state of these immigrant patients make an organic cause unlikely, since they were well-orientated and in clear consciousness. Littlewood & Lipsedge are left grappling with the same problem of classification that we discussed in Chapter 14, and have been unable to resolve it. It is of interest that their West Indian patients were predominantly women, in view of the above-average rate of "other psychoses" among first-admitted West Indian women in the study by Dean *et al* (1981), who were probably picking up the same clinical phenomenon.

Another clinical study that has highlighted this group was conducted by Richardson & Henryk-Gutt (1982). They examined all patients admitted to Shenley Hospital during a 12-month period, who were resident in the London Borough of Brent but born in the West Indies, the Indian sub-continent, or to Indian parents in East Africa. A PSE was administered within 48 h of admission, with the help of an interpreter for some of the Asian patients. The authors compared the ward doctor's diagnosis with the Catego classification based on the PSE data. Agreement between these two methods was 80% for the 21 Asian patients, 70% for the 20 West Indian men, but only 25% for the 36 West Indian women. The largest single discrepancy in this group related to seven women given a ward diagnosis of affective disorder, but a Catego class equivalent to paranoid schizophrenia. This appeared to be generated by abnormal motor and verbal activity exhibited by these women. Of the group of 36, as many as 31 women displayed over- or under-activity in motor and/or verbal behaviour. The level of activity often fluctuated from one extreme to the other, and was interpreted by ward doctors as a disturbance of mood. This raised uncertainty as to whether delusions and hallucinations present might have an affective basis, and in combination with a caution about cultural issues, led doctors to diagnose an affective condition.

These two studies of the diagnostic process in West Indian immigrants reach different conclusions. Littlewood & Lipsedge emphasise the emotional turmoil and transient course of the disturbances and suggest that they belong with affective illnesses rather than schizophrenia. Richardson & Henryk-Gutt consider that ward doctors are already classifying these conditions as affective illnesses, and avoiding the diagnosis of schizophrenia even when the symptoms point clearly to it. Either tendency fails to solve the epidemiological puzzle. If the very high incidence of schizophrenia in West Indian immigrants is due to misclassification of affective illness, then reclassification will produce a high rate of affective disorders, since as we shall see, the incidence of mania in West Indians is already several times that in British natives. If ward doctors are leaning over backwards not to diagnose schizophrenia, then the incidence of schizophrenia in West Indians is even higher than it appears. The only way in which reclassification could eliminate an excess rate is if two out of every three West Indians admitted to hospital are actually psychiatrically normal or neurotically ill, but are wrongly considered to be suffering from some psychotic condition. Only four of Littlewood & Lipsedge's 20 West Indian patients had first-rank symptoms, which would automatically place them in Catego class S + (see p. 36). However 13 of the other 16 were given Catego classes, which were as follows: S + , 5; M + , 4; P + and P?, 3; O + 1. No patient was assigned to a neurotic or normal class, so that on this evidence the above explanation is not tenable.

In Chapter 6, it was concluded that the predilection shown by patients in developing countries for a bodily expression of their distress could also influence the form in which schizophrenia presented. It seems possible that the abnormalities in bodily activity that dominate the clinical picture in these psychotic West Indian women may be another manifestation of the same phenomenon. Evidence supporting this hypothesis derives from studies of involuntary admission of psychiatric patients in the UK.

It has been known for some years that West Indian patients are over-represented among compulsory admissions. For instance, Rwegellera (1980) showed that the police or Mental Welfare Officers were much more frequently involved in the admission of West Indian patients than of British patients. He also found a strong association between disturbed behaviour and involuntary admission among West Indian patients ($P < 0.0001$), which did not apply to British patients. These findings were amplified by Ineichen *et al* (1984) and Harrison *et al* (1984), who examined in-patient psychiatric admissions from the city of Bristol during 1978–1981. Whereas 28% of white British in-patients were admitted involuntarily, the figure for West Indians was 63%. A detailed study of patients admitted compulsorily corroborated Rwegellera's finding that the police were much more often involved in the admission of West Indian patients than of white suburban patients. However, this was not because the West Indians were the stereotyped threatening, aggressive young men. The West Indian patients admitted compulsorily were predominantly women who had drawn attention to themselves by acting strangely in public; taking off their clothes, conducting traffic, and behaving in other conspicuously inappropriate ways. We propose that the tendency to express psychotic experiences in bodily forms of behaviour accounts both for the increased involvement of the police in admission of West Indian patients and for the difficulty psychiatrists have in making a diagnosis. We cannot explain why West Indian women should choose this form of expression more than men, but this female preponderance is reflected in first-admission rates for "other psychoses". Furthermore, if the findings of Richardson & Henryk-Gutt (1982) can be generalised, these abnormalities of physical activity lead psychiatrists to misdiagnose schizophrenic conditions in West Indian women as affective disorders. Hence, the occurrence of acute transient psychoses in West Indian immigrants and the consequent diagnostic problems do not account for their increased levels, ranging from three- to sixfold, of hospital admissions for schizophrenia.

This conclusion is supported by an important study conducted in Nottingham by Harrison *et al* (1988). As noted above (p. 113) Nottingham was the British centre in the WHO study of the incidence of schizophrenia (Sartorius *et al*, 1986). Harrison *et al* applied the rigorous research techniques of the WHO project to a study of the incidence of psychotic disorders in Afro-Caribbean patients. Their work was novel because a high proportion of second-generation immigrants was included in their sample, due to their collecting data in 1984–1986. A wide net was cast for screening and detecting potential patients of "likely Afro-Caribbean ethnic origin". The existence of the Nottingham Case Register was an additional security against missed cases. Assessment was by the WHO schedules, including the PSE. A variety of approaches to diagnosis was adopted, which included the Catego program (Wing *et al*, 1974), the application of DSM–III criteria, and a consensus by the research team.

The most problematic issue was the estimation of the size of the Afro-Caribbean population in Nottingham. Individuals born in the Caribbean can be enumerated from the 1981 census, but not those of Afro-Caribbean ethnic origin who were born in the UK. However, it is possible to make a reasonable estimate of the latter from the age structure of residents in households headed by a person born in the Caribbean. The age band 16–29 must contain a high proportion of second-generation Afro-Caribbeans, as well as a number of immigrants who came to the UK as small children. There is inevitably a degree of inaccuracy involved in using these figures, but they are the best currently available.

Over the 2 years of the study, 45 patients met the screening criteria, and a full PSE could be completed in 39 of these. Evidently the problems experienced by Littlewood & Lipsedge (1981*b*) in assessing the mental state of their patients were much less prominent in the Nottingham sample. Furthermore, when Harrison *et al* compared their Afro-Caribbean patients given a definite diagnosis of schizophrenia with the same diagnostic grouping from the WHO sample in Nottingham, they found an almost identical proportion with an onset of symptoms within a week (14 and 16% respectively). This was after the exclusion of six patients with unspecified psychoses and drug-induced states (Rottanburg *et al*, 1982). The clinical differences between this sample and the Hackney patients studied by Littlewood & Lipsedge are explained by Harrison *et al* on the basis that the former workers concentrated on acute transient conditions that gave rise to diagnostic problems, whereas the Nottingham study was epidemiologically based. They also entertain the possibility that such conditions may be presented less commonly by second-generation Afro-Caribbeans.

When Harrison *et al* restricted themselves to patients who were considered as "certain" or "very likely" cases of schizophrenia, the incidence rates per 10 000 population were 29.1 for the age group 16–29, and 19.7 for the age group 30–44. The corresponding rates for non-Afro-Caribbean Nottingham residents were 2.0 and 1.6. Application of DSM–III criteria reduced the rates considerably for both populations, but made little or no impact on the proportionate differences between them. Afro-Caribbean patients born in the UK had *higher* rates than those born in the Caribbean.

One further finding is worth emphasising. As in previous studies, the Afro-Caribbean patients with definite schizophrenia included a much higher proportion with both overactivity and underactivity than did their British counterparts. We have proposed above a cultural explanation for this difference in motor behaviour.

The findings from the various studies of rates of schizophrenia in West Indian immigrants are displayed in Table XVII for ease of comparison. It is noteworthy that the ratio of West-Indian to UK-native rate ranges from

TABLE XVII

West Indian immigrants and UK natives incidence rates per 10 000 for schizophrenia

Study	Location	Diagnosis	Age standardisation	UK natives	West Indians	Ratio
Hemsi (1967)	Camberwell and Lambeth	Own from case-notes	+	2.7	13.1	4.9
Cochrane (1977)	England and Wales	Mental Health Enquiry	0	M, 8.7[1] F, 8.7[1]	29.0 32.3	3.3 3.7
Cochrane & Bal (1987)	England and Wales	Mental Health Enquiry	+	M, 1.2 F, 1.2	3.9 3.3	3.3 2.8
Carpenter & Brockington (1980)	Manchester	Hospital	+	2.0[2]	11.1	5.6
Dean *et al* (1981)	SE England	Own from assessment	+	M, 1.1 F, 1.0	5.5 5.3	5.0 5.3
Littlewood & Lipsedge (1981)	Hackney	Own from case-notes	+	1.9	4.5	2.4
Harrison *et al* (1988)	Nottingham	Own from assessment	+	Age 16–29 2.0 30–44 1.6	29.1 19.7	14.6 12.3

[1] Prevalence rates.
[2] West Indians and West Africans.

2.4 up to 14.6. The remarkably high rate of schizophrenia found by Harrison *et al* in second-generation Afro-Caribbeans is most unlikely to be explained by diagnostic procedures in view of the stringency of their psychiatric examination and diagnostic techniques. The problem of enumerating the Afro-Caribbean population in Nottingham might introduce an error factor as great as two. Even if the rate they found was halved, however, it would still exceed the native rate by more than seven times. The fact that these patients were born in the UK absolutely rules out the experience of migration as a stress factor. If selective migration were to be invoked as an explanation, one would have to argue that the personality factors responsible were transmitted to the next generation. My view is that the disadvantages afflicting the West Indian population in the UK constitute the most plausible explanation for the Nottingham finding. However, why then do Asians in the UK not also show such extraordinarily inflated rates? As the possibility of an ethnic liability to schizophrenia has not been effectively ruled out by Royes' (1961) incidence study in the West Indies, it would be particularly informative to mount a careful study of the incidence of psychoses in an island such as Trinidad, which is inhabited by a mixture of peoples of African and Asian origin. Until such a project has been completed, the question must remain open.

The last hospital-based study to be discussed focused on one non-schizophrenic illness, mania. In a cross-national epidemiological study that was stimulated by the findings of the IPSS (p. 33 ff.) (World Health Organization, 1973), Leff *et al* (1976) determined the incidence of mania in London and Aarhus, Denmark. A major part of the study was a retrospective collection of first-admitted patients, satisfying research criteria for mania, from case registers. In London, the Camberwell Register was used, and a period of 9 years was covered, from 1965 to 1973. It was noted that a high proportion of the London sample of cases came from overseas. In fact only 21 (55%) of the 38 were born in the UK, the largest single group of immigrants originating in the Caribbean. Five of the six West Indian patients were men, which gives some basis for calculating an incidence rate, although the number is still uncomfortably small.

It was seen above that the West Indian population of Camberwell had virtually stabilised by 1966, so that the 9-year period covered by this study is one of slow growth. Therefore, there can be little error involved in taking the 1971 census figure as representative of the whole period. With regard to the age distribution, it was found that all five West Indian male patients were between the ages of 25 and 49. This was reflected in the make-up of the male West Indian population of Camberwell, in which the 25- to 49-year-old group formed 62% of the total age distribution. This contrasted markedly with the equivalent figure for England and Wales of 32%. However, this was still not a fair comparison, for an interesting reason. Camberwell, like other inner-London areas, had been subject to progressive depopulation over a number of years. The very factor that attracts immigrants, the availability of low-rent accommodation, was an integral part of a constellation of poor social conditions that drove out the more enterprising natives. As the quality of life in Western cities deteriorates, there is a selective migration of the most able-bodied citizens. These tend to be men at the peak of their earning capacity, who in terms of their age structure, are equivalent to the incoming migrants from overseas. Thus, the native emigrants leave a gap in the age distribution of inner-city populations which is filled by the foreign immigrants. As a consequence, the age distribution of the native inner-city dwellers is also skewed, but in the opposite direction to that of the immigrants. In Camberwell, for example, 25–49-year-old men form only 26% of the native population compared with the national figure of 32%. A comparison of rates of psychiatric disorder calculated on the basis of the total population of males would result in a spurious increase of more than twofold for the West Indians. This is an even greater bias than Ödegaard (1932) found in comparing Norwegian immigrants with native Minnesotans. When age-specific rates were calculated for the Camberwell population, the incidence of mania for native-born males between the ages of 25 and 49 was found to be 3.7 per 100 000. The corresponding rate for West Indian males was 23.9 per 100 000, an increase of more than sixfold.

Leff *et al* (1976) investigated the possibility that this difference might be a consequence of a diagnostic bias on the part of native-born psychiatrists, who might be more likely to diagnose mania than schizophrenia in psychotic immigrants. The ratio of the diagnoses of schizophrenia and mania among UK-born and non-UK-born first admissions from Camberwell was derived from the Register over the same period as the study. The ratio of schizophrenia to mania was found to be 4.7:1 for the UK-born and 4.6:1 for the non-UK-born. Hence, there is no evidence of a diagnostic bias of the kind postulated. The fact that these ratios are virtually identical indicates that West Indians must show a similar excess over the native-born for schizophrenia as they do for mania, thus corroborating the findings presented above.

A further possible explanation of these findings could be that there is a lower threshold for admitting immigrants with a manic illness than for natives. A greater intolerance for disturbed behaviour in immigrants would result in an apparently higher admission rate, but should also be reflected in milder forms of illness among admitted immigrants compared with native hospital in-patients. In fact, when the symptomatic pictures of non-UK patients in the London sample were compared with the natives, the former were found to be more severely ill. Significantly more of the immigrants showed delusions of special abilities, of grandiose identity, and of a special mission than the natives. A delusion of one kind or another was held by 16 of the 17 immigrants compared with 12 of the 21 natives ($P < 0.02$). Hence, the higher incidence of mania in immigrants cannot be ascribed to a greater ease of admission.

The immigrant group as a whole showed considerable variation in the duration of stay in the UK before the first admission to hospital with mania.

The shortest interval was represented by a Nigerian immigrant who was admitted within a few days of his arrival in London. His relatives reported that he arrived without warning and brought no luggage with him, so it is likely that his flight to London was part of the manic episode. The longest duration of stay was shown by a French immigrant of 22 years' standing, and the second longest by a West Indian male who had emigrated 17 years earlier. Length of residence before the onset of symptoms was over 2 years in 65% of the immigrant sample.

A study by Bebbington *et al* (1981) of immigrant patients included in the Camberwell Register confirms these findings. The Camberwell Register records out-patient and in-patient contacts with the psychiatric services by people resident in Camberwell (see p. 61). The age-corrected incidence rates for a variety of diagnostic groups were calculated. The rate for mania was found to be three times the native rate in West Indian men and nearly five times in West Indian women.

These hospital-based studies indicate that West Indian immigrants to the UK show a significant excess in the incidence of schizophrenia and mania and in the prevalence of schizophrenia compared with the native-born. These differences cannot be ascribed to the immediate stress of the process of emigration, but may be due to living for some time among foreigners or to selective migration of the illness-prone. For the latter to be acceptable as an explanation, it must be postulated that both people prone to schizophrenia, and those liable to mania, are more likely to emigrate than West Indians without these propensities.

The focus can now be shifted from hospital to general practice, two relevant studies of which have been conducted. We should expect to find the clinical material in general practice dominated by neurotic conditions, since not only are they many times more common in the populace than psychoses, but GPs refer only a tiny proportion of neurotic patients to psychiatric hospitals. Pinsent (1963) studied a general practice in the north of Birmingham, an area of West Indian immigration since 1952. He found 127 West Indians, 66 men and 61 women, on the GP's list and matched them on age and sex with a sample of the native-born Birmingham population. He determined the rates of consulting the GP for a variety of conditions, and compared them between the two matched groups. He did not apply tests of statistical significance, but found that slightly more English men consulted for psychiatric conditions than did West Indian men. For women, the ratio was dramatically reversed, with more than twice as many psychiatric consultations by West Indian than by English women. The absence of a definition of a psychiatric consultation and the method of handling the data prevent much weight being given to these findings.

A more rigorously conducted study is that by Kiev (1965) of a group general practice in Brixton. This borough contained 18% of all West Indians living in London. Kiev drew a one-in-six sample of people registered with the practice over a 6-month period from January to July 1962. He excluded children born after 1950, and immigrants other than West Indians. The categories he used were: psychosis; dementia; mental deficiency; neurosis; personality disorder; and psychological factors contributing to or complicating physical illness or symptoms. This is a methodological advance on Pinsent's study, although Kiev's last category must have involved some difficult judgements, which were the responsibility of the doctors in the group practice. The presence of any one of these disorders was taken to be evidence of conspicuous psychiatric morbidity (CPM). To determine the validity of the data, 50 West Indian patients were randomly selected from the 476 in the sample population and were interviewed by the author at home using a semi-structured schedule, which took 1–3 h to administer. An additional 50 West Indian patients were interviewed for briefer periods in the GPs' surgery. The author does not report on the results of these personally conducted interviews, so that the validity of the GPs' judgements cannot be assessed.

Kiev found the 6-month prevalence rate for CPM to be 17.4% in West Indian clients of the practice compared with 12.6% in the Brixton natives. The prevalence was significantly higher in West Indian men than in native-born men, but the difference failed to reach significance among the women. This finding is opposed to that of Pinsent, but can be given greater weight because of the more stringent assessments carried out. However, one must have reservations about Kiev's wide category of psychological symptoms complicating physical disorders, particularly in view of his observation that English patients frequently expressed complaints in psychological terms, whereas West Indian complaints were often vague statements such as "I ache all over". In Part I, an extended argument was presented concerning the expression of emotional distress in somatic rather than psychological terms by people in developing cultures. West Indian immigrants fall into this group, and considerable difficulty would be expected in distinguishing physical from minor psychiatric illness in the context of a general practice. This may account for the contradiction in the findings from these two studies, particularly in view of Kiev's inclusion of mixtures of psychological and physical symptoms. In any event, the dramatic differences in incidence rates between West Indians and natives evident in hospital statistics are not echoed in these prevalence studies of general practice.

Finally, the only general population study in the UK that has included a substantial number of West Indians should be considered. This is the epidemiological survey of psychiatric morbidity in Camberwell by Bebbington *et al* (1981*b*) referred to in Chapter 9 (p. 106). These workers conducted a survey of a random sample of 800 subjects aged 18–64 living in Camberwell. All subjects were given a screening interview with a 40-item version of the PSE by trained lay interviewers. All subjects identified by this means as psychiatrically ill and a random sample of those not were interviewed 4 weeks later by research workers using the full PSE. Cases of psychiatric disorder were defined as those of level five and above on the Index of Definition

(Wing *et al*, 1978). Of the initial 800 interviewees, 611 were British-born and 69 were West Indians. Of the 310 subjects successfully reinterviewed by the research workers, 31 were West Indians and 233 British-born (Bebbington *et al*, 1981*a*).

From the lay interviewers' ratings, 8.8% of the British-born males were identified as psychiatrically ill compared with 3.2% of West Indian men. The prevalence rates among women were almost identical, being 18.1% for British-born and 18.4% for West Indians. One would expect the research workers to be rather more stringent in their ascertainment of pathology, and indeed the prevalence rates derived from their interviews were somewhat lower. However, the pattern remained the same, with 6.2% among British males as compared with none among West Indians, and 14.7% and 10.9%, respectively, among British and West Indian women. None of these differences reached statistical significance.

Hence, this carefully conducted population study did not show up any above-average psychiatric morbidity in West Indians living in the community. This provides backing for the two general-practice studies, which, while showing some increase in neurotic illness among West Indians, failed to reflect the dramatic excesses in rates of psychosis apparent from hospital statistics. The evidence suggests that whatever stresses are implicit in settling in a foreign land, or whatever selection factors operate in migration, they are not responsible for a general increase in psychiatric morbidity. Rather, specific links must exist between the aetiological factors involved and the psychotic conditions of schizophrenia and mania. There is growing evidence for the aetiological effect of environmental stress on schizophrenia, although equivalent work on mania is sparse. One must wait for firm conclusions to develop from this area of study and for pioneering work on the selection factors in migration. Only then can it be decided whether the marked susceptibility of West Indian migrants to schizophrenia and mania is a specific feature of migration, or one example of a more general principle in the aetiology of the psychoses.

16 Asians in the UK

Like the West Indian immigrants, the bulk of the Asians in the UK travelled there to find a better life for themselves and their families. However, one group of Asians arrived *en masse* after their expulsion from Uganda by Idi Amin. There are other important differences between these two groups of immigrants, both in language and culture. West Indians speak English, albeit a distinctive dialect, whereas for Asians, English is a second or even a third language. The culture in the West Indies is oriented towards Britain, which many consider as the mother country, although judging from the novels of V. S. Naipaul, the West Indian image of Britain is that of its heyday in the Edwardian era, rather than today's austere reality. British culture has also had an impact on India and Pakistan, but not to the same pervasive extent as it has in the West Indies. It has been claimed that India has absorbed each of its conquerors in turn without its basic culture being affected. There would seem to be a considerable amount of truth in this assertion. Furthermore, family structure and relationships in Asian immigrants differ fundamentally from those in West Indian immigrants, which have been deeply affected by generations of slavery.

As with the West Indians, studies carried out on hospital statistics will first be considered. Cochrane's (1977) analysis of psychiatric admissions throughout England and Wales during the year 1971, which was summarised above, is drawn on again. The total prevalence of psychiatric-hospital admissions was determined separately for Indians and Pakistanis and both figures, 403 and 336, respectively, per 100 000 population over 15 years, were found to be considerably lower than the rate for British natives, which was 494. This is in marked contrast to the total prevalence rate for West Indians, which was higher than the native rate. However, when the total rate was broken down into rates for individual diagnoses, which were not standardised for age, the prevalence for admission for schizophrenia was higher for both men and women from India and Pakistan than for British natives, although the excess among the immigrant Asians was not as marked as in the West Indians. In fact, the Asian prevalence rates for schizophrenia

197

are half or less of the West Indian rates, and almost entirely account for the difference in total prevalence rates between the groups. Unfortunately, Cochrane chose to concentrate on the total rates, emphasising "low rates of mental illness among Asians" and contrasting them with "intermediate rates" among the West Indians. This is a misleading approach, and the issue of real relevance is to determine why the Asians do not show such high levels compared with the British-born in the prevalence of schizophrenia as do the West Indians.

Cochrane's findings on schizophrenia in Asian immigrants were confirmed by Pinto (1970) in another study based on the Camberwell Register. In his thesis, Pinto gave some basic information about Asian immigrants which is of considerable interest. He quotes figures from the 1966 Census of England and Wales to show that West Indians numbered 450 000, while Indians and Pakistanis amounted to 360 000 and constituted the second largest immigrant group from the New Commonwealth. He divides Asian immigrants into three main groups: Punjabis, the majority of whom are Sikhs; Pakistanis, who are strict Muslims; and Gujeratis, who are mostly Hindus, and who represent the most Westernised and literate of the three.

Pinto studied all Asian-born patients over the age of 15 who were recorded in the Camberwell Register from 1965 to 1969 inclusive. Patients were included in the Register if they lived in Camberwell and made contact with the in-patient or out-patient psychiatric services or a psychiatric social worker. Thus, although Pinto calculated prevalence rates, as did Cochrane, he covered a much broader spectrum of contact with the services. He identified a total of 49 Asian immigrant patients over the 5-year period, of whom six were Caucasians who happened to be born in Asia. He attempted to trace all 49 in the sample and found that 30 were still living in Camberwell and another three in other parts of London. He interviewed these 33 patients personally, using a mixture of Hindi and Urdu.

He calculated the prevalence rates for the year 1966 based on the census data for Camberwell. He points out that in the census, children born in the UK to natives of another country are counted as British and are not identified by their ethnic origin. Nevertheless, in making comparisons between the immigrants and the English-born, he made no attempt to standardise the figures for age. Thus, his rates for the Asian immigrants are biased by the paucity both of the young and the elderly in this population group and should probably be reduced by something like 50% to give more accurate estimates of prevalence. The total prevalence rates were found to be 238 per 10 000 for Asian men and 108 per 10 000 for English men. Even if the Asian rate were halved to adjust for the difference in age distribution, it would still be above the English rate. For women, the prevalence rates were 174 and 176 per 10 000 for Asians and English, respectively. In the case of women, halving the Asian rate would result in a considerably lower figure than in the English.

Pinto went on to look at the rates for individual diagnoses. Here the small scale of his study gave him an advantage over Cochrane, as he was able to check the majority of the diagnoses recorded on the Register by personal interviews with the patients. As he came from the same cultural background as the patients, his diagnoses are likely to be more accurate than those of the hospital psychiatrists faced with patients from an alien culture who often spoke poor English. Of the 33 patients, usually interviewed in their mother tongue, Pinto decided on a major change in diagnosis in five, four of which involved schizophrenia. He changed one case from depression to schizophrenia, and three cases from schizophrenia to other diagnoses. Thus, the net alteration to the category of schizophrenia was an overall loss of two cases out of ten, representing a reduction of 20% in the prevalence rate for this condition. Before making this adjustment, the rate for schizophrenia was calculated as 55 per 10 000 for Asians, compared with 13 per 10 000 for natives of Camberwell. Even when we halve the Asian figure and reduce it by a further 20% for misdiagnoses, it remains substantially above the native rate. Pinto found the rates for affective illness to be 82 and 46 per 10 000 for Asians and natives, respectively, and for neuroses to be 26 and 9 per 10 000. In the case of these diagnostic categories, halving the Asian rates would bring them close to the native rates. Thus, when we make a rough adjustment to Pinto's rates to account for the bias due to differing age distributions, the results fail to confirm Cochrane's figures showing unusually low prevalence rates compared with the English-born for diagnoses other than schizophrenia. This may in part be due to the wider definition of prevalence in Pinto's study, which included out-patient treatment and contact with a psychiatric social worker in addition to in-patient admission.

In an attempt to determine factors leading to contact with the psychiatric services, Pinto compared the 49 Asian immigrant patients derived from the Camberwell Register with 49 Asians selected from GPs' lists in the Camberwell area who had had no psychiatric contacts. The comparison group was paired with patients with regard to country of origin, 5-year age group, sex, and duration of stay in the UK. All members of the control group were visited and interviewed by the author in the relevant Asian languages. He found no significant difference between the Asian patients and the matched control subjects in terms of marital status, housing conditions, or social class. However, significantly more of the patients had a family history of psychiatric illness than the control subjects, a feature that evidently transcends culture, and a greater proportion of the patients (70%) showed marked or moderate social isolation than the control subjects (43%). This last feature could be interpreted equally well as a cause or a consequence of psychiatric illness. Hence, this comparison failed to identify beyond doubt any social factor in the migrants' environment that accounted for their development of psychiatric illnesses. Nevertheless, the role of social isolation merits further study, particularly as Pinto found that it was associated with a poorer outcome of the psychiatric condition.

These two hospital-based studies by Cochrane and Pinto present considerable difficulties in interpretation owing to the use of prevalence rather than incidence rates, a failure to standardise most figures for age, and the likelihood of quite a high proportion of misdiagnoses. Pinto's findings indicate that Asian immigrants in Camberwell use the psychiatric services as frequently as English natives, whereas Cochrane's analysis of national figures reveals an underutilisation by Asians. Even if Cochrane's data were shown to provide a more accurate picture, it would not necessarily follow that Asian immigrants suffered less from psychiatric illness than the British-born. Underutilisation of psychiatric services could also result from a number of other factors including reluctance to bring sufferers to the attention of doctors because of the stigma, the attitudes of GPs to Asian immigrants, the existence of traditional treatment facilities within the Asian community, and the presentation of psychological distress in the form of somatic complaints. Some of these possibilities could be explored by studying general practices, others by community surveys.

Two further studies of hospital admission statistics, which were reviewed in the previous chapter, give first-admission data for Asian patients and thus clarify some of the issues raised by Cochrane's and Pinto's findings. Carpenter & Brockington (1980) analysed first-admission rates for immigrants living in Manchester. They treated all immigrants from the Indian sub-continent as a homogeneous group, and found that their rate for schizophrenia was six times that of the native British, a rate comparable to that of the West Indians. Unlike the West Indians, though, the Asians showed a significantly higher first-admission rate than the British for a number of other diagnoses, namely personality and sexual disorders, depressive neurosis, and other neuroses. When stratified by age, the total first-admission rate for Asians was significantly greater than that for British in the bands 25–34 and 35–44. These results are closer to Pinto's than Cochrane's.

Dean *et al* (1981) have produced a more fine-grain analysis, in that they treated Indians and Pakistanis as separate categories, and also gave sex-specific rates. Their study of first-admission rates to hospitals in south-east England revealed that whereas Indians, both men and women, had three times the expected rate for schizophrenia, Pakistani immigrants had a rate that did not differ from the native-born. Furthermore, while the Indians did not show an excess or deficit in any other single diagnostic category, the Pakistanis had significantly *lower* rates than the native British for a number of diagnoses. These included alcoholism, neuroses, and personality disorders for men, and neuroses for women. These intriguing differences between Indian and Pakistani immigrants need to be followed up in detail, but they indicate the importance of treating these groups separately in any epidemiological analysis.

There is one recent study of morbidity in Asian immigrants in the context of general practice, which bridges the gap between the psychiatric hospital studies and community surveys. Brewin (1980) carried out a survey of a group general practice in Oxford, which is similar in method to the study by Pinsent (1963) discussed in the previous chapter. He was stimulated to do so by Cochrane's finding of a generally lower psychiatric admission rate in Asian immigrants, suspecting that this might be due to differing referral practices with regard to immigrants and natives on the part of GPs. Brewin drew a random sample of 200 Indian and Pakistani patients from the medical records of a group practice in Oxford. The sample consisted predominantly of Pakistanis living in the area. A sample of 200 patients of other nationalities was selected at random and matched individually for age and sex with the Asian group. The control sample did include a small number of Irish and West Indian patients, but consisted predominantly of white English-born people. It is not clear why Brewin did not eliminate the non-English born from his control sample.

From the records of each patient, the number of consultations with the GP over the previous year was abstracted. Unlike Pinsent, Brewin did not categorise consultations by the type of symptoms presented, so that it was not possible to calculate the consultation rate for psychiatric conditions separately. On the other hand, he did present the consultation rates for 10-year age blocks, thus compensating for any bias due to different age distributions in his two samples. No significant difference emerged between the Asian and English samples for either sex or any age group in the average number of consultations per year. Brewin argues from this result that Asians present psychological distress to the GP to a similar extent as do native English, but it is not so easily recognised, and consequently they are less often referred to a psychiatric facility. In pursuing this line of argument, he makes the implicit assumption that consultations for psychological symptoms are directly proportional to the overall consultation rate. He presents no evidence for this and there is no *a priori* reason why it should be true, so that Brewin's case is consequently weakened.

There are no other general-practice studies of relevance, but Cochrane & Stopes-Roe (1977) have carried out a population survey of a limited number of Indian and Pakistani residents of Birmingham, which deserves detailed consideration. These workers screened for the presence of psychological disturbance with a form of the Langner 22-item scale (Langner, 1962) which originated in the Midtown Manhattan Study. Cochrane *et al* (1977) chose this questionnaire in the absence of an instrument specifically validated for use with immigrant groups in Britain. They tested its validity on a sample of Asian and British respondents, some of whom were picked out from an out-patient clinic of a psychiatric hospital, while others were selected from the general population. The questionnaire was translated into Hindi, Punjabi, Bengali, Urdu, and Gujerati, and subjects were interviewed in their first language even if they could speak English as well. The Langner scale successfully distinguished patients from non-patients in each of the ethnic and language groups studied, confirming its validity for a survey of psychiatric morbidity among Asian immigrants.

In addition to assessing psychological disturbance, Cochrane & Stopes-Roe included questions on possible disruptions to daily life, demographic data, personal and family relationships, employment, housing, and satisfaction with living conditions. They selected from a high immigration area of the West Midlands 50 Indian and 50 Pakistani immigrants. They were chosen in terms of age and sex to be representative of the total Indian and Pakistani immigrant communities in Britain. Subjects were included who were actually born in India or Pakistan, were of appropriate ethnic origin, and were aged over 20 years. For every immigrant respondent, a matched British respondent was selected who fulfilled the criteria of being born in England, Scotland, or Wales, having parents from these areas, being white, and living in the same locality as the Asians. The authors make the point that as the British control subjects were matched with the Asians on age, sex, and area of residence, the sample is not representative of native Britons. The process of emigration of able-bodied natives from inner-city areas was stressed above (p. 193).

The respondents were interviewed in their homes by lay interviewers who were all experienced and trained and who asked the questions in the respondents' first language, regardless of the fluency of their English. Questions were read to all subjects to prevent differential treatment of the illiterate. The success rate in interviewing subjects was 78% for the British, 90% for Pakistanis, and 94% for Indians. Pakistani and Indian immigrants have different demographic characteristics, so that each ethnic sample had a quite separate, matched, British comparison group. The Asians were more likely to be married, and more poorly educated than their British counterparts, but showed no differences in occupational status, the great majority in all groups being manual workers.

The median score on the Langner scale was found to be lower in Pakistanis than in Indians, and lower in both Asian groups than in their British control groups; however, the difference only reached significance in the comparison between Pakistani and British men. Both Asian samples reported fewer disruptions in their lives in the previous year than the British control subjects did, and were more likely to be in employment, and to have stable employment histories, than their British counterparts were. Greater stability was also shown in housing by the Asians, who were more likely to be owner-occupiers, and less likely to have moved during the preceding 12 months. Reflecting these social indices, the Asians showed more satisfaction with their present financial position than did the British control subjects.

Cochrane & Stopes-Roe explain the lower prevalence of psychiatric morbidity and the greater social stability of the Asian immigrants when compared with the matched British samples in terms of the unrepresentative nature of the latter. The British-born who remain in inner-city areas of high immigrant density are likely to be "socially incompetent or psychologically disturbed'' compared with the natives who move out to more desirable areas. These considerations make it likely that the comparison between the Asian groups and their matched British counterparts from the same location is an invalid one. Therefore, more interest lies in a comparison between the Indian and Pakistani immigrants, and in associations between psychological and social measures within the Asian samples. In terms of scores on the Langner scale, the Indian and Pakistani men were very similar, while the Indian women scored much higher than the Pakistani women, although no significance level for the difference was given. The difference shown by the women may be connected with overcrowding. Both Indian and Pakistani subjects had significantly more crowded homes than their British control subjects, but it was only for Indian females that the degree of crowding was highly correlated ($P < 0.01$) with their Langner scale score. Overcrowding was brought about largely by the immigrants having almost twice as many children as the native group. Furthermore, both groups of immigrants were more likely to be sharing their homes with other people who were not members of their nuclear family than were the British. This does not, however, explain why Indian women should be more susceptible to the stressful effect of overcrowding than Pakistani women.

Another significant correlation with psychological disturbance shown by Indians and not by Pakistanis is that between the Langner scale scores in the men and the length of time their spouses have resided in the UK. The longer the wives have been in Britain, the lower are their husbands' scores. This suggests that the wife plays a more significant supportive role for Indian immigrants than for Pakistanis. The differences found between the two Asian samples are explained tentatively by the authors on the basis that Indian immigrants are drawn from more educated and advantaged sectors of their society than are Pakistani immigrants. They put foward the evidence that 64% of Indians but only 36% of Pakistanis interviewed had at least secondary education. This view corresponds with the statement made by Pinto, quoted above, that the Gujeratis are the most Westernised and literate of Asian immigrants. Gujeratis formed 62% of Cochrane & Stopes-Roe's (1977) Indian sample and were absent from their Pakistani sample. These authors consider that the act of migration may have been somewhat easier for the Indians than for the Pakistanis because of their higher educational level, possible financial superiority, and greater familiarity with Western culture. On the other hand, they may have brought expectations of higher achievement and better living conditions with them to Britain than did the Pakistanis, which could explain the greater susceptibility of Indian women to overcrowding. These explanations must remain speculative on the basis of the available data and require more focused studies before they can be accepted.

Cochrane & Stopes-Roe (1981) proceeded to extend their research with a more detailed survey of Indian immigrants in four cities: London; Birmingham; Coventry; and Slough. They used the same instrument and interview techniques as in their previous study. The comparison group of British natives was selected in working-class residential areas comparable to those in which the immigrants lived, and matched to them on age and sex. As in the earlier study, the Indians were more likely to be employed than the natives, and many more of them owned their own houses. The Indians scored significantly lower on the Langner scale than the British ($P < 0.001$) and their scores showed a contrasting relationship with social class. Whereas the natives showed the expected social-class gradient of higher scores in lower social classes, the Indians exhibited the reverse association. This was entirely due to high-scoring Indian women in the non-manual group. Upward social mobility was associated with higher scores in Indian women, while for Indian men, the link was with downward mobility. It appears that moving out of their traditional roles is particularly stressful for Indian women immigrants. This is supported by the data on employed women. In the British sample, employment outside the home was significantly related to lower symptom scores, as the body of work built up by Brown & Harris (1978) has shown. However, among the Indian women, employment did not appear to exert this protective function. In the samples as a whole, marital status was unrelated to symptom scores, but unmarried Indian women had significantly higher scores than their married compatriots. However, even those Indian women at highest risk, the unmarried performing non-manual work outside the home, had symptom scores which were no greater than the average for all English women.

This second study by Cochrane & Stopes-Roe represents a methodological advance on the first, as the comparison group of British natives was selected from areas where immigrants had not settled and is therefore likely to be a more valid yardstick. As before, a lower morbidity in Indian immigrants compared with British control subjects was obtained. However, the group of Indian women who were in transition between a traditional and a Western lifestyle, exhibited a level of morbidity equivalent to that of the British women.

Before accepting these results, we need to consider the methodological issues that could affect responses to the Langner scale. The first, we have already discussed at length, namely the presentation of distress in terms of bodily complaints, which are not included in scales such as Langner's, developed for use with a Western population. It is conceivable, for example, that the most Westernised Indian women had not experienced an increase in distress, but, unlike their more traditional compatriots, had learned to express it in psychological complaints which registered on the Langner scale.

The other issue was raised by Krause & Carr (1978) in connection with Langner's 22-item scale, so is of great relevance to our discussion. They used Langner's questionnaire in a survey of Puerto Rican immigrants to the USA. In addition to the 22 items, which were translated into Spanish, they included two questions designed to measure "acquiescence to health-related items". They defined this as *the tendency to agree with health-associated statements which appear to be physiologically improbable.* The two items they included to assess this form of suggestibility in respondents were taken from Phillips & Clancy (1970) and were as follows: "My heart sometimes stops beating for a few minutes. My lungs sometimes feel empty".

Krause & Carr (1978) found that positive answers to these questions were significantly related to scores on psychiatric symptoms ($P < 0.001$), and that this form of response-set bias accounted for 29% of the variation in the symptom scores of Puerto Rican migrants. This form of suggestibility particularly affects questionnaires administered by lay interviewers, however experienced they may be in interviewing techniques. It is much less likely to exert an influence on instruments such as the PSE, which depend on a cross-questioning approach by interviewers who are attempting to match respondents' descriptions of their experiences against a comprehensive definition of each item. Under these circumstances a simple *yes* would never be accepted as sufficient evidence that an item was present. These two forms of bias operate in opposite directions, suggestibility raising the score on a psychiatric questionnaire, somatisation reducing it, so that the findings of Cochrane & Stopes-Roe may not be that wide of the mark.

From this review of studies on Asian immigrants to the UK, we can conclude that the picture is similar to that for West Indian immigrants. Both groups show above-average levels of schizophrenic admissions to psychiatric hospitals. This is not reflected in an increase in the amount of psychiatric morbidity in the community, either as it presents to the GP or as is detected in population surveys. Studies of psychiatric morbidity in the West Indies do not currently exist, but they abound in Asia. Virtually all the major epidemiological studies have been reviewed in Chapter 8, where it was concluded that the enormous variations found in the prevalence of neurotic conditions were attributable to differences in methodology. By contrast, there was close agreement on the prevalence of schizophrenia, which did not differ from that in the West. Hence, we have solid evidence that the high level of schizophrenia in Asian immigrants to the UK is not due to a constitutional liability to develop that condition. The alternative explanations, as with any immigrant group, are selective migration and the stress of living in an alien country. The findings of the studies that have been conducted to date indicate that it would be more profitable to attempt to identify the causes of the high admission rate for schizophrenia than to embark on further surveys of psychiatric morbidity among the clientele of GPs or in the general population.

17 Doctors abroad

This chapter concentrates on doctors, a particular class of immigrants, and will pay special attention to immigrant psychiatrists. The reasons for this include both my experience in looking after overseas psychiatrists in training, and the way in which the problems of immigrant doctors crystallise many of the themes explored in this book. Some of the difficulties they face are common to all immigrants, while others are peculiar to their profession. The common problems are discussed first.

Differences in climate between the home country and the host country can adversely affect immigrants. The person accustomed to tropical heat and predictable sunshine can be made quite miserable by cold, grey weather and unpredictable, but frequent rain. The recurrent bouts of 'colds' and flu that accompany such a climate only increase the misery. Another source of homesickness is food. Once an immigrant colony is well established, ways are found of obtaining the raw ingredients of their particular cuisine. A stroller through the markets in West Indian areas of London will see many unfamiliar fruits and vegetables which have been imported to fulfil local demand. However, the first wave of immigrants is deprived of familiar foods and has to adapt to native produce. The situation is worse for immigrant doctors who, while in training, have little choice but to accept food provided by the hospital in which they work.

Separation from members of the family is a burden commonly borne by immigrants. When emigration is for economic reasons, it is usual for the man of the family to travel over first and establish some modicum of security, a job, and a place to live, before sending for his wife, children, and other relatives. Examples of this practice are documented by Cochrane & Stopes-Roe (1977), who found that the wives of Indian immigrants to Birmingham joined them after an average period of 5 years, while the delay in the case of Pakistani immigrants' wives was 8 years. Apart from the deprivation of emotional support and companionship this entails, there is an obvious problem in finding an acceptable outlet for sexual needs. Ödegaard (1932) pointed this out in describing the plight of the Norwegian

206

immigrant to the USA (p. 182). In addition to the loneliness occasioned by separation from spouse and children, there are the worries about their financial position and health. Many immigrants regularly send home money to the relatives they have left behind, but it is difficult, if not impossible, to cope with crises at a distance. News is always delayed, and sudden demands for extra amounts of money may be difficult to meet at short notice. It is often the case that the solitary male immigrant is the shining hope, not only of his wife and children, but of a large extended network of ever more distant relatives, at least one of whom, at any point in time, is likely to be ill or unemployed. The immigrant is obliged, by his cultural norms, to honour his ties to a large clan of dependents.

The pressure of this invisible, but ever-present, extended family weighs heavily on the doctor in training, as on any student abroad. His professional status is the guarantee of security to an army of relatives, so that failure to come home with a degree is unthinkable. It is a fact of life that doctors, and other students, do fail examinations, and that they are given a second chance at least. However, any delay in qualifying is an added strain in terms of prolonged separation, financial considerations, and a build-up of greater anxiety each time the examination is faced again.

The solitary immigrant who has come to another country to work can always find compatriots to ease his loneliness and homesickness. This is not true of the foreign doctor who, while in training, may have very little time to spend away from the hospital, and anyway is likely to find problems in mixing with his or her compatriots who have settled on a permanent basis, who have families and social networks of their own, and who mostly come from a different social stratum. Some doctors in training attempt to curtail these separation problems by bringing over their spouses and children once they have had time to settle down. Unfortunately, few hospitals provide suitable accommodation for whole families, and it is difficult to find private lodgings. Prejudice against foreigners often compounds a reluctance to accept small children, and furthermore, rents are extremely high for accommodation of sufficient size for a family. If the wife wishes to work in order to supplement the family income, there are considerable problems in finding someone suitable to look after small children, or in placing them in a day nursery.

In many developing countries, young married women depend a great deal on women from an older generation to teach them mothering and housewifely skills, and to act as a source of emotional support. Cut off from these assets, and often separated from her new neighbours by a language barrier, the wife of an immigrant doctor, or student, may develop anxiety and depression herself, adding to the problems of her husband.

Language is, of course, a source of numerous problems for immigrant doctors, and psychiatrists in particular. Apart from the obvious need to develop an extensive vocabulary, immigrant doctors have to be able to cope with accents as different as Irish and Cockney, and if they work in a metropolis, they are likely to come up against immigrants from parts of the world other than their own. Furthermore, they have usually learned their English in school or college on the basis of textbooks and find that the English spoken by the person in the street is considerably different. Even when their command of English is excellent, there are still subtleties in the way questions are asked, which, if not appreciated, can leave the patient with an impression of rudeness. Many immigrants counteract their loneliness by spending all their leisure time with compatriots, conversing in their native language. Unfortunately, this tends to retard the development of their English.

Another factor which infuences communication between doctor and patient is that of relative status. In many developing countries, society has a more hierarchical structure than in the West today, and doctors have a particularly elevated status, both in relation to the patient and to other members of the medical team. Consider the following vignette: a psychiatrist in a developing country drives up to the psychiatric hospital of which he or she is the head. An orderly is waiting in the parking area and as the psychiatrist gets out of the car, the orderly receives a rolled-up newspaper from the psychiatrist's hand. The orderly, walking a pace or two behind the psychiatrist, carries the newspaper into the office and deposits it on the desk. The psychiatrist settles down to interview the first patient of the day. The rest of the staff have gathered in his or her office and, a mixed group of men and women, they stand in a semicircle behind his or her desk. The psychiatrist and the patient are the only seated people. After some preliminary questions, the psychiatrist is ready to make notes. He or she signals this by lifting the right hand, fingers positioned as if holding a pen. A member of staff hurriedly picks up a pen from the desk and slips it between the poised fingers.

This sequence of events, which we have witnessed, would be unthinkable in a Western country. Hierarchies do exist in the medical profession in the West, but not to such a pronounced degree. They also vary in rigidity within the profession, such that surgeons tend to be more hierarchical than physicians, among whom psychiatrists are the most egalitarian. This is probably because of their professional concern with distinctions between individuals and the roles they occupy. When doctors from a developing country come to the West to train or to work, they have to learn to make do with less deferential treatment from their colleagues and from patients. If they attempt to maintain the superior position which they are used to at home, they will be very unpopular. Immigrant doctors are also likely to be disconcerted by the questioning attitudes of patients and their relatives. They want to be informed about the illness, its likely course, and details of treatment – questions that clients rarely ask doctors in a developing country. Furthermore, they may occasionally challenge doctors over their management of the case.

The drop in status which results from coming to a Western country is compounded in the case of doctors on postgraduate courses by changes in their working conditions. The lack of staff that is usual in a developing country means that relatively junior doctors are often given full responsibility for the management of the most difficult cases. In addition, the enormous workload means that they are vastly more experienced than doctors of the same vintage in the West. Yet when they arrive here, they are invariably treated with a certain amount of condescension, since they have not had the same excellent academic training as their Western colleagues. A further discriminating feature which puts them at a disadvantage in relation to indigenous trainees is the issue of payment. The overseas doctors in training are almost certain to be on scholarships from some funding body and have to pay fees for the privilege of being trained. By contrast, their Western colleagues, working alongside them and undergoing the same training, are receiving a salary commensurate with their labours.

When we focus on overseas psychiatrists training in the West, it is obvious that fluency in language of the host country is a prerequisite for the practice of their profession. However, due to understandable pressures in their country of origin, not all trainees have reached an acceptable standard of fluency on arrival at the training institution. It is not possible to give such candidates full responsibility for looking after patients until their command of the language is more satisfactory, which inevitably adds to their frustrations. Even when their fluency is sufficient to take a reasonable history and examine a patient's psychiatric state, the subtleties of psychotherapy are well beyond their communication abilities. It could be argued that psychotherapeutic skills are a luxury for a developing country, but it seems regrettable that so few overseas trainees gain any experience of such skills.

When the language of the host country is effectively mastered, considerable problems still remain in assessing the social situation of patients. This aspect of a patient's circumstances is often crucial in determining admission and discharge policies. Yet the ability to weigh up the relative contribution to a patient's psychiatric condition made by the marital relationship, financial problems, and poor housing, for example, demands an intimate familiarity with the culture which is likely to take years to acquire.

The final problem we shall discuss is that of psychiatric illness in trainee doctors from overseas. Doctors are by no means immune to psychiatric illness. For example, their suicide rate is among the highest of any occupational group (Sakinofsky, 1980). The variety of stresses acting on immigrant doctors have been dealt with. It is hardly surprising that they develop psychiatric conditions at times during their postgraduate training, although no study of the actual prevalence has been conducted. The whole range of diagnoses is encountered, from examination 'nerves' to schizophrenia. Neurotic conditions are treated in the same way as in a lay clientele, although the issue of who should provide the treatment requires some thought. It is advisable, in order to avoid embarrassment and to preserve confidentiality, that sick doctors be treated by psychiatrists from outside their training institutions. More difficult problems are posed by immigrant doctors who develop a psychosis. It is obviously inadvisable to allow psychotic doctors to carry on treating patients, yet if they lack insight into their mental condition, they may insist that they are not ill and refuse treatment. Legal provisions exist for compelling psychiatrically ill people to have treatment, but the reluctance to use these, which characterises psychiatry in the UK, is naturally increased in the case of colleagues.

Once treatment has been effective and the psychotic symptoms are under control, a further dilemma has to be faced: whether to allow doctors to continue their training or to send them home. It might seem that the kindest approach would be repatriation, relieving doctors of all the stress associated with an unfamiliar environment, separation from family and friends, and taxing examinations. However, this is a trap for the unwary, as was discovered by Burke (1973) in a study of Jamaicans repatriated from the UK because of psychiatric illness, mostly schizophrenia. In an unselected series of 110 readmitted patients seen at Bellevue Hospital, the only psychiatric institution in Jamaica, Burke found 16 who had been repatriated from England after being admitted to psychiatric hospitals there. Most of them claimed that they had not wanted to leave England, and ten had other family members there. It appeared that severe stigma was attached to those repatriated on psychiatric grounds. Burke points out that: ''For most people emigration involved family sacrifice and the expectation of economic and social success. Thus when failure in both areas is realized, with eventual repatriation, self-esteem is severely lowered. This is borne out by the findings of unmotivated, depressed chronically ill patients who remained ambivalent to being home''. The shame of returning home without a qualification clearly exacerbates this reaction in the case of students, but there are further complications. Some governments insist on scholarships being paid back if the student is unsuccessful in obtaining the required qualification, a daunting prospect for the psychiatrically ill emigrant returning home. Furthermore, in the case of doctors, their careers would certainly be placed in jeopardy once the fact of a psychotic illness was revealed to their employers. This raises the issue of confidentiality, in which there is a conflict of interest involved. From the viewpoint of patients' welfare, it would be advisable for employers to be aware of a doctor's susceptibility to serious psychiatric illness. From the doctor's point of view, the passing on of this information would be potentially damaging to career prospects. In the case of a postgraduate trainee, another conflict surrounds the question of examinations. If failure or delay in sitting examinations is due to a psychiatric illness, advising the doctor's sponsors will gain him or her time or a second chance, but may again indelibly stigmatise a future career.

Many of the issues discussed in this chapter are relevant to immigrants in general and to manual workers abroad, but students, doctors, and student doctors in particular give rise to problems which stretch to the limit the resources of those responsible for their welfare. Nevertheless, as I have argued elsewhere (Leff, 1980), the benefits of training doctors from overseas greatly outweigh the cost in human terms.

Epilogue

This book began by asking four questions. Reasonably complete answers to some and only partial answers to others have been provided. For instance, it has emerged that schizophrenia is recognisable as the same illness in a diverse variety of cultures, although the catatonic form is considerably more common in developing countries than in the West. However, while it has been established that the outcome for schizophrenia is outstandingly better in developing countries, the reasons for this are still inadequately understood. Where there are gaps in knowledge, at least the questions that need to be asked have been formulated. In many instances, the appropriate techniques have already been developed and it only needs someone with sufficient curiosity and time to tackle the issues.

Throughout this book I have been concerned to stress the concept of cultural relativity and to avoid an ethnocentric stance. By this point, you should readily appreciate that our subculture is as exotic to the Tswapong as theirs is to us. If you are a psychiatrist, then you share many of the beliefs and assumptions of our subculture. If not, then you may have been surprised by some of those that have been made explicit here. Once it is realised that we each inhabit a specific cultural niche, it becomes possible to examine our beliefs and assumptions relative to those of other cultures. One of the principal values of a transcultural approach to psychiatry is to bring to light the assumptions underlying the psychiatrist's view of illness and its treatment and to question them. Perhaps this book has achieved that.

References

ABSE, D. W. (1950) *The Diagnosis of Hysteria*. Bristol: John Wright.
AL-ISSA, I. (1977) Social and cultural aspects of hallucinations. *Psychological Bulletin*, **84**, 570–587.
ALLEN, N. J. (1976) Approaches to illness in the Nepalese Hills. In *Social Anthropology and Medicine* (ed. J. B. Loudon). ASA Monograph No. 13. London: Academic Press.
AMERICAN PSYCHIATRIC ASSOCIATION (1980) *Diagnostic and Statistical Manual of Mental Disorders* (3rd edn). Washington, DC: APA.
ANDRONICOS, M., CHATZIDAKIS, M. & KARAGEORGHIS, V. (1974) *The Greek Museums*, pp. 153–154. New Rochelle: Caratzas Brothers.
ANG, P. C. & WELLER, M. P. I. (1984) Koro and psychosis. *British Journal of Psychiatry*, **145**, 335.
ASUNI, T. (1967) Tropical neuropathy and psychosis. *British Journal of Psychiatry*, **113**, 1031–1033.
—— (1971) Vagrant psychotics in Abeokuta. *Journal of the National Medical Association*, **63**, 173–180.
BAGSHAW, V. E. & McPHERSON, F. M. (1978) The applicability of the Foulds and Bedford hierarchy model to mania and hypomania. *British Journal of Psychiatry*, **132**, 293–295.
BARBER, T. X. (1969) *Hypnosis, a Scientific Approach*. New York: Van Nostrand Reinhold.
BAZZOUI, W. (1970) Affective disorders in Iraq. *British Journal of Psychiatry*, **117**, 195–203.
BEBBINGTON, P. HURRY, J. & TENNANT, C. (1981a) Psychiatric disorders in selected immigrant groups in Camberwell. *Social Psychiatry*, **16**, 43–51.
——, ——, ——, STURT, E. & WING, J. K. (1981b) The epidemiology of mental disorders in Camberwell. *Psychological Medicine*, **11**, 561–579.
BEEMAN, W. O. (1985) Dimensions of dysphoria: the view from linguistic anthropology. In *Culture and Depression: Studies in the Anthropology and Cross-Cultural Psychiatry of Affect and Disorder* (eds A. Kleinman & B. Good). Berkeley: University of California Press.
BEISER, M., RAVEL, J-L., COLLOMB H., & ENGELHOFF, C. (1972) Assessing psychiatric disorder among the Serer of Senegal. *Journal of Nervous and Mental Diseases*, **154**, 141–151.
BEN-TOVIM, D. I. (1987) *Development Psychiatry: Mental Health and Primary Health Care in Botswana*. London: Tavistock Publications.
—— & CUSHNIE, J. M. (1986) The prevalence of schizophrenia in a remote area of Botswana. *British Journal of Psychiatry*, **148**, 576–580.
BERNSTEIN, B. (1958) Some sociological determinants of perception. *British Journal of Sociology*, **9**, 159–174.
BERRIOS, G. E. & MORLEY, S. J. (1984) Koro-like symptom in a non-Chinese subject. *British Journal of Psychiatry*, **145**, 331–334.
BLEULER, E. (1911) *Dementia Praecox oder Gruppe der Schizophrenien*. Leipzig: Denticke.
BORELLI, J. (1890) *Ethiopie Méridionale*. Quoted in Oesterreich T. K. (1930) *Possession Demoniacal and Other Among Primitive Races in Antiquity the Middle Ages and Modern Times*. London: Kegan Paul, Trench.

BOURGIGNON, E. (1976) Possession and trance in cross-cultural studies of mental health. In *Culture-Bound Syndromes, Ethnopsychiatry, and Alternate Therapies* (ed. W. P. Lebra). Honolulu: University Press of Hawaii.

BREUER, J. & FREUD, S. (1956) *Studies on Hysteria*. London: Hogarth Press.

BREWIN, C. (1980) Explaining the lower rates of psychiatric treatment among Asian immigrants to the United Kingdom: a preliminary study. *Social Psychiatry*, **15**, 17–19.

BRIQUET, P. (1859) *Traité Clinique et Thérapeutique de l'Hystérie*. Paris: Ballière.

BROWN, G. W., BIRLEY, J. L. T. & WING, J. K. (1972) Influence of family life on the course of schizophrenic disorders: a replication. *British Journal of Psychiatry*, **121**, 241–258.

—— BONE, M., DALISON, B. & WING, J. K. (1966) *Schizophrenia and Social Care*. Maudsley Monograph No. 17. London: Oxford University Press.

—— & HARRIS, T. (1978) *Social Origins of Depression: A Study of Psychiatric Disorders in Women*. London: Tavistock.

—— MONCK, E. M., CARSTAIRS, G. M. & WING J. K. (1962) Influence of family life on the course of schizophrenic illness. *British Journal of Preventive and Social Medicine*, **16**, 55–68.

BRUNER J. S. & POSTMAN, L. (1949) On the perception of incongruity: a paradigm. *Journal of Personality*, **18**, 206–223.

BUCHAN, T. & GREGORY, L. D. (1984) Anorexia nervosa in a Black Zimbabwean. *British Journal of Psychiatry*, **145**, 326–330.

BUCKLEY, A. D. (1976) The secret – an idea in Yoruba medicinal thought. In *Social Anthropology and Medicine* (ed. J. B. Loudon). ASA Monograph No. 13. London: Academic Press.

BURKE, A. W. (1973) The consequences of unplanned repatriation. *British Journal of Psychiatry*, **123**, 109–111.

CAROTHERS, J. C. (1951) Frontal lobe function and the African. *Journal of Mental Science*, **97**, 12–48.

CARPENTER, L. & BROCKINGTON, I. F. (1980) A study of mental illness in Asians, West Indians and Africans living in Manchester. *British Journal of Psychiatry*, **137**, 201–205.

CARSTAIRS, G. M. (1977) Protective elements in traditional cultures. *Journal of Psychosomatic Research*, **21**, 307–312.

—— & KAPUR, R. L. (1976) *The Great Universe of Kota*. London: Hogarth Press.

CHANDRASENA, R. & RODRIGO, A. (1979) Schneider's first rank symptoms: their prevalence and diagnostic implications in an Asian population. *British Journal of Psychiatry*, **135**, 348–351.

CHAPMAN, J. (1966) The early symptoms of schizophrenia. *British Journal of Psychiatry*, **112**, 225–251.

CHEETHAM, W. S. & CHEETHAM, R. J. (1976) Concepts of mental illness amongst the Xhosa people in South Africa. *Australian and New Zealand Journal of Psychiatry*, **10**, 39–45.

CHIU, T. L. TONG, J. E. & SCHMIDT, K. E. (1972) A clinical and survey study of latah in Sarawak, Malaysia. *Psychological Medicine*, **2**, 155–165.

COCHRANE, R. (1977) Mental illness in immigrants to England and Wales: An analysis of mental hospital admissions, 1971. *Social Psychiatry*, **12**, 25–35.

—— & BAL, S. S. (1987) Migration and schizophrenia: An examination of five hypotheses. *Social Psychiatry*, **22**, 181–191.

—— HASHMI, F. & STOPES-ROE, M. (1977) Measuring psychological disturbance in Asian immigrants to Britain. *Social Science and Medicine*, **11**, 157–164.

—— & STOPES-ROE, M. (1977) Psychological and social adjustment of Asian immigrants to Britain: a community survey. *Social Psychiatry*, **12**, 195–206.

——, —— (1981) Psychological symptom levels in Indian immigrants to England – a comparison with native English. *Psychological Medicine*, **11**, 319–327.

COHEN, A. (1968) *Everyman's Talmud*. London: Dent and Sons.

COLLOMB, H. (1965) Bouffées délirantes en psychiatrie africaine. *Psychopathologie Africaine*, **1**, 167–239.

COOPER, J. E., KENDELL, R. E., GURLAND, B. J., SHARPE, L., COPELAND, J. R. M. & SIMON, R. (1972) *Psychiatric Diagnosis in New York and London*. Maudsley Monograph No. 20. London: Oxford University Press.

CRISP, A. H. (1980) *Anorexia Nervosa: Let Me Be*. London: Academic Press.

CULPIN, M. (1920) *Psychneuroses of War and Peace*. London: Cambridge University Press.

DAY, R., NEILSEN, J. A., KORTEN, A., ERNBERG, G., DUBE, K. C., GEBHART, J., JABLENSKY, A., LEON, C., MARSELLA, A., OLATAWURA, M., SARTORIUS, N., STRÖMGREN, E.,

TAKAHASHI, R., WIG, N. & WYNNE, L. C. (1987) Stressful life events preceding the acute onset of schizophrenia: a cross national study from the World Health Organization. *Culture Medicine and Psychiatry*, **11**, 123–205.

DEAN, G., WALSH, D., DOWNING, H. & SHELLEY, E. (1981) First admissions of native-born and immigrants to psychiatric hospitals in South-East England 1976. *British Journal of Psychiatry*, **139**, 506–512.

DOUGLAS, M. (1973) *Natural Symbols*. Harmondsworth: Penguin Books.

DRINKA, G. F. (1984) *The Birth of Neurosis: Myth, Malady, and the Victorians*. New York: Simon and Shuster.

DUBE, K. C. (1970) A study of prevalence and biosocial variables in mental illness in a rural and an urban community in Uttar Pradesh – India. *Acta Psychiatrica Scandanavica*, **46**, 327–359.

DUPRÉ, M-C. (1976) The Mukisi women of the Teke Tsaayi. *Transcultural Psychiatric Research Review*, **13**, 67–70.

DUTTA, D. (1983) Koro epidemic in Assam. *British Journal of Psychiatry*, **143**, 309–310.

EATON, J. W. & WEIL, R. J. (1955) *Culture and Mental Disorders: A Comparative Study of the Hutterites and Other Populations*. Glencoe, Illinois: Free Press.

EBIGBO, P. (1982) Development of a cultural specific screening scale for somatic complaints indicating psychiatric disturbance. *Culture, Medicine and Psychiatry*, **6**, 29–43.

EISENBERG, L. (1977) Disease and illness. *Culture, Medicine and Psychiatry*, **1**, 9–23.

EKMAN, P., LEVENSON, R. W. & FRIESEN, W. V. (1983) Autonomic nervous system activity distinguishes among emotions. *Science*, **221**, 1208–1210.

EL-ISLAM, M. F. (1979) A better outlook for schizophrenics living in extended families. *British Journal of Psychiatry*, **135**, 343–347.

—— (1982) Rehabilitation of schizophrenics by the extended family. *Acta Psychiatrica Scandanavica*, **65**, 112–119.

ELNAGAR, M. N., MAITRA, P. & RAO, M. N. (1971) Mental health in an Indian rural community. *British Journal of Psychiatry*, **118**, 499–503.

ELSARRAG, M. E. (1968) Psychiatry in the Northern Sudan: a study in comparative psychiatry. *British Journal of Psychiatry*, **114**, 945–948.

EY, H., BERNARD, P. & BRISSETT, C. (1960) *Manuel de Psychiatrie*, p. 245. Paris: Masson.

FARMER, A. E. & FALKOWSKI, W. F. (1985) Maggot in the salt: The snake factor and the treatment of atypical psychosis in West African women. *British Journal of Psychiatry*, **146**, 446–448.

FIELD, M. J. (1968) Chronic psychosis in rural Ghana. *British Journal of Psychiatry*, **114**, 31–33.

FIELD, T. M., WOODSON, R., GREENBERG, R. & COHEN, D. (1982) Discrimination and imitation of facial expression by neonates. *Science*, **218**, 179–181.

FORSYTH, D. (1920) Hysterical paralysis in a soldier. *The Lancet*, **ii**, 794.

FORTES, M. (1936) Culture contact as a dynamic process. *Africa*, **9**, 24–55.

FOULDS, G. A. & BEDFORD, A. (1975) Hierarchy of classes of personal illness. *Psychological Medicine*, **5**, 181–192.

FRANKENBERG, R. & LEESON, J. (1976) Disease, illness and sickness: social aspects of the choice of healer in a Lusaka suburb. In *Social Anthropology and Medicine* (ed. J. Loudon). ASA Monograph No. 13. London: Academic Press.

FUKUDA, K., MORIYAMA, M., CHIBAT, T. & SUZUKI, T. (1980) Hysteria and urbanisation. *British Journal of Psychiatry*, **137**, 300–301.

GATERE, S. (1980) Patterns of psychiatric morbidity in rural Kenya. M.Phil. Thesis, University of London.

GELFAND, M. (1964) Psychiatric disorders as recognized by the Shona. In *Magic, Faith and Healing* (ed. A. Kiev). London: Collier-Macmillan.

—— (1967) *The African Witch*. London: Livingstone.

GIEL, R., GEZAHEGN, Y. & VAN LUIJK, J. N. (1968) Faith-healing and spirit-possession in Ghion, Ethiopia. *Social Science and Medicine*, **2**, 63–79.

—— & VAN LUIJK, J. N. (1969a) Psychiatric morbidity in a small Ethiopian town. *British Journal of Psychiatry*, **115**, 149–162.

——, —— (1969b) Psychiatric morbidity in a rural village in South-Western Ethiopia. *International Journal of Social Psychiatry*, **16**, 63–71.

GILLEARD, E. (1983) A cross-cultural investigation of Foulds' hierarchy model of psychiatric illness. *British Journal of Psychiatry*, **142**, 518–523.

GILLIS, L. S., ELK, R., BEN-ARIE, O. & TEGGIN, A. (1982) The Present State Examination: Experiences with Xhosa-speaking psychiatric patients. *British Journal of Psychiatry*, **141**, 143–147.

—— LEWIS, J. B. & SLABBERT, M. (1968) Psychiatric disorder amongst the Coloured people of the Cape Peninsula. *British Journal of Psychiatry*, **114**, 1575–1587.

—— & STONE, G. L. (1973) A follow-up study of psychiatric disturbance in a Cape Coloured community. *British Journal of Psychiatry*, **123**, 279–283.

GILMORE ELLIS, W. (1897) Latah. A mental malady of the Malays. *Journal of Mental Science*, **43**, 32–40.

GOLDBERG, D. P. & BLACKWELL, B. (1970) Psychiatric illness in general practice. *British Medical Journal*, ii, 439–443.

GOOD, B. J. (1977) The heart of what's the matter: The semantics of illness in Iran. *Culture, Medicine and Psychiatry*, **1**, 25–58.

—— GOOD, M. & MORADI, R. (1985) The interpretation of human depressive illness and dysphoric affect. In *Studies in Anthropology and Cross-Cultural Psychiatry of Affect and Disorder* (eds A. Kleinman & B. Good). Berkeley: University of California Press.

GUTHRIE, G. M. & SZANTON, D. L. (1976) Folk diagnosis and treatment of schizophrenia: bargaining with the spirits in the Philippines. In *Culture-Bound Syndromes, Ethnopsychiatry and Alternate Therapies* (ed. W. P. Lebra). Honolulu: University Press of Hawaii.

HADFIELD, J. A. (1942) War neurosis. *British Medical Journal*, i, 281–285.

HAGNELL, O. (1966) *A Prospective Study of the Incidence of Mental Disorder*. Stockholm: Norstedts.

HALLOWELL, A. I. (1934) Culture and mental disorder. *Journal of Abnormal and Social Psychology*, **29**, 1–9.

HARDING, T. (1973) Psychosis in a rural West African community. *Social Psychiatry*, **8**, 198–203.

HARRINGTON, J. A. (1982) Epidemic psychosis. *British Journal of Psychiatry*, **141**, 98–99.

HARRISON, G., INEICHEN, B., SMITH, J. & MORGAN, H. G. (1984) Psychiatric hospital admissions in Bristol. II. Social and clinical aspects of compulsory admission. *British Journal of Psychiatry*, **145**, 605–611.

—— OWENS, D., HOLTON, A., NEILSON, D. & BOOT, D. (1988) A prospective study of severe mental disorder in Afro-Caribbean patients. *Psychological Medicine*, **18**, 643–657.

HARVEY, Y. K. (1976) The Korean *Mudang* as a household therapist. In *Culture-Bound Syndromes, Ethnopsychiatry and Alternate Therapies* (ed. W. P. Lebra). Honolulu: University Press of Hawaii.

HARWOOD, A. (1977) Puerto Rican spiritism. *Culture, Medicine and Psychiatry*, **1**, 69–95.

HEAD, H. (1922) The diagnosis of hysteria. *British Medical Journal*, i, 827–829.

HELGASON, T. (1964) Epidemiology of mental disorders in Iceland. *Acta Psychiatrica Scandinavica* (suppl. 173), **40**, 258.

HELMAN, C. G. (1978) "Feed a cold; starve a fever"–folk models of infection in an English suburban community, and their relation to medical treatment. *Culture, Medicine and Psychiatry*, **2**, 107–137.

HEMSI, L. K. (1967) Psychiatric morbidity of West Indian immigrants. *Social Psychiatry*, **2**, 95–100.

HENRY, J. (1936) The linguistic expression of emotion. *American Anthropologist*, **38**, 250–256.

HES, J. P. (1964) The changing social role of the Yemenite Mori. In *Magic, Faith and Healing* (ed. A. Kiev). London: Collier-Macmillan.

HSU, J. (1976) Counselling in the Chinese temple: a psychological study of divination by *Chien* drawing. In *Culture-Bound Syndromes, Ethnopsychiatry and Alternate Therapies* (ed. W. P. Lebra). Honolulu: University Press of Hawaii.

HURRY, J. TENNANT, C. & BEBBINGTON, P. E. (1980) The selective factors leading to psychiatric referral. *Acta Psychiatrica Scandinavica* (suppl. 285), **61**, 315–323.

HURST, A. F. (1919) Hysteria in the light of the experience of war. *The Lancet*, ii, 771–775.

—— & SYMNS, J. L. M. (1918) The rapid cure of hysterical symptoms in soldiers. *The Lancet*, ii, 139–141.

HUXLEY, A. (1952) *The Devils of Loudon*. London: Chatto and Windus.

INEICHEN, B., HARRISON, G. & MORGAN, H. G. (1984) Psychiatric hospital admissions in Bristol. I. Geographical and ethnic factors. *British Journal of Psychiatry*, **145**, 600–604.

JANET, P. (1965) *The Major Symptoms of Hysteria.* New York: Hafner.

JASPAN, M. A. (1976) Health and illness in highland South Sumatra. In *Social Anthropology and Medicine* (ed. J. B. Loudon). ASA Monograph No. 13. London: Academic Press.

JENKINS, J. H., KARNO, M., DE LA SELVA, A. & SANTANA, F. (1986) Expressed emotion in cross-cultural context: Familial responses to schizophrenic illness among Mexican Americans. In *Treatment of Schizophrenia: Family Assessment and Intervention* (eds. M. J. Goldstein, I. Hand & K. Hahlweg). Berlin: Springer-Verlag.

JILEK, W. G. & JILEK-AALL, L. (1970) Transient psychoses in Africans. *Psychiatrica Clinica,* **3,** 337-364.

KARNO, M., JENKINS, J. H., DE LA SELVA, A., SANTANA, F., TELLES, C., LOPEZ, S. & MINTZ, J. (1987) Expressed emotion and schizophrenic outcome among Mexican-American families. *Journal of Nervous and Mental Disease,* **175,** 143-151.

KATCHADOURIAN, H. & RACY, J. (1969) The diagnostic distribution of treated psychiatric illness in Lebanon. *British Journal of Psychiatry,* **115,** 1309-1322.

KATO, M. (1969) Psychiatric epidemiological surveys in Japan: the problem of case finding. In *Mental Health Research in Asia and the Pacific* (eds. W. Caudill & T. Lin). Hawaii: East-West Center Press.

KATZ, M., COLE, J. O. & LOWERY, H. A. (1969) Studies of the diagnostic process: the influence of symptom perception, past experience and ethnic background on diagnostic decisions. *American Journal of Psychiatry,* **125,** 937-947.

KEDWARD, H. (1969) The outcome of neurotic illness in the community. *Social Psychiatry,* **4,** 1-4.

KENNEDY, J. G. (1967) Nubian Zar ceremonies as psychotherapy. *Human Organization,* **26,** 185-194.

KERCKHOFF, A. C. & BACK, K. W. (1968) *The June Bug.* New York: Appleton-Century-Crofts.

KIEV, A. (1965) Psychiatric morbidity of West Indian immigrants in an urban group practice. *British Journal of Psychiatry,* **III,** 51-56.

KLEINMAN, A. (1986) *Social Origins of Distress and Disease: Depression Neurasthenia and Pain in Modern China.* New Haven: Yale University Press.

—— & GOOD, B. (1985) *Culture and Depression: Studies in the Anthropology and Cross-Cultural Psychiatry of Affect and Disorder.* Berkeley: University of California Press.

KLINE, N. S. (1954) Use of *Rauwolfia serpentina* Benth. in neuropsychiatric conditions. *Annals of the New York Academy of Science,* **59,** 107-132.

KRAEPELIN, E. (1893) *Psychiatrie* (4th edn). Leipzig: Abel.

KRAMER, M. (1961) Some problems for international research. In *Proceedings of the Third World Congress of Psychiatry,* vol. 3, Montreal: University of Toronto Press.

—— (1969a) Cross-national study of diagnosis of the mental disorders: origin of the problem. *American Journal of Psychiatry,* **125,** (suppl.), 1-11.

—— (1969b) Statistics of mental disorders in the United States: Current status and future goals. In *Comparative Epidemiology of the Mental Disorders* (eds. P. Hoch & J. Zubin). New York: Grune and Stratton.

KRAUSE, N. & CARR, L. G. (1978) The effects of response bias in the survey assessment of the mental health of Puerto Rican migrants. *Social Psychiatry,* **13,** 167-173.

KROEBER, A. L. & KLUCKHOHN, C. (1952) *Culture: A critical review of concepts and definitions.* Papers of the Peabody Museum, Cambridge: Massachusetts.

KULHARA, P. & WIG, N. N. (1978) The chronicity of schizophrenia in North West India: Results of a follow-up study. *British Journal of Psychiatry,* **132,** 186-190.

LAMBO, T. A. (1960) Further neuropsychiatric observations in Nigeria. *British Medical Journal,* ii, 1696-1704.

LANGNER, T. S. (1962) A twenty-two item screening score of psychiatric symptoms indicating impairment. *Journal of Health and Social Behaviour,* **3,** 269-276.

LEBRA, T. S. (1976) Taking the role of supernatural "other": spirit possession in a Japanese healing cult. In *Culture-Bound Syndromes, Ethnopsychiatry and Alternate Therapies* (ed. W. P. Lebra). Honolulu: University Press of Hawaii.

LEFF, J. P. (1973) Culture and the differentiation of emotional states. *British Journal of Psychiatry,* **123,** 299-306.

—— (1974) Transcultural influences on psychiatrists' rating of verbally expressed emotion. *British Journal of Psychiatry,* **125,** 336-340.

—— (1977) International variations in the diagnosis of psychiatric illness. *British Journal of Psychiatry*, **131**, 329–338.

—— (1978) Psychiatrists' vs patients' concepts of unpleasant emotions. *British Journal of Psychiatry*, **133**, 306–313.

—— (1980) Overseas trainees in psychiatry. *British Journal of Psychiatry*, **137**, 288–289.

—— FISCHER, M. & BERTELSEN, A. (1976) A cross-national epidemiological study of mania. *British Journal of Psychiatry*, **129**, 428–437.

—— TRESS, K. & EDWARDS, B. (1988) The clinical course of depressive symptoms in schizophrenia. *Schizophrenia Research*, **1**, 25–30.

—— & VAUGHN, C. (1972) Psychiatric patients in contact and out of contact with services: a clinical and social assessment. In *Evaluating a Community Psychiatric Service* (eds. J. K. Wing & A. M. Hailey). London: Oxford University Press.

——, —— (1985) *Expressed Emotion in Families: Its Significance for Mental Illness*. New York: Guildford Press.

—— WIG, N. N., GHOSH, A., BEDI, H., MENON, D. K., KUIPERS, L., KORTEN, A., ERNBERG, G., DAY, R., SARTORIUS, N. & JABLENSKY, A. (1987) Expressed emotion and schizophrenia in North India. III. Influence of relatives' expressed emotion on the course of schizophrenia in Chandigarh. *British Journal of Psychiatry*, **151**, 156–173.

LEIGHTON, A. H. (1959) *My Name is Legion: Foundations for a Theory of Man in Relation to Culture*. New York: Basic Books.

—— LAMBO, T. A., HUGHES, C. C., LEIGHTON, D. C., MURPHY, J. M. & MACKLIN, D. B. (1963) *Psychiatric Disorder Among the Yoruba*. New York: Cornell University Press.

LEVENTHAL, H. & SCHERER, K. (1987) The relationship of emotion to cognition: A functional approach to a semantic controversy. *Cognition and Emotion*, **1**, 3–28.

LEWIS, A. (1967) Problems presented by the ambiguous word 'anxiety' as used in psychopathology. *Israel Annals of Psychiatry and Related Disciplines*, **5**, 105–121.

LEWIS, G. (1976) A view of sickness in New Guinea. In *Social Anthropology and Medicine* (ed. J. Loudon), ASA Monograph No. 13. London: Academic Press.

LI, Y-Y. (1976) Shamanism in Taiwan: An anthropological enquiry. In *Culture-Bound Syndromes, Ethnopsychiatry and Alternate Therapies* (ed. W. P. Lebra). Honolulu: University Press of Hawaii.

LIN, K-M., KLEINMAN, A. & LIN, T-Y. (1980) Overview of mental disorders in Chinese cultures: Review of epidemiological and clinical studies. In *Normal and Abnormal Behaviour in Chinese Culture* (eds A. Kleinman & T-Y Lin). New York: Reidel.

LIN, T. (1953) A study of the incidence of mental disorder in Chinese and other cultures. *Psychiatry*, **16**, 313–336.

—— RIN, H., YEH, E., HSU, C. & CHU, H. (1969) Mental disorders in Taiwan fifteen years later: A preliminary report. In *Mental Health Research in Asia and the Pacific* (eds W. Caudill & T. Lin). Hawaii: East–West Center Press.

LITTLEWOOD, R. & LIPSEDGE, M. (1978) Acute psychotic reactions in Africans. *British Journal of Psychiatry*, **132**, 106–107.

—— & —— (1981*a*) Some social and phenomenological characteristics of psychotic immigrants. *Psychological Medicine*, **11**, 289–302.

—— & —— (1981*b*) Acute psychotic reactions in Caribbean-born patients. *Psychological Medicine*, **11**, 303–318.

LO, W. H. & LO, T. (1977) A ten-year follow-up study of Chinese schizophrenics in Hong Kong. *British Journal of Psychiatry*, **131**, 63–66.

LOW, S. M. (1981) The meaning of *nervios*: A sociocultural analysis of symptom presentation in San Jose, Costa Rica. *Culture, Medicine and Psychiatry*, **5**, 25–47.

LUTZ, C. (1985) Depression and the translation of emotional worlds. In *Culture and Depression: Studies in the Anthropology and Cross-Cultural Psychiatry of Affect and Disorder* (eds A. Kleinman & B. Good). Berkeley: University of California Press.

MACLEAN, U. (1969) Community attitudes to mental illness in Edinburgh. *British Journal of Preventive and Social Medicine*, **23**, 45–52.

—— (1971) *Magical Medicine*. Harmondsworth: Penguin.

—— (1976) Some aspects of sickness behaviour among the Yoruba. In *Social Anthropology and Medicine* (ed. J. B. Loudon). ASA Monograph No. 13. London: Academic Press.

MAKANJUOLA, R. O. A. & ADEDAPO, S. A. (1987) The DSM–III concepts of schizophrenic disorder and schizophreniform disorder: A clinical and prognostic evaluation. *British Journal of Psychiatry*, **151**, 611–618.

MARSELLA, A. J. (1979) Depressive experience and disorder across cultures. In *Handbook of Crosscultural Psychology* (eds H. Triandis & J. Draguns), Vol. 5. Boston: Allyn and Bacon.

MAVREAS, V. G., BEIS, A., MOUYIAS, A., RIGONI, F. & LYKETSOS, G. C. (1986) Prevalence of psychiatric disorders in Athens. *Social Psychiatry*, **21**, 172–181.

McEVEDY, C. P. & BEARD, A. W. (1970) Royal Free epidemic of 1955: A reconsideration. *British Medical Journal*, *i*, 7–11.

—— & —— (1973) A controlled follow-up of cases involved in an epidemic of "benign myalgic encephalomyelitis". *British Journal of Psychiatry*, **122**, 141–150.

McPHERSON, F. M., ANTRAM, M. C., BAGSHAW, V. E. & CARMICHAEL, S. K. (1977) A test of the hierarchical model of personal illness. *British Journal of Psychiatry*, **131**, 56–58.

MEDICAL STAFF OF THE ROYAL FREE HOSPITAL (1957) An outbreak of encephalomyelitis in the Royal Free Hospital Group, London in 1955. *British Medical Journal*, *ii*, 895–904.

MEGGITT, M. J. (1974) *Desert People*. Sydney: Angus and Robertson.

MILLER, C. W. (1942) Factors affecting the prognosis of paranoid disorders. *Journal of Nervous and Mental Diseases*, **95**, 580–588.

MINER, H. (1952) The folk–urban continuum. *American Sociological Review*, **17**, 529–537.

MODAI, I., MUNITZ, H. & AIZENBERG, D. (1986) Koro in an Israeli Male. *British Journal of Psychiatry*, **149**, 503–505.

MOREY, L. C. (1985) A comparative validation of the Foulds and Bedford hierarchy of psychiatric symptomatology. *British Journal of Psychiatry*, **146**, 424–428.

MORICE, R. (1978) Psychiatric diagnosis in a transcultural setting: the importance of lexical categories. *British Journal of Psychiatry*, **132**, 87–95.

MORRISON, J. R. (1974) Changes in subtype diagnosis of schizophrenia: 1920–1966. *American Journal of Psychiatry*, **131**, 674–677.

MOSS, P. D. & McEVEDY, C. P. (1966) An epidemic of overbreathing among schoolgirls. *British Medical Journal*, *ii*, 1295–1300.

MUKHERJEE, S. (1983) Reducing American diagnosis of schizophrenia: Will the DSMIII suffice. *British Journal of Psychiatry*, **142**, 414–418.

MURPHY, H. B. M. (1982) *Comparative Psychiatry: The International and Intercultural Distribution of Mental Illness*. Berlin: Springer-Verlag.

—— & RAMAN, A. C. (1971) The chronicity of schizophrenia in indigenous tropical peoples. *British Journal of Psychiatry*, **118**, 489–497.

—— & TAUMOEPEAU, B. M. (1980) Traditionalism and mental health in the South Pacific: A re-examination of an old hypothesis. *Psychological Medicine*, **10**, 471–482.

MURPHY, J. M. (1964) Psychotherapeutic aspects of shamanism on St. Laurence Island, Alaska. In *Magic, Faith and Healing* (ed. A. Kiev). London: Collier-Macmillan.

NADEEM, A. A. & YOUNIS, Y. O. (1977) Physical illness and psychiatric disorders in Tigani El-Mahi Psychiatric Hospital (Sudan). *East African Medical Journal*, **54**, 207–210.

NANDI, D. N., AJMANY, S., GANGULI, H., BANERJEE, G., BORAL, G. C., GHOSH, A. & SARKAR, S. (1975) Psychiatric disorders in a rural community in West Bengal – an epidemiological study. *Indian Journal of Psychiatry*, **17**, 87–99.

NANDI, D. N., AJMANY, S., GANGULI, H., BANERJEE, G., BORAL, G. C., GHOSH, A. & SARKAR, S. (1976) A clinical evaluation of depressives found in a rural survey in India. *British Journal of Psychiatry*, **128**, 523–527.

—— MUKHERJEE, S. P., BORAL, G. C., BANERJEE, G., GHOSH, A., SARKAR, S. & AJMANY, S. (1980) Socio-economic status and mental morbidity in certain tribes and castes in India. *British Journal of Psychiatry*, **136**, 73–85.

NEUTRA, R., KEVY, J. E. & PARKER, D. (1977) Cultural expectations versus reality in Navajo seizure patterns and sick roles. *Culture, Medicine and Psychiatry*, **1**, 255–275.

NGUBANE, H. (1976) Some aspects of treatment among the Zulu. In *Social Anthropology and Medicine* (ed. J. B. Loudon). ASA Monograph No. 13. London: Academic Press.

NGUI, R. W. (1969) The koro epidemic in Singapore. *Australian and New Zealand Journal of Psychiatry*, **3**, 263–266.

NICHTER, M. (1981*a*) Idioms of distress: alternatives in the expression of psycho-social distress: A case study from South India. *Culture, Medicine and Psychiatry*, **5**, 379–408.

—— (1981*b*) Negotiation of the illness experience: Ayurvedic therapy and the psychosocial dimension of illness. *Culture, Medicine and Psychiatry*, **5**, 5–24.

OBEYESEKERE, G. (1985) Depression, Buddhism and the work of culture in Sri Lanka. In *Studies in the Anthropology and Cross-Cultural Psychiatry of Affect and Disorder* (eds A. Kleinman & B. Good). Berkeley: University of California Press.

ÖDEGAARD, Ö. (1932) Emigration and insanity. *Acta Psychiatrica et Neurologica Scandinavica* (suppl. 4), **7**, 206.

—— (1967) Changes in the prognosis of functional psychoses since the days of Kraepelin. *British Journal of Psychiatry*, **113**, 813–822.

OFFICE OF HEALTH ECONOMICS (1968) *Without Prescription*. London: HMSO.

OKASHA, A. (1966) A cultural psychiatric study of El-Zar cult in UAR. *British Journal of Psychiatry*, **112**, 1217–1221.

—— KAMEL, M. & HASSAN, A. H. (1968) Preliminary psychiatric observations in Egypt. *British Journal of Psychiatry*, **114**, 949–955.

ONYANGO, P. P. (1976) The views of African mental patients towards mental illness and its treatment. *MA Thesis*, University of Nairobi, Kenya.

ORBACH, S. (1978) *Fat is a Feminist Issue*. London: Hamlyn.

ORLEY, J. H. (1970) *Culture and Mental Illness*. Nairobi: East African Publishing House.

—— & LEFF, J. P. (1972) The effect of psychiatric education on attitudes to illness among the Ganda. *British Journal of Psychiatry*, **12**, 137–141.

—— & WING, J. K. (1979) Psychiatric disorders in two African villages. *Archives of General Psychiatry*, **36**, 513–520.

OYEBODE, F., JAMIESON, R., MULLANEY, J., & DAVISON, K. (1986) Koro–a psychophysiological dysfunction? *British Journal of Psychiatry*, **148**, 212–214.

PARSONS, C. D. F. (1984) Idioms of distress: Kinship and sickness among the people of the Kingdom of Tonga. *Culture, Medicine and Psychiatry*, **8**, 71–93.

PHILLIPS, D. & CLANCY, K. (1970) Response biases in field studies of mental illness. *American Sociological Review*, **35**, 503–514.

PILOWSKY, I. (1975) Dimensions of abnormal illness behaviour. *Australian and New Zealand Journal of Psychiatry*, **9**, 141–147.

PINSENT, R. J. F. H. (1963) Morbidity in an immigrant population. *The Lancet*, **i**, 437–438.

PINTO, R. T. (1970) A study of psychiatric illness among Asians in the Camberwell area. *MPhil Thesis*, University of London.

PLOWDEN, W. C. (1868) *Travels in Abessinia and the Galla Country*. London.

PRINCE, R. (1960) The use of Rauwolfia for the treatment of psychoses by Nigerian native doctors. *American Journal of Psychiatry*, **117**, 147–149.

—— (1964) Indigenous Yoruba psychiatry. In *Magic, Faith and Healing* (ed. A. Kiev). London: Collier-Macmillan.

—— & TCHENG-LAROCHE, F. (1987) Culture-bound syndromes and international disease classifications. *Culture, Medicine and Psychiatry*, **11**, 3–19.

PU, T., MOHAMED, E., IMAM, K. & EL-ROEY, A. M. (1986) One hundred cases of hysteria in Eastern Libya: A socio-demographic study. *British Journal of Psychiatry*, **148**, 606–609.

RACY, J. (1980) Somatization in Saudi women: A therapeutic challenge. *British Journal of Psychiatry*, **137**, 212–216.

RAWNSLEY, K. (1968) An international diagnostic exercise. In *Proceedings of the Fourth World Congress of Psychiatry* vol. 4. Amsterdam: Excerpta Medica Foundation.

REES, W. D. (1971) The hallucinations of widowhood. *British Medical Journal*, **iv**, 37–41.

RICHARDSON, E. & HENRYK-GUTT, R. (1982) Diagnosis of psychiatric illness in immigrant patients. *British Journal of Clinical and Social Psychiatry*, **1**, 78–81.

RIN, H. & LIN, T. (1962) Mental illness among Formosan Aborigines as compared with the Chinese in Taiwan. *Journal of Mental Science*, **108**, 134–146.

RISSO, M. & BÖKER, W. (1968) Delusions of witchcraft: a cross cultural study. *British Journal of Psychiatry*, **114**, 963–972.

RITCHIE, J. E. (1976) Cultural time out: generalised therapeutic socio-cultural mechanisms among the Maori. In *Culture-Bound Syndromes, Ethnopsychiatry and Alternate Therapies* (ed. W. P. Lebra). Honolulu: University Press of Hawaii.

ROLLIN, H. R. (1965) Unprosecuted mentally abnormal offenders. *British Medical Journal, i*, 831–835.

ROTTANBURG, D., ROBINS, A. & BEN-ARIE, O. (1982) Cannabis associated psychosis with hypomanic features. *The Lancet, i*, 1364–1365.

ROYES, K. (1961) The incidence and features of psychosis in a Caribbean community. In *Proceedings of the Third World Congress of Psychiatry, Montreal 1961* pp. 1121–1125. University of Toronto Press and McGill University Press.

RWEGELLERA, G. G. C. (1980) Differential use of psychiatric services by West Indians, West Africans and English in London. *British Journal of Psychiatry*, **137**, 428–432.

SAKINOFSKY, I. (1980) Suicide in doctors and their wives. *British Medical Journal, ii*, 386–387.

SARGANT, W. (1957) *Battle for the Mind*. London: Heinemann.

SARTORIUS, N., JABLENSKY, A., KORTEN, G., ERNBERG, G., ANKER, M., COOPER, J. E. & DAY, R. (1986) Early manifestations and first-contact incidence of schizophrenia in different cultures. *Psychological Medicine*, **16**, 909–928.

SCHIEFFELIN, E. L. (1985) The cultural analysis of depressive affect: An example from New Guinea. In *Culture and Depression: Studies in the Anthropology and Cross-Cultural Psychology of Affect and Disorder* (eds A. Kleinman & B. Good). Berkeley: University of California Press.

SCHLAUCH, M. (1943) *The Gift of Tongues*. London. George Allen and Unwin.

SCHNEIDER, K. (1957) Primäre und sekundäre Symptome bei der Schizophrenie. *Fortschritte der Neurologie und Psychiatrie*, **25**, 487–490.

SCHWAB, M. E. (1977) A study of reported hallucinations in a Southeastern County. *Mental Health and Society*, **4**, 344–354.

SETHI, B. B., GUPTA, S. C. & KUMAR, R. (1967) 300 urban families – a psychiatric study. *Indian Journal of Psychiatry*, **9**, 280–291.

——, —— & KUMARI, P. (1972) A psychiatric survey of 500 rural families. *Indian Journal of Psychiatry*, **14**, 183–196.

——, —— MAHENDRU, R. K. & KUMARI, P. (1974) Mental health and urban life: a study of 850 families. *British Journal of Psychiatry*, **124**, 243–247.

SHEPHERD, M., BROOKE, E. M., COOPER, J. E. & LIN, T. (1968) An experimental approach to psychiatric diagnosis. *Acta Psychiatrica Scandinavica* (suppl. 201), **44**, 89.

—— COOPER, B., BROWN, A. C. & KALTON, G. W. (1966) *Psychiatric Illness in General Practice*. London: Oxford University Press.

SHWEDER, R. A. (1985) Menstrual pollution, soul loss, and the comparative study of emotions. In *Culture and Depression: Studies in the Anthropology and Cross-Cultural Psychiatry of Affect and Disorder* (eds A. Kleinman & B. Good). Berkeley: University of California Press.

SIMÕES, M. & BINDER, J. (1980) A socio-psychiatric field study among Portuguese emigrants in Switzerland. *Social Psychiatry*, **15**, 1–8.

SIMONS, H. J. (1957) Tribal medicine. *African Studies*, **16**, 85–92.

SIMONS, R. C. (1980) The resolution of the Latah paradox. *Journal of Nervous and Mental Disease*, **168**, 195–206.

SIMPSON, C. J. (1984) Doctors and nurses use of the word confused. *British Journal of Psychiatry*, **145**, 441–443.

SKULTANS, V. (1974) *Intimacy and Ritual*. London: Routledge and Kegan Paul.

SKULTANS, V. (1976) Empathy and healing: Aspects of spiritualist ritual. In *Social Anthropology and Medicine* (ed. J. Loudon). ASA Monograph No. 13. London: Academic Press.

SLATER, E. (1943) The neurotic constitution. A statistical study of two thousand neurotic soldiers. *Journal of Neurology and Psychiatry*, **6**, 1–16.

—— (1965) Diagnosis of "Hysteria". *British Medical Journal, i*, 1395–1399.

SMARTT, C. G. F. (1964) Short-term treatment of the African psychotic. *Central African Journal of Medicine*, **10** (suppl.), 1–12.

SNAITH, R. P., BRIDGE, G. W. K. & HAMILTON, M. (1976) The Leeds scale for self-assessment of anxiety and depression. *British Journal of Psychiatry*, **128**, 156–165.

SPECK, R. V. & REUVENI, V. (1969) Network therapy – a developing concept. *Family Process*, **8**, 182–191.

SPENCER, J. (1975) The mental health of Jehovah's Witnesses. *British Journal of Psychiatry*, **126**, 556–559.

STEFANIS, C., MARKIDIS, M. & CHRISTODOULOU, G. (1976) Observations on the evolution of the hysterical symptomatology. *British Journal of Psychiatry* , **128**, 269–275.

STEVENS, J. R. & WYATT, R. J. (1987) Similar incidence worldwide of schizophrenia: Case not proven. *British Journal of Psychiatry*, **151**, 131-132.

STURT, E. (1981) Hierarchical patterns in the distribution of psychiatric symptoms. *Psychological Medicine*, **11**, 783-794.

—— BEBBINGTON, P. E., HURRY, J. & TENNANT, C. (1981) The Present State Examination used by interviewers from a Survey Agency. Report from the MRC Camberwell Community Survey. *Psychological Medicine*, **11**, 185-192.

SUWANLERT, S. (1976) *Phii Pob*: Spirit possession in rural Thailand. In *Culture-Bound Syndromes, Ethnopsychiatry and Alternate Therapies* (ed. W. P. Lebra). Honolulu: University Press of Hawaii.

SWARTZ, L., BEN-ARIE, O. & TEGGIN, A. F. (1985) Subcultural delusions and hallucinations: Comments on the Present State Examination in a multi-cultural context. *British Journal of Psychiatry*, **146**, 391-394.

TAMBIAH, S. J. (1977) The cosmological and performative significance of a Thai cult of healing through meditation. *Culture, Medicine and Psychiatry*, **1**, 97-132.

TAN, E. K. & CARR, J. E. (1977) Psychiatric sequelae of amok. *Culture, Medicine and Psychiatry*, **1**, 59-67.

TARNOPOLSKY, A., CAETANO, R., LEVAV, I., DEL OLMO, G., CAMPILLO, C. & PINHEIRO, H. (1977) Prevalence of psychiatric morbidity in an industrial suburb of Buenos Aires. *Social Psychiatry*, **12**, 75-88.

THACORE, V. R., GUPTA, S. C. & SURAIYA, M. (1975) Psychiatric morbidity in a North Indian community. *British Journal of Psychiatry*, **126**, 364-369.

TIDMARSH, D. & WOOD, S. (1972) Psychiatric aspects of destitution: a study of the Camberwell Reception Centre. In *Evaluating a Community Psychiatric Service* (eds J. K. Wing & A. M. Hailey). London: Oxford University Press.

TOOTH, G. (1950) *Studies in Mental Illness in the Gold Coast*. London: HMSO.

TORREY, E. F. (1987) Similar incidence worldwide of schizophrenia: Case not proven. *British Journal of Psychiatry*, **151**, 132-133.

—— TORREY, B. B. & BURTON-BRADLEY, B. G. (1974) The epidemiology of schizophrenia in Papua New Guinea. *American Journal of Psychiatry*, **131**, 567-573.

TSENG, W. S. (1972) Psychiatric study of shamanism in Taiwan. *Archives of General Psychiatry*, **26**, 561-565.

—— (1975) The nature of somatic influences among psychiatric patients: The Chinese case. *Comprehensive Psychiatry*, **16**, 237-245.

—— (1976) Folk psychotherapy in Taiwan. In *Culture-Bound Syndromes, Ethnopsychiatry and Alternate Therapies* (ed. W. P. Lebra). Honolulu: University Press of Hawaii.

TSUANG, M. T., BUCHER, K. D. & FLEMING, J. A. (1982) Testing the monogenic theory of schizophrenia. *British Journal of Psychiatry*, **140**, 595-599.

TURNER, V. (1967) *The Forest of Symbols*. London: Cornell University Press.

VAUGHN, C. E. & LEFF, J. P. (1976) The influence of family and social factors on the course of psychiatric illness: A comparison of schizophrenic and depressed neurotic patients. *British Journal of Psychiatry*, **129**, 125-137.

—— SNYDER, K. S., JONES, S., FREEMAN, W. B. & FALLOON, I. R. H. (1984) Family factors in schizophrenic relapse: A California replication of the British research on expressed emotion. *Archives of General Psychiatry*, **41**, 1169-1177.

VERMA, S. K. & WIG, N. N. (1976) PGI Health Questionnaire N-2: Construction and initial try outs. *Indian Journal of Clinical Psychology*, **3**, 135-142.

WALSH, D. (1985) Case register for monitoring treatment outcome in chronic functional psychoses. In *The Long-term Treatment of Functional Psychoses* (ed. T. Helgason). Cambridge: Cambridge University Press.

WARNER, R. (1985) *Recovery from Schizophrenia: Psychiatry and Political Economy*. London: Routledge and Kegan Paul.

WAXLER, N. E. (1979) Is outcome for schizophrenia better in nonindustrial societies? The case of Sri Lanka. *Journal of Nervous and Mental Diseases*, **167**, 144-158.

WERBNER, R. P. (1973) The superabundance of understanding: Kalanga rhetoric and domestic divination. *American Anthropologist*, **75**, 1414-1440.

WESTERMEYER, J. (1984) Economic losses associated with chronic mental disorder in a developing country. *British Journal of Psychiatry*, **144**, 475-481.

—— & KROLL, J. (1978) Violence and mental illness in a peasant society. *British Journal of Psychiatry*, **133**, 529–541.

WIG, N. N., MENON, D. K., BEDI, H., GHOSH, A., KUIPERS, L., LEFF, J., KORTEN, A., DAY, R., SARTORIUS, N., ERNBERG, G. & JABLENSKY, A. (1987) Expressed Emotion and schizophrenia in North India. 1. Cross-cultural transfer of ratings of relatives' Expressed Emotion. *British Journal of Psychiatry*, **151**, 156–173.

——, —— LEFF, J., KUIPERS, L., GHOSH, A., DAY, R., KORTEN, A., ERNBERG, G., SARTORIUS, N., JABLENSKY, A., NIELSEN, J. A. & THESTRUP, G. (1987) Expressed Emotion and schizophrenia in North India. II. Distribution of Expressed Emotion components among relatives of schizophrenic patients in Aarhus and Chandigarh. *British Journal of Psychiatry*, **151**, 156–173.

——, & PERSHAD, D. *Triennial Statistical Report* (1975, 1976 and 1977). Chandigarh, India: Department of Psychiatry, Postgraduate Institute of Medical Education and Research.

WIJESINGHE, C. P., DASSANAYAKE, S. A. W. & DISSANAYAKE, P. V. L. N. (1978) Survey of psychiatric morbidity in a semi-urban population in Sri Lanka. *Acta Psychiatrica Scandinavica*, **58**, 413–441.

—— DISSANAYAKE, S. A. W. & MENDIS, N. (1976) Possession trance in a semi-urban community in Sri Lanka. *Australian and New Zealand Journal of Psychiatry*, **10**, 135–139.

WILLIAMS, A. H. (1950) A psychiatric study of Indian Soldiers in the Arakan. *British Journal of Medical Psychology*, **23**, 130–181.

WILSON-BARNETT, J. & TRIMBLE, M. R. (1985) An investigation of hysteria using the Illness Behaviour Questionnaire. *British Journal of Psychiatry*, **146**, 601–608.

WING, J. K., COOPER, J. E. & SARTORIUS, N. (1974) *The Measurement and Classification of Psychiatric Symptoms*. London: Cambridge University Press.

—— & HAILEY, A. M. (1972) *Evaluating a Community Psychiatric Service*. London: Oxford University Press.

—— MANN, S. A., LEFF, J. P. & NIXON, J. M. (1978) The concept of a case in psychiatric population surveys. *Psychological Medicine*, **8**, 203–217.

WOOFF, K., FREEMAN, H. L. & FRYERS, T. (1983) Psychiatric service use in Salford. *British Journal of Psychiatry*, **142**, 588–597.

WORLD HEALTH ORGANIZATION (1967) *Manual of the International Statistical Classification of Diseases, Injuries, and Causes of Death*, 1965 revision (8th edn) (ICD-8). Geneva: WHO.

—— (1973) *The International Pilot Study of Schizophrenia*, vol. 1. Geneva: WHO.

—— (1979) *Schizophrenia. An International Follow-up Study*. Chichester: John Wiley and Sons.

WYATT, J. L. & WYATT, G. B. (1967) An analysis of the patients seen at Igbo-Ora Rural Health Centre Western Nigeria during the year from July 1964 to June 1965. *Annals of Tropical Medicine and Parasitology*, **61**, 224–233.

YANPING, Z., LEYI, X. & QIJIE, S. (1986) Styles of verbal expression of emotional and physical experiences: a study of depressed patients and normal controls in China. *Culture, Medicine and Psychiatry*, **10**, 231–243.

YAP, P. M. (1965) Koro - a culture-bound depersonalization syndrome. *British Journal of Psychiatry*, **111**, 43–50.

Index

OSTEOPATHY
Is it for you?

Biography

Chris Belshaw first became interested in osteopathy
whilst studying medicine. After qualifying as a doctor
he spent several years in hospital work which included
some time in Nigeria with the Church Missionary
Society and in Rheumatology and Orthopaedics in
Harrogate. A short spell in general practice was
followed by postgraduate training at the London
College of Osteopathic Medicine. He runs his own
practice, which has been established for over twelve
years, and enjoys teaching at the London College.

He is convinced that osteopathy forms one part of
the wholeness of healing and will play an increasing
role within medicine as we approach the year 2000 and
beyond.

He has wide interests in music, sailing, hockey,
travel, reading, writing and good company.

OSTEOPATHY
Is it for you?

Dr Chris Belshaw

MB BCh BAO MLCOM

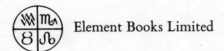 Element Books Limited

First published 1987 by
Element Books Limited, Shaftesbury, Dorset

Printed and bound in Great Britain by
Billings, Hylton Road, Worcester

Designed by Humphrey Stone
Illustrations by Ray Smith
Cover illustration by Ariane Dixon

British Library Cataloguing in Publication Data
Belshaw, Chris
   Osteopathy: is it for you?
   1. Osteopathy
   I. Title
   615.5′33   RZ341
   ISBN 0-906540-95-X

Contents

This book is dedicated to the memory of
TED DUNHAM DO
Osteopath, Friend and Mentor

Acknowledgements

I express my grateful thanks to all those who have helped me in various ways, including my patients, to make this book happen. I have enjoyed researching and writing it and have learnt more about osteopathy as a result.

In particular I thank Jean Makepeace and Roddy McDonald for their useful suggestions and comments; Evelyn Hunter for her clarity in criticism of the whole typescript to ensure that my explanations were understood; Elizabeth Hedgecock who patiently and thoroughly completed all the typing and added a few comments on the writing; John Rolles for his encouragement; my publisher Michael Mann for his patience and guidance enabling me to express a professional subject in a readable way (not without its difficulty!) and most importantly for completing the project; Rebecca Smith for her clear indexing and Maggie for her support at home throughout the book's gestation and growth.

Introduction

Dare to be different. So many would rather be orthodox than right.
H. H. FRYETTE DO

The first school of osteopathy was opened by Dr Andrew Taylor Still in Kirksville, Missouri in 1892 and will shortly celebrate its centenary. This was the culmination of many years of study beginning in 1874 when Still first outlined his basic osteopathic principles. Since those early days countless people have benefited with improved health, relief from pain and prevention of disability. The principles and practice of osteopathy are just as important for good health today as they ever were.

Osteopathy is found throughout America and is gaining ground in Canada. It has also spread as far as Britain, Australia and New Zealand. Europe is not as yet well represented apart from several individual practitioners, a similar situation to several other countries world wide. However some osteopathic methods have been incorporated within medical manipulation in many European states.

In this century we have seen a rapid development of orthodox medical practice with increasing use of powerful drugs to combat disease, and technological advances that threaten to engulf us – yet disease and pain have not gone away. We are continually frustrated and troubled by the side-effects of the medicines used today just as Andrew Taylor Still was over 100 years ago. Osteopathy then as now is successful in treating a wide variety of painful conditions, particularly those related to the muscles and joints.

Nowadays we would not use osteopathy to treat chest infections because we have antibiotics, yet in preantibiotic days when pneumonia was a fatal disease, osteopathic manipulation of the ribs and spine aided recovery of many people who would otherwise have died. However, we can and do use this principle today in treatment for maintaining rib and spinal movements in the elderly, and thus minimise the risk of an opportune infection in a weakened chest. Similar principles apply in the use of chest physiotherapy in hospitals.

The increasing public antagonism to the widespread use of tranquillisers and painkillers has resulted in the search for alternatives. The predominance of orthodox medicine is being challenged by the increasing use of many older therapies, among them homeopathy, acupuncture, hypnosis, and herbal medicine. A steady increase in the use of osteopathy has been seen. In America there are now fifteen accredited colleges of osteopathic medicine of which several are colleges within universities. In Britain osteopathy has recently received favourable comment in the British Medical Association's report on complementary therapies. In Australia there are now two colleges of osteopathy in Victoria and Sydney. In New Zealand there are exciting developments with an 'Osteopathic Bill' to be presented to parliament. Osteopathy is already recognised under the New Zealand Register of Osteopaths Incorporated Act 1978.

A distinct shift of power is taking place between doctors and their patients. More and more people are taking responsibility for their own health and questioning the meaning behind their illness. This is reflected in the rise of 'alternative' or 'complementary' therapies, and the inevitable conflict with orthodox medicine denies the common ground and the integration of different perspectives which form a new whole.

I believe that all forms of medicine and healing complement each other along a healing spectrum with validity for different people at different times. Osteopathy is one indispensable spoke in the wheel of wholeness.

Most diseases are caused by a variety of factors, and more than one form of treatment is usually needed. An alteration in lifestyle or attitude is often necessary to achieve optimum health. I envisage an integration of medical healing in the broadest sense to include spiritual, social, nutritional, environmental, ecological, psychological and physical aspects.

Each person's needs may encompass one or several of these aspects at any one time, and these needs may change at different times. Our value systems, social attitudes, beliefs and conditioning play their part in leading both to our unique illness pattern and to the adoption of a particular treatment form.

Osteopathy is a very important form of treatment, and when used with the highest intentions, in good hands, for the right people, excellent improvement in health results. It is not, however, a panacea for all ills. It does not seek to replace traditional medicine but it does offer a valuable, effective and whole person therapy by which the body condition is stimulated to heal itself. The final common pathway for each individual is his/her own innate ability to get well. Hippocrates, often referred to as the father of medicine, said 'nature is the first physician', which is what osteopathy has always claimed. A physician never cures but *relieves*.

Osteopathy, like orthodox medicine, works with hypotheses and theories expressed through reliable and satisfactory treatment methods. There is a continuous evaluation process of scientific searching for data through research and clinical experience which results in new forms of treatment.

Osteopaths are always willing to discuss new developments and absorb further knowledge in which factual evidence is sought. Only by extending our minds and thoughts to embrace and live the spiritual, physical and environmental aspects of the whole person will we make illness and disease less destructive and move towards actively preventing them.

Osteopathy has always held this deeper philosophy from its origin with Andrew Taylor Still to the present day; its many expressions through the art of manipulation and the science of understanding are dynamic and still growing. I can only show you in this book a glimpse of what osteopathy is all about, but if it can lead to relief of pain and healthy improvement in your life or in another's it will have done its work.

CHRIS BELSHAW
Guildford, 1987

1 *What is Osteopathy?*

Osteopathy is the law of mind over matter and motion.
ANDREW TAYLOR STILL, 1892

Osteopathy is not just a form of manipulation, clicking bones and joints back into place. It is not replacing 'slipped discs'. Neither is it a series of steps, like commands for a computer program, which must be followed to remove symptoms of pain and distress. In common with all healing systems it involves the interaction of two people, osteopath and patient, with the aim of improving the patient's wellbeing. This depends on the attitude, skills and experience of the osteopath, and the attitude and trust of the patient.

The philosophy behind osteopathy is concerned with the whole person, how various parts of our body affect each other, and how emotions and attitudes can affect our physical body, while our lifestyles, both at work and play, affect our health. It is a system of health care that emphasizes the belief in the body's own healing potential. By restoring our own physiological self-regulating mechanisms with osteopathic treatment we can find a way of releasing that healing power. This recognition and encouragement of the healing power within us lies behind the use of other therapies, among them homeopathy, herbal medicine and naturopathy. Sadly orthodox medicine has moved away considerably from this important truth.

SCIENCE AND ART

Osteopathy requires and follows both a scientific and artistic approach. Science provides the basis of osteopathy through knowledge of anatomy, our circulatory and nervous systems and how these systems interact with our environment. On the

I

artistic side the importance of touch is fundamental. This is expressed in the subtlety of an innumerable number of manual techniques for moving joints, freeing the skull bones, stretching ligaments, stimulating circulation, and affecting reflexes. Those who have an intuitive ability in the art of touch have a special gift of nature beyond what is learnt.

AIM OF TREATMENT

The aim of treatment is to achieve a balance and harmony in the body: for joints to regain their normal position and movement in the back and limbs; muscles to be balanced; posture improved; circulation restored; elimination of waste body fluids encouraged; breathing improved; and the ability to relax made easier. The result is a feeling of wellbeing that creates energy for living – and we could all do with more energy!

In applying the principles of osteopathy to treatment needed for any one individual the osteopath's most important ability is to understand what a patient's tissues are expressing. In the same way that a trained mechanic can tell what is wrong with a car, or a surveyor that subsidence has occurred, a trained osteopath interprets the messages and signals of the body to make a diagnosis. Through a combination of listening to details of the complaint, looking, and particularly through touch, he or she will apply knowledge to say what is wrong. It is mainly through the use of the hands that treatment is given and also shown to be completed.

The healing forces, although incompletely understood, are undoubtedly present within all of us and act to bring about change. Healing often demands our time and energy and involves our deepest emotions – feelings that may be buried deep in our minds or consciousness. Sometimes an emotional release of crying or unexplained tiredness after treatment is followed by improved benefit.

The emotional, mental and spiritual aspects of ourselves are focused through our physical body as health or disease. By recognizing these aspects we do not remove the importance of understanding and treating, in the more orthodox way, specific pathological processes of infection, degeneration and accidents that damage our body and cause pain and disability. It is rather seeking to acknowledge that these processes themselves can be linked to further deeper causes that may need to be removed to achieve good health. These deeper causes lie within our thoughts and feelings – some we will be aware of, while others lie deep in our subconscious. For example, there was a woman suffering from migraine whose condition was improved but not cured with treatment, and who suddenly expressed the real reason for her migraines; she was still upset about her husband's affair nineteen years before and had not yet been able to forgive him.

A SYSTEM WITHIN MEDICINE

Anatomical, physiological and biological knowledge, in common with conventional medicine, are the building blocks of osteopathy. These are not distinct systems of medicine but part of the same whole. The trained osteopath applies this knowledge to detect the difference between body tissues of skin, muscles, ligaments etc., both when these are normal, and when affected by injury, strain or disease. He or she knows what is normal and therefore can detect the abnormal. Osteopathy is a system of health care that has expanded and developed over the years as our knowledge of the functions and behaviour of the human body has grown. The emphasis is that of the link between a person's pain, disability and symptoms to faulty function of the body structures such as joints, muscles and tendons. This contrasts with the conventional medical approach that attempts to link pain and symptoms to specific structural damage confirmed by tests such as blood analysis and X-rays, from which a name for the problem is given – for example, the diagnosis of osteoarthritis in the lower spine or cervical spondylosis (wear and tear in the neck). However, doctors will admit that in most back pain a definite physical cause cannot always be proved with these tests, so inappropriate drug therapy or possibly surgery may be used. Osteopathy looks at these diagnostic labels in a different way by assessing the body's various reactions to resist the particular injury or disease. A range of manual and other techniques are then used to

3

encourage our own natural ability to recover. In this way osteopathy can be used on its own or successfully combined with orthodox treatment.

Osteopathy concerns itself with the whole person within his or her environment. The osteopath is *health*-oriented as well as *disease*-oriented. Treatment is aimed at the *patient with the disease* and not the disease alone. Good health needs, among other things, individual responsibility, a political and social environment that encourages a healthy lifestyle, an adequate diet, exercise, emotional satisfaction and a positive feeling of self-worth.

A significant part of osteopathy deals with the movement patterns of the joints of the back, arms and legs together with their muscular and ligament attachments, and their effect on what we can (function) or cannot do (dysfunction). A growing part of osteopathy is the use of cranial techniques which apply osteopathic principles to the diagnosis and treatment of the cranium (the skull bones that surround and protect our brain). Head injuries both at birth and later in life can produce many local and distant symptoms which will benefit from osteopathic techniques applied to the skull bones. More about this later in the chapter.

Osteopathy deals directly with the state of the easily reached body tissues of skin, muscles, joints etc. that have caused symptoms of pain and disruption. By examination through observation and touch, combined with placing the body in certain positions, osteopaths aim to detect those areas of the body that show tension, spasm, restriction, excess movement or positions of compensation. These body reactions are always observed in relation to the normal range that might be expected for each person whether child or adult. Knowledge of the ageing process and any disease process is taken into account when assessing the likely amount and type of treatment.

I am always mindful of those people who say 'Well, what can you expect at my age?' or 'I don't expect you can help much, I'm just wearing out', because I believe a lot *can* be done to help those people live more comfortably using gentle osteopathic treatment, and encouraging certain adaptations in lifestyle and change of attitudes. Don't give up if you are told there is nothing more that can be done for you. Any one doctor, nurse or therapist won't know all the possible ways of healing. Talk with your friends, look up some information, get a second opinion. Trust yourself a little more. Think positive.

CAUSES OF DISEASE AND INJURY

Typically, we see the cause of disease as coming from *outside* ourselves, or as happening to us. We 'catch' a cold, we 'go down with pneumonia', we are 'struck by' a heart attack or we had 'bad luck' being involved in a road traffic accident. Yes, viruses and bacteria do invade our bodies to produce illness, and anyone can break a leg in an accident. Likewise we often strain our backs by lifting something awkwardly. Most of us know of someone who has strained their back through lifting, possibly when angry. But what about our condition when we get a cold or severe infection? We are usually overtired, not eating properly, working too hard or inappropriately, or emotionally upset.

Those who are gardeners know that the condition of the soil is crucial to a healthy plant, and no matter what care is given to the plant above ground, if something is wrong with the soil the plant is less likely to remain healthy. Top sports people pay as much, if not more, attention to their inner state of mind as to physical fitness – they 'psych' themselves up to do well. Similarly, healthy bodies depend on a balance between our inner thoughts and emotions and our outer environment. If these are out of balance, so to speak, we are then open to the effects of organisms and accidents from outside. Louis Pasteur, who discovered micro-organisms, claimed towards the end of his life that if he could live over again he would study the environment in which the organisms thrive, namely the soil to the gardener, inner thoughts and feelings to the human.

In osteopathic teaching, repeated manual or machine-produced manipulation will not always result in cure on its own if other continuing factors (both internal and external) are not recognized and removed or coped with in some way. By internal I mean our thoughts, feelings, attitudes and expectations; by external, factors like posture, work, accidents,

5

relationships etc. Both internal and external aspects interlink so that usually one is not present without the other. For example, if we experience an unhappy relationship or a boring job our feelings will respond and might (if not otherwise expressed) result in tense muscles, a sore back or headaches. Of course these interactions are complex and open to different interpretations but the links are there nevertheless. However, the very complexity of such links means that self-diagnosis is difficult, even if we accept that the mental, emotional and physical are interdependent. It is very difficult for us to accept that we might have some responsibility for our illness, but if we can then it also means we can take the responsibility for getting better.

A man once came to me for treatment of a painful low back. He was the foreman in a small factory run by a rather retiring yet authoritarian man who kept in the background and did not relate to his staff. My patient was expected to deal with the men, do the hiring and firing and general administrative duties to the extent that he felt he was really running the factory. Although this may have suited some people, he also felt that he had no support or help from his boss. The pressure was too much for him and he reacted by straining his back. He needed direct osteopathic manipulation, but he also needed to deal with his feelings about his boss by talking them over.

Osteopathy therefore concerns itself with the underlying cause or causes, as well as physical aches and pain in the joints and muscles. Are we using our bodies correctly when lifting, carrying, doing housework, or specific jobs, enjoying hobbies? Does our physical strength match our job? Are we making repetitive movements, particularly twisting and bending, that produce a strain on our tissues at work or in sport? Are we under emotional stress in our family with spouse, children, in-laws or parents? Has there been some sudden shift in life's circumstances with which we find it difficult to cope such as unemployment, the death of someone close to us, an affair, a job move, an examination failure, divorce, becoming a step-parent? Often there is delay between the life event and the development of a physical complaint. Have we just too much to do and need to reorganize our lives? Do we have enough relaxation? What about our diet? There are many more questions we might ask

6

about our lifestyle and its effect on our physical health.

CAN WE DEFINE OSTEOPATHY?

It will have become clear by now that a simple definition of osteopathy is not possible. Osteopathy is not a fixed concept with definite limits, but a dynamic expanding one which continues to grow as man's awareness of the human potential in health and disease increases. To this end it is a healing system that uses the body's own natural resources to lead to cure and harmony within the body mechanism, always seeking to apply and understand the scientific knowledge that is available at any one time. The most obvious manifestation of osteopathy is its use of manipulation, and to many medical and lay people this has probably been their only understanding of it.

Osteopathy is thus a form of manipulation but one that has developed and is still developing its specific ways of handling and treating. It is the *intention* behind a manipulative treatment that makes it unique. In osteopathy this is the restoration of joint and tissue abnormalities that leads to normal functioning of the body which is also encouraged to use its own recuperative powers. The skill is in the diagnostic and therapeutic ability of touch and the application of manipulative forces in the right dose, in the right place and at the right time for each particular individual.

CRANIAL TECHNIQUES

The cranium is made up of the bones that form our skull which in turn surrounds and protects our brain. In the 1920s William Sutherland, a teacher at the Kirksville Osteopathic College, had a sudden inspiration. He had stopped to look at a collection of skull bones in the College when he suddenly thought of the possible movement of the skull bones and their effect on the rest of the body. In order to prove or disprove this strange idea he set about studying it. He found that the skull bones were designed for rhythmic movement linked to the base of the spine by the dura mater, the protective sleeve covering the spinal cord as it lies within the backbone.

The skull is formed by several separate pieces of bone which allow for slight movement between them. This makes it possible for a newborn baby's head to come more easily through the birth canal. All mothers will know of the soft spot at the front of their baby's head at birth (fontanelle), the bones closing over shortly after birth. In the same way that a builder or plumber uses silastic as a seal between a bath and the wall to allow some slight movement, the sutures joining the skull bones together allow for extremely small movements of hundredths of a millimetre. Sutherland experimented on himself to test this minimal movement and created small distortions in his own skull to the extent that his wife saw her husband go through startling changes of personality as the brain tissues were affected. He did this by applying pressure to his head using various devices and carefully recording all the changes produced. His knowledge of anatomy and osteopathic manipulation enabled him to correct all the changes he made on himself. Sutherland named this system the *primary respiratory mechanism*, because it is essentially the powerhouse of the body that gives life and includes the brain and spinal cord with the skull bones above and the sacrum at the base of the spine below. The *secondary respiratory mechanism* is made up of our lungs, diaphragm and chest wall which quietly get on with the job of breathing – we know all about it when we get out of breath running for the bus or after a hard game of tennis.

Life is characterized by rhythms, movements and patterns. The tides rise and fall, night follows day, salmon leap up rivers to spawn. We have our own rhythms that maintain our body in balance and health, among these a normal physiological pattern of the skull bones and spinal cord just like the normal working activity of the joints and muscles. The skill of the osteopath using cranial techniques is in using these patterns for diagnosis and treatment.

A whole range of problems around the head and neck as well as in distant parts of the body can have their origin within the skull. These may include headaches, high blood pressure, skin rashes, pain in the face and problems with the teeth. Due to slight pressure on nerves originating in the skull possible heart complaints, stomach ulcer and irritable bowel syndrome may

8

also have their origin here. This all seems highly unusual, and is by no means generally known about or accepted by the medical profession at large, but for those working in the field the reality is already present.

The cranial aspect of osteopathy is a potent tool in treatment and I believe will continue to expand in its application and usefulness over the years to come. Cranial treatment is covered more fully in chapter 2.

COMPARATIVE MANIPULATION

I have been asked many times the difference between osteopathy and chiropractic – and similarly, though less often, physiotherapy. I will attempt to give some answers that I hope give a balanced view. All these approaches to health care essentially aim to relieve distress and discomfort and regain normal physiological function. It is the extent of the philosophy behind each, and the scope and skills needed to practise them that are different.

Chiropractic and osteopathy both use highly developed skills of sight and touch in diagnosis of abnormal spinal problems and both aim to restore joints to normal, thus removing symptoms. However, the method and rationale in achieving these aims is different, and each is likely to appeal to different types of people.

Chiropractic lays most emphasis on the joint itself, while osteopathy lays equal emphasis on the joint and adjacent muscles, fascia (fibrous supporting tissues) and ligaments that make up each spinal vertebra. All areas of the spine are interdependent in functioning as a whole unit, though perhaps chiropractic lends more weight to the neck region in restoring balance to the whole unit. In osteopathy the attainment of a level pelvic mechanism at the base of the spine is felt essential in maintaining equilibrium both above and below in the legs. In practice both ends of the spine are equally important. In diagnosis chiropractors lay major emphasis on X-ray evidence in directing their attention to spinal derangements, whereas the osteopath is more aware of his/her diagnostic skill of touch in following the dynamic changes of the body tissues as they begin to work properly and return to normal.

9

The ways of giving manipulation are often in contrast. Chiropractic uses sharp, short thrusting pressure on the spine with the patient face down on an elaborate couch which lowers him/her from the standing to lying position. Osteopathy uses treatment with a more rhythmical and gentle pressure on the whole body including the spine. Both need careful application to bring about change. Chiropractic treatment is generally more uncomfortable than that used in osteopathy.

Physiotherapy also uses some manipulative techniques, but they comprise a relatively small part of a physiotherapist's training in the United Kingdom and are mainly different from those used in osteopathy. Physiotherapists follow the medical model of symptoms leading to a named diagnosis based on structural pathological changes. They use a range of 'physical' therapies including machines of various types applying heat, and various electrical wave stimuli such as shortwave diathermy and ultrasound. They concentrate on rehabilitation after surgery to facilitate breathing, muscle strength and movement. Some physiotherapists in private practice concentrate on manipulation and acquire some chiropractic and osteopathic techniques.

Despite some overlap in aims, theory and the application of several manipulative techniques, the distinction is readily apparent between osteopathy and both chiropractic and physiotherapy. Nevertheless each of the three disciplines, among others, is necessary for health care. The important thing is for a patient to see a trained and competent practitioner whom he/she can trust and who restores them to health.

2 Can Osteopathy Help Me?

To find health should be the object of the doctor.
Anyone can find disease.
ANDREW TAYLOR STILL

Find it, fix it and leave it alone.
ANDREW TAYLOR STILL

The first question about osteopathy is often 'What does it treat and can it cure *my* complaint?' Since you may have turned to this chapter first to see if your complaint is listed, I will summarize what osteopathy is. However, do read Chapter 1 for a fuller picture.

Osteopathy is a system of health care based on scientific enquiry about how and why the body reacts to disease and injury. It seeks to understand the many interconnections between the body structures, and believes in our self-regulating and healing abilities. Osteopaths treat by various types of manipulation with the hands on the most easily reached parts of the body: our joints, muscles and the fascial membrane that surrounds our nerves and blood vessels as a protective envelope. Treatment can also affect deeper body organs such as stomach, bowel or lung by way of known nerve connections. Osteopathy is aware of the value of a sensible diet, a good posture, the benefits of exercise and aims to prevent problems returning.

LOW BACK PAIN AND SCIATICA

It is probable that some 80 per cent of us will at one time or another experience back pain. That adds up to many millions of people. Fortunately, for most of us this will be a single episode or two with no lasting effects. Others of us will not be so lucky. We will get repeated attacks of back pain, but only a very small percentage, around 1 per cent, will need more drastic treatment in the form of surgery. Even surgery has improved with more accurate diagnosis from special types of X-ray examination and surgical procedures using high-powered binoculars and very small instruments – microsurgery. Recovery here is more rapid because the surgery is less disruptive.

Osteopathy is particularly effective in helping the great majority of people with low back pain which provides about 50 per cent of an osteopath's work. The low back area together with the hips and thighs are of crucial importance in keeping our upright posture, and failure to hold this position is one cause of pain. Other causes are hereditary, repeated lifting or overstretching, and falls or accidents. The back and hips also provide a stable and secure base or support for many movements, from walking and turning to playing sport of all kinds. The hips and pelvis act as a central point of balance in our body, so injury or pain in these areas is extremely restrictive, limiting and depressing. Treatment will improve blood flow, relax muscles, free any joints that are not moving properly and restore normal nerve activity.

Treatment is effective for so-called 'slipped discs', arthritis in the low back or hip, and pain down the leg, commonly known as sciatica. Sciatica is not a cause of pain but only a description of pain felt along the pathway of the sciatic nerve that extends down the back of the leg to the ankle and foot. It is usually caused from the lower part of the back.

In my experience the range of medical words and labels used by doctors, nurses and other health workers are not always clear in their meaning to a patient. Because of fear and misunderstanding of words like 'arthritis', 'slipped disc' and 'trapped nerve' always ask your doctor or osteopath to clarify their meaning for your particular condition.

Several structures in the back produce pain when irritated or disrupted in some way, and these include skin, joints, bone, muscle, ligaments, blood vessels as well as the nerves themselves (Figures 2.1 and 2.2). A message is registered by small nerve endings which then carry this message along nerve pathways to the brain via the spinal cord, the main nerve inside the backbone, and is felt as pain.

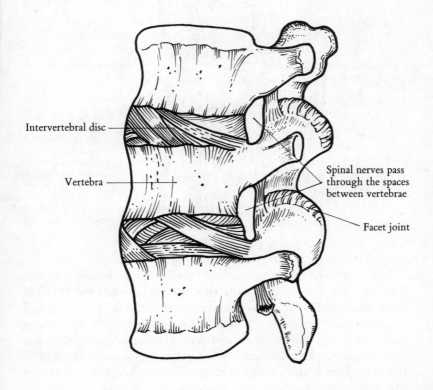

Intervertebral disc

Vertebra

Spinal nerves pass
through the spaces
between vertebrae

Facet joint

Figure 2.1 THE SPINE *(side view)*

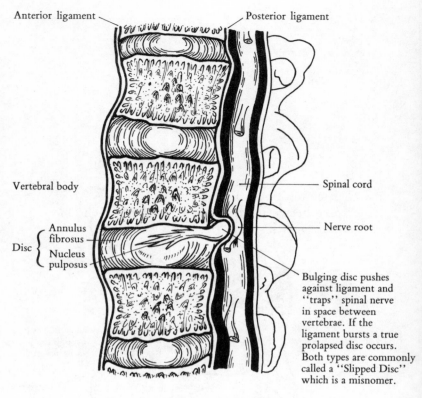

Anterior ligament

Posterior ligament

Vertebral body

Spinal cord

Disc {
  Annulus fibrosus
  Nucleus pulposus
}

Nerve root

Bulging disc pushes against ligament and "traps" spinal nerve in space between vertebrae. If the ligament bursts a true prolapsed disc occurs. Both types are commonly called a "Slipped Disc" which is a misnomer.

Figure 2.2 THE SPINE *(cross-section view)*

For example a blow to the body will produce bruising in the skin or pain deeper down in the muscle. A strained joint is particularly common. The nerve endings in the skin, muscle and joint capsule respectively will send messages via the nerve pathways to the spinal cord and then the brain where they are represented as the experience of pain, stiffness, etc. The skill of the osteopath is to find out what part of the body is producing the pain, give treatment if suitable, or refer the patient to someone who can help if osteopathy is not indicated (in Chapter 6 medical problems not suitable for osteopathy are listed).

The word 'slipped disc', although widely used, is a misnomer that incorrectly describes what happens. Adjacent vertebrae (Figures 2.3 and 2.4) in the back are separated by discs that act like shock absorbers (Figure 2.5). The discs are formed of an outer harder fibrous material that surrounds a much softer substance containing a high proportion of water. The whole disc softens as we age and becomes less resilient and less able to absorb shocks. The water content is also reduced in ageing and accounts for the shrinkage and loss of height in some old people. As shown in Figure 2.2 the disc can:

(1) bulge;
(2) prolapse totally with a tear of the supporting ligament.

Both these conditions will press or 'trap' the nerve where it lies in the space between the adjacent vertebrae. The bulge will usually heal with rest and treatment, but total prolapse will usually require surgery to remove the offending bits of tissue. Remember only a very small number of people overall need an operation.

Other factors, such as bone disease, growth of extra bone, tumours or arthritis, can interfere with the nerves in the spine. If these are suspected from the history and/or X-rays a further medical opinion will be sought. The facet joint (see Figure 2.2) is similar to other joints in the body and can be affected by a wide range of disease. However, pain from the mechanical blockage of these joints is quite usual and is very well treated with osteopathic manipulation.

The two large pelvic joints, the sacroiliac joints, are a common source of pain from twists and strains (Figure 2.6). They can also be affected by certain types of arthritis. They are big joints and transfer the weight of our upper body through the hip joints to our feet, acting as a pivot. The osteopath will lay particular emphasis on having a level pelvis. A short leg is a common finding in low back pain, perhaps a true short leg, from birth or a response to trouble in the back which tilts one hip higher than the other. Sometimes a small raise for the shoe is recommended for a true short leg. But if the leg difference is a result of problems in the back and pelvis, treatment will usually produce legs of equal length again. Other more serious medical conditions, most usually from hip disease in children and following hip surgery in adults, can give a short leg, and

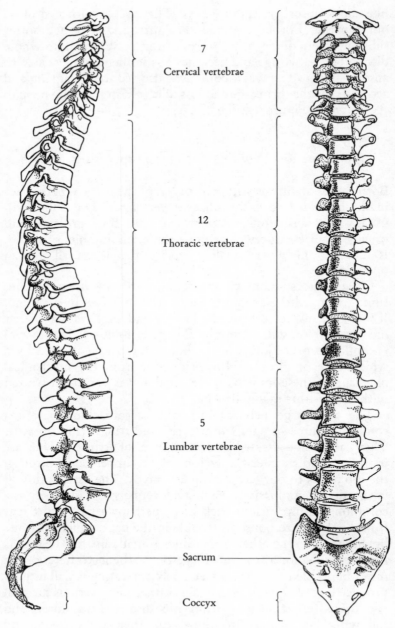

7

Cervical vertebrae

12

Thoracic vertebrae

5

Lumbar vertebrae

———————— Sacrum ————————

Coccyx

Figure 2.3 THE SPINE

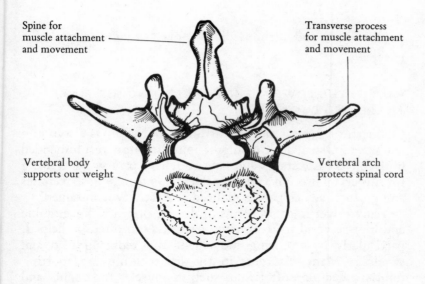

Spine for
muscle attachment
and movement

Transverse process
for muscle attachment
and movement

Vertebral body
supports our weight

Vertebral arch
protects spinal cord

Figure 2.4 FUNCTIONS OF A SPINAL VERTEBRA

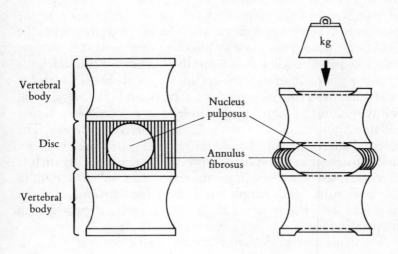

Vertebral
body

Disc

Vertebral
body

Nucleus
pulposus

Annulus
fibrosus

kg

Figure 2.5 INTERVERTEBRAL DISC SHOWING CUSHIONING
VALUE OF THE NUCLEUS PULPOSUS

17

paediatricians and orthopaedic doctors are familiar with the problem.

PAIN IN THE LOWER LIMBS, INCLUDING HIP, KNEE, ANKLE AND FOOT

Osteoarthritis (wear and tear arthritis) of the hip is a common condition. Osteopathic manipulation is strongly recommended both for its early stages and later to relieve pain while waiting for surgery. Through a series of stretching techniques, exercises and postural advice pain is reduced and activity maintained.

Many lower limb problems of diverse origin in knee, ankle and foot respond to treatment. Arthritis can often be helped, particularly by restoring movement and reducing pain and swelling. Many disorders in the lower limbs are sporting injuries affecting soft tissues such as muscles, ligaments and tendons. These respond well to osteopathy. In sporting injuries co-operation with sports trainers or coaches regarding training and technique is essential to prevent the return of problems.

Successful management of these lower limb problems, particularly the feet, brings significant benefit to posture, ease of standing and walking. Our feet symbolically provide the platform or base on which we stand in life, together with the facility to move from place to place; so they need to provide a firmness and flexibility to last our lives. They are the recipients of many minor injuries from sprains to simple abuse: with the ankle they are a common site for fractures; and the several small joints within the foot are affected by a wide range of arthritic inflammation, and by pressure from incorrect footwear. The feet and ankles are also the site for referred pain caused by bony maladjustment in the spine and pressure on nerve roots such as in a prolapsed disc. Foot problems themselves will also result in low back pain. Many people put up with foot discomfort in the mistaken belief nothing can be done, yet osteopathy can frequently help.

The manipulative element of treatment is often used alone, or after appropriate surgery or drug therapy if indicated. The natural stresses on the feet during life result in slight stiffness in joints, tension in muscles and sluggish circulation, all of which

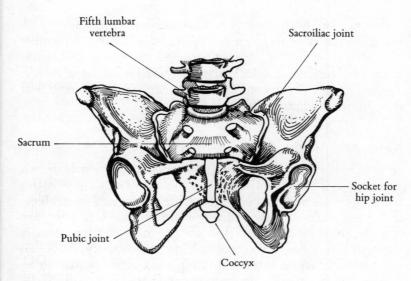

Fifth lumbar vertebra

Sacroiliac joint

Sacrum

Socket for hip joint

Pubic joint

Coccyx

PELVIS FROM FRONT

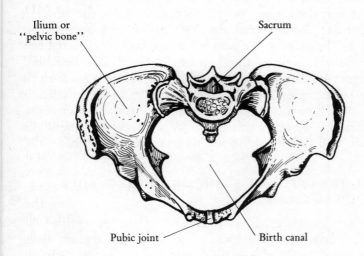

Ilium or "pelvic bone"

Sacrum

Pubic joint

Birth canal

PELVIS FROM ABOVE

Figure 2.6 THE PELVIS

19

are improved with osteopathic manipulative techniques. A wonderful sense of freedom and lightness is felt after treatment – 'walking on air' is often mentioned by patients. Regular preventive treatment is particularly required for those of middle age and above. When combined with chiropody an overall foot care programme can be followed.

NECK AND UPPER BACK PAIN

'A pain in the neck' is an expression some of us use to describe a person who is being a nuisance or troublesome. For those with a real pain in the neck and upper back life can be very unpleasant. It is soon realized how much we use our neck in everyday activity. It is no wonder that we get into trouble, usually through lifting heavy weights or lifting awkwardly, from bad posture both when inactive (sitting) and when active doing various jobs like gardening, or in playing a wide range of sports.

Most commonly the neck is sprained with locking of the joints and limited movement. More severe is whiplash injury from a car accident. Osteopathy is successfully used for both. Don't be surprised when your osteopath looks at the joints in the upper back between the shoulder blades. It is because this area can be the cause of the pain felt in the neck. Restricted ribs are often a source of pain and will be checked. The neck and upper back also cause pain felt in the arm and hand. As with all problems the osteopath will use his skill to find out what is wrong and whether osteopathic treatment is suitable on its own or combined with other treatment. When it is not suitable the osteopath will always advise you to go to your doctor.

PAIN IN THE UPPER LIMBS INCLUDING SHOULDER, ELBOW, WRIST AND HAND

Pain in the joints, muscles, ligaments of the upper limbs – shoulder, elbow, wrist and hand whether diagnosed as arthritis, trapped nerve, muscle strain, inflammation, fibrositis or brachalgia – will commonly respond favourably to osteopathic manipulation. Obviously acute infection, loss of use or fracture are not suitable for treatment. Three of the most often seen conditions are tendonitis of the shoulder ('frozen shoulder'), tennis elbow and carpal tunnel syndrome (trapped nerve at the wrist). Because of the nature of the reflex nerve links in the body the osteopath will direct his or her attention to the neck and upper spine, as well as the actual area of pain, when treating these problems. This concept of referred pain is discussed in Chapter 7. Persistent pain from carpal tunnel syndrome will need a small surgical operation.

MIGRAINE AND HEADACHES

All migraines are headaches, but not all headaches are migraine. Migraine is diagnosed on a distinct pain pattern. Headache, mainly related to tension, is one of the commonest complaints that responds to treatment. A large number of migraines or simple headaches are related to problems in the skull and neck, and manipulative treatment either alone or combined with other treatments such as acupuncture or diet change will often be successful.

In common with many medical problems, migraine is caused by several linking factors such as tension, more severe stress, circulation changes, hormonal changes, injury and strains to the head and neck and reaction to food. The assessment of the most significant causal factor is part of the osteopath's skill in helping a patient achieve optimum health.

I recently saw a 40-year-old man who had suffered persistent migraine since a teenager. He had mainly used drug therapy with only minimal improvement. A bad fall at the age of 11 had resulted in slight displacement of the neck joints with reflex pain felt in the head. After treating him weekly for a month, normal function was restored and his migraine disappeared.

ARTHRITIS

The words 'arthritis' and 'rheumatism' are commonly used by the lay public as meaning a specific disease or problem associated with pain and stiffness in joints and muscles. However, these only touch the tip of the iceberg that represents a wide range of conditions causing arthritis. Several different types of therapy are therefore needed, apart from simple pain relief. Arthritis generally causes inflammation and degeneration of joints. Inflammation is the process of cellular activity in a joint (or other tissue) that produces swelling, redness, pain and restriction. Degeneration is simply described as 'wear and tear' in our joints as we grow older, but of course this process is more complex.

The many causes of arthritis in joints include infections both bacterial (such as streptococcal) and viral (rubella or German measles), rheumatic fever, gout, blood disorders such as haemophilia, rheumatoid arthritis of unknown cause, and occupational arthritis (such as wicket keeper's fingers). The list is a long one. Many conditions, such as arthritis caused by infection, are unsuitable for osteopathic treatment. But when in doubt a good osteopath will always ask you to see your own doctor.

The common form of osteoarthritis – 'wear and tear' – will respond well to osteopathic treatment with its encouragement of movement, freeing of stuck joints, relaxing of muscles and stimulation of the circulation. A wide number of joints are affected. Apart from the neck and low back, the hip and knee are most often in trouble, mainly because they are weight-bearing joints and take a lot of strain. Exercise will be encouraged to strengthen the muscles that act on the joints. Prolonged rest will be discouraged and reduction of overweight discussed. Occupational habits may need to be changed. The use of osteopathic treatment can coexist quite happily with medicines such as painkillers (analgesics) and anti-inflammatory tablets (NSAIDs).

The use of drug treatment is more usual in rheumatoid arthritis than osteoarthritis. Gentle osteopathic treatment can also ease the stiffness and pain of rheumatic joints particularly when the disease is less active or burnt out. When very acute and painful local treatment should be avoided. Active and continuing joint disease must receive specialist advice because joint problems have many causes for which most osteopaths will not have had training and experience. This in no way lessens an osteopath's skill but recognizes the skill of other specialists.

TREATING CHILDREN

Children of all ages respond well to osteopathy for a range of problems from feet to skull. Apart from the more general strains and stresses, several specific problems need to be mentioned, including asthma and other chest complaints, spastic paralysis, foot deformities, mental handicap, scoliosis. Babies with certain head or face deformities from birth can benefit from cranial osteopathic treatment to the skull. There are specialist children's clinics at both the British School of Osteopathy and the Maidstone School of Osteopathy. They will advise and treat these and many other problems. The addresses are listed at the back of the book (p. 101).

USE IN PREGNANCY

During pregnancy women can suffer low back pain from several causes. These include: a silent lesion or old back problem preceding pregnancy which may then flare up due to the extra weight of the growing baby; postural imbalance; a fall or strain; or vascular, the natural increase in circulation overfills the veins producing an ache. It is possible to use osteopathic treatment throughout pregnancy and pain need not be a problem. So don't suffer when something can be done. Period pains can also be reduced by treatment to the lower spine.

OSTEOPATHY AND SURGERY

Osteopathy is successfully employed in aiding recovery after surgery, particularly of joint surgery. It is also useful in helping lung and heart function following general surgery. This link with surgery is evident in the United States where osteopathic doctors are fully trained in all branches of medicine with the additional knowledge of osteopathic principles and skills to use in treatment. However, in Britain the majority of osteopaths are not medically trained (except for the doctor osteopaths trained at the London College of Osteopathic Medicine), so the opportunities for a more widespread use in this manner are limited. Historical development has also resulted in osteopaths being omitted from National Health Service hospitals.

Traditionally our physiotherapists provide this rehabilitation after surgery, and although a few are aware of the osteopathic concepts and use them, the majority of physiotherapists do not.

GENERAL MEDICAL COMPLAINTS

The above limitation is also evident in the acceptance and use of osteopathy in Britain to treat disease of internal organs. In most instances osteopathy is not even considered relevant for such disease. No true osteopath would deny necessary drugs or surgery which, quite rightly, provide our main line of therapy for many people. Tremendous advances have been made in understanding drugs and their usage, anaesthetics have improved beyond all recognition and surgical techniques continue to develop all the time. Nursing developments complement these changes. Nevertheless the positive part that osteopathic therapy can play in the spectrum of treatment methods must be recognized and used responsibly. For example, chest infections can recover more quickly combining manipulative therapy with antibiotics, as treatment helps breathing and circulation. Certain types of asthma will respond favourably both to general treatment of the neck and upper spine, and to cranial treatment. This does not deny specific removal of allergens and treatment directed to relaxation and other coping mechanisms, all of which may be necessary.

Hayfever and sinus trouble can be distressing and painful. The increased secretion of fluid comes from the tissue lining the nose and sinuses which is swollen and inflamed. General treatment applied to the skull and face is often very successful and avoids the constant use of tablets and sprays which sometimes aggravate rather than help the problem.

Attention to the rib cage is beneficial in many chest conditions such as asthma and bronchitis. The normal rib movement during breathing can become restricted because of these conditions and also from twists or overstretching in sport or other activity. Treatment improves movement and position which is essential for good breathing and circulation. Pain is therefore eliminated. Older people are particularly likely to sag in the rib cage which then reduces normal breathing activity and produces muscular aches in the shoulders and upper back. Treatment restores the correct movement and gives relief from discomfort, and that aimed at relaxing the diaphragm aids these chest complaints by ensuring a free flow of body fluids in those arteries, veins and lymphatic channels that pass through the diaphragm from chest to abdomen.

Pain in the stomach from indigestion or ulcers is significantly helped. Persistent chronic conditions of irritable bowel, constipation, heartburn and vague feelings of tiredness and illhealth can be traced to inappropriate nerve reflex activity from joint dysfunction in the spine and/or blockage of fluid circulation of blood or body cells. Removing this nerve activity or fluid blockage by osteopathy leads to improved physiological function with reduction and hopefully removal of symptoms. The links between the spinal joints and muscles and disease of internal body organs is covered more fully in Chapter 7.

High blood pressure is a common and often severe disability related to increased narrowing and thus resistance in the arterial blood vessels. The centre in the brain for controlling blood pressure is affected by cranial techniques. The use of cranial osteopathy together with the release of tension in the upper neck is beneficial in lowering the pressure. The longer high blood pressure is present and the more severe it becomes, the less likely that osteopathy will be beneficial.

The skull contains, supports and protects many of the vital centres that control our physiological function throughout the body such as breathing, heart rate, blood flow, digestive function, glandular secretion and muscular activity. Several chronic persistent problems that have either failed to show an organic cause, or are in themselves treated unsatisfactorily by currently known treatments, will improve with treatment from those who are properly trained in cranial techniques. These may include many so-called neurotic patients, some mental neuroses and personality problems, some respiratory diseases and cerebral palsy.

DENTAL PROBLEMS INCLUDING FACIAL PAIN

Cranial technique has a significant role to play treating many problems in dentistry. This comes about through the understanding that structural problems in the skull cause disturbed function in the head, face and jaw.

Developmental problems usually related to trauma during or after birth can alter bony plates in the skull leading to deformities in the jaw, face and teeth. Incorrect positioning of upper and lower teeth and bite problems are more likely an effect of facial deformities rather than a cause, and much of the difficult and skilful reconstruction work of dentists would become less needed if osteopathic correction techniques were used first. These techniques will release tight meningeal membranes around the brain and help to mould warped skull plates back towards their normal position. The cranial bones that make up the skull are known to move very slightly and are not totally rigid. Trauma such as blows to the face, including the common extraction of teeth, can lead to restriction of facial and cranial bones, resulting in facial pain, overbiting, circulation disturbances with possible effects in the ears and eyes. The possible damaging effects of birth forceps on the face and skull of newly born babies needs further study and understanding.

Many jaw joint problems resulting in facial neuralgia, headaches and arthritis can be traced back to structural lesions in the skull. And the fitting of dentures may be more satisfactorily completed following osteopathic treatment to the skull.

Only a very few dentists in Britain have acknowledged the usefulness of osteopathic treatment for dental and facial problems, and some now integrate both approaches to the benefit of their patients. Further opportunities must be created for osteopathic manipulative treatment to be combined with that of dentists and orthodontists. It will produce a whole new development area for dentistry with many satisfied patients.

VERTIGO, TINNITUS, DIZZINESS

Cranial osteopathy is strongly indicated in many people suffering from vertigo and dizziness. Slight shifts of the temporal bone at the side of the skull alter the orientation of the semicircular canals, the organs of balance situated in the middle ear, resulting in these distressing symptoms. Tinnitus may also respond to early treatment of the temporal bones and many facial pains will also benefit, for example, trigeminal neuralgia. Some cases of Bell's palsy also respond to cranial manipulation, particularly if trauma, commonly dental extraction, was the cause.

CAN CRANIAL TECHNIQUES WITHIN OSTEOPATHY BE USED FOR OTHER PROBLEMS?

Let us be reminded at this point that the integrity of anatomical structures in any part of the body is a prime necessity for normal healthy functioning of that part. Osteopathic cranial theory has profound significance. Theoretically all problems in the body may have some links to abnormal function of the skull, brain and brain tissues. For example, irritation of cranial nerves is commonly due to bone shifts and increased tension in brain tissues. Many of these, particularly if early treatment is given, will benefit from treatment. With further research and understanding of the brain and skull this form of treatment will undoubtedly expand, but progress needs to be matched by careful assessment and application by highly skilled operators.

UNDERLYING FACTORS IN DISEASE

The bases for many disease states are dependent on the effects on the body of neurological control, of arterial blood supply and venous drainage, and of tissue nutrition; many of these can be treated using osteopathic techniques including those to the cranial mechanism in the skull.

Osteopathic medicine is in the forefront of advancement of knowledge about the human body, its diseased states and treatment to maintain health. Structure and function cannot be separated. Osteopathic philosophy directed through its manipulative therapy is a system which does not *make* the patient well, but helps the patient *achieve* optimum health.

Osteopathic treatment aims to restore and maintain normal physiological function in body tissues. This may include advice about posture, work positions, inappropriate activity; or discussion on emotional upsets, nutrition and exercise. The basic body responses to insult or injury and the resulting tissue changes are well recognized in both medicine and osteopathy. It is in the recognition of the means of restoring to normal function that opinions differ between orthodox medicine and osteopathic medicine. Further discussion of differences can lead to better medicine, although I believe there is more common ground than is generally realized.

Osteopathic principles and treatment need to be more fully appreciated and understood by the medical profession as a whole, and seen not as a threat but as a way forward to bring medicine into the twenty-first century, approaching illness in a more comprehensive manner.

3 Historical Perspective

Man should study and use drugs compounded in his own body.
ANDREW TAYLOR STILL

ANDREW TAYLOR STILL

Osteopathy developed in America towards the end of the last century through the efforts of one man, Andrew Taylor Still (1828 – 1917).

Still was born near Jonesboro, West Virginia, around the period of frontier exploration when the early pioneers opened up the western seaboard. His varied experiences on the frontier and working on his parents' farm and as a millwright taught him many practical skills. His mother was naturally very practical and an excellent homemaker who, in Still's own words, 'made cloth, clothing and pies to perfection'.

His father was a strong man also of many skills – farmer, millwright, doctor and minister; he rode as a circuit-rider around the Missouri countryside with one saddlebag containing his bible and hymn book, the other a wallet full of medicines in sections of cane because bottles were likely to break. Thus armed, his main aim was for the comfort of both body and soul.

As a young man Still worked as a doctor with his father among the Indians in mid-west America. Living close to animals as a boy he almost perfected the knowledge of anatomy from the great book of nature. His skinning of squirrels showed him muscles, nerves and veins. He took a keen interest in bones long before he learned the names given to them scientifically.

A simple incident occurred in Andrew's boyhood which may be said to be his first discovery in the science of osteopathy. One day when he was about ten years old he felt sick with a headache. He made a swing of his father's plough-line between two trees, but his head was too painful for swinging so he let the

29

rope down to about eight inches off the ground and put a blanket over it. He then lay down flat on his back placing his neck against the rope as a swinging pillow. He went to sleep and woke up with the headache gone. He knew nothing of anatomy at that time so did not think how his headache and sick stomach had been cured. Nevertheless this discovery enabled him to use this technique for himself when he felt these spells coming on. It was not until twenty years later that he realized what had happened physiologically – the pressure on the occipital nerves had increased the circulation and relaxed the muscles thus easing the pain.

He became a widower, married a second time and had seven live children, three by his first wife and four by his second. During the political disruption around slavery in the years 1835 – 60 Still remained an ardent abolitionist despite danger to himself as he went about his duties as a doctor. During the slave wars he was a scout surgeon, his surgeon's outfit complete when it contained calomel, quinine, whisky, opium, rags and a knife.

He saw active service during the Civil War which ended in 1865 with victory for the North over the South. He and his family came through the war unscathed, but then a disastrous event overtook his family. Two of his children and one adopted child all died from spinal meningitis despite their doctor's good intentions and care. He felt sure that the doctor's pills and the minister's prayers would save the children, but they didn't. In his grief Still felt that God did not give life simply for the purpose of destroying it prematurely, and this convinced him there was something surer and stronger with which to fight sickness than drugs, and he vowed to search until he found it.

This crisis stands out as an event which determined Still to study and explore the human body. He came to believe that God in all his wisdom was not a guessing God, one who would guess what illness was present and pick a dose of medicine at random; but he believed he was a God of truth who had provided within man's own body all that was needed to combat disease. His study and application of the new science of osteopathy showed him that many factors relevant to health already existed in the human mind and body if only recognized and used. His many successes proved this and laid the foundation for preventive medicine.

He became dissatisfied and later very angry at the 'old-established' theories and treatments which failed to explore the underlying causes and so effect a cure. He himself had followed this path for many years, being content to accept the opinions and customs of older and more experienced physicians. These included an emphasis on symptoms, a requirement to name the disease, and the use of treatments, often through the rule of 'cut and try', which had little success and resulted in a high death rate.

He knew a cause and a cure could be found, but how? He believed that up to a particular point (after which decline is beyond the inner vitality) all diseases are curable by nature's own ingenious remedies, so the solution must be to harness these energies.

Throughout his life the seed of osteopathy had been germinating, starting in the early days when he learnt anatomy by digging up Indian graves and handling and studying the bones. Despite the existence of this information in printed books he followed the poet's dictum 'The greatest study of mankind is man' and dissected numerous bodies. This was only the forerunner of later patterns in medical school anatomy departments.

His passion for physiological truth and a deeper understanding of the body mechanisms took him beyond the narrow confines of the then medical approach. His theories were radical and brought much opposition. He pioneered a more scientific approach and applied careful observation with individual insight.

During the time of Still's discoveries and achievements in America around the late nineteenth century the medical environment was in great upheaval. The few drugs available like morphia and quinine were commonly overused with disastrous results. Surgery was crude and often fatal. In the centres of medical learning the relationship of germs (bacteria and viruses) to disease was not established, the cellular structure of the body not accepted and the nature of the immune system unknown (it is this system of body protection that is destroyed by the AIDs virus). Still was a contemporary of Lister and antisepsis theory, and also Koch who postulated that germs caused certain diseases and who also discovered organisms such as tuberculosis, typhoid, tetanus and diphtheria.

In the late nineteenth century and early twentieth century drug treatment was recognized by physicians of the day as useless for pneumonia. There were no antibiotics. So osteopaths provided a means of direct manipulative treatment on the ribs and joints in the spine which reduced the death rate for pneumonia by increasing the blood supply and improving breathing. The results at the time were considered miraculous. Indeed, Dr C.L. Johnston, who still practises in London, was inspired to train in osteopathy following a cure from pneumonia as a child.

Still was very much an explorer, striving after the truth with little to guide him but his own inner desire to understand illness and use this knowledge to produce health. Like all pioneers he had to overcome opposition to his ideas and theories but that did not stop his enquiry. When he first believed that drugs would not cure disease since they were not specifics he spent twelve years ostracized by his own relatives who gave no assistance or support for his, as they saw it, 'lunatic views'.

He maintained that the basis of all osteopath's work is, first, a thorough knowledge of anatomy; second, it is an understanding of the difference between normal and abnormal. It is essential to be familiar with the normal before approaching the abnormal. Only the minimal force that is necessary should be used in treatment. To work by force with a great number of treatments will only bring discomfort and bruising. In contrast, an intelligent person will soon learn that a soft hand and a gentle move is the way to obtain the desired result.

Still's practical experience as a farmer and millwright led him to compare the human body to a machine that needs constant attention, summed up with his words 'The living person is the engine, nature the engineer and you (the osteopath) the master mechanic.' He laid emphasis on the heart and lungs since a healthy system depends on normal heart and lungs. As an osteopath, to achieve a healthy blood and nerve supply was his first and last duty: 'The rule of the artery is supreme,' he said 'remove the cause which stops or clogs the blood flow or blocks the nerve which controls the blood flow and the blood itself will work the cure.'

Still talked of the importance of the lymphatic system, regarding it as equal to that of the arteries and veins, and of vital importance in flushing away impurities as they accumulate in our tissues. The lymphatics are tubes like veins and arteries which carry waste products from the body organs.

In osteopathic treatment turning attention to the fascia brought great cures. The fascia sheath is a thin fibrous sleeve or membrane which permeates, divides and subdivides all parts of the body surrounding muscles, arteries, veins and lymphatics, and supports a network of nerves around these body tissues. If it becomes trapped, bruised, overstretched, or loses its nutrition pain and other symptoms will arise linked to the organ or part of the body next to the affected fascia. By stimulating the fascia with manipulation the blood supply and nerve messages will return and healing take place. Find and remove the cause, then the effect will disappear, sums up the basic philosophy behind osteopathy. 'Find it, fix it and leave it alone' was Still's famous dictum.

The drugs (medicines) used in the latter part of the nineteenth century were mainly quinine, opium (morphine) and whisky, and it was more a matter of luck than skill that people were cured. Set against this background the cures of osteopathy were not far short of miraculous. Still, however, was not prepared to accept his cures as miracles and was always striving to improve his diagnosis and treatment to know precisely what he was doing. He was particular to avoid any well-worn routine and was uncompromising in seeking the best and precise movement of muscle, bone, ligament and nerve that would allow the body to heal.

He was very much a believer in the link between the spiritual, mental and physical sides of life. He practised holistic medicine long before its present day re-emergence. He was very intuitive, a quick thinker and it was felt by some that he was so gifted a healer using osteopathy that no one else would be able to learn. He did not accept this and strongly maintained that any intelligent person would be able to learn and use osteopathy, that his followers must continue to develop and enlarge it. His three sons, Harry, Charles and Herman, all studied with him and in a few years they had more work than they could cope with. Having reached this point Dr Still then said he must start a school. In 1887 he began to teach a few people, but it was only in 1892, when he felt he had fully established osteopathy on a scientific basis and demonstrated its efficacy, that he consented to organize a school.

Within twenty-five years of the opening of Kirksville in 1894 eight further colleges were active in the United States, each fully equipped with laboratories for study and research with an attached hospital for inpatients. Des Moines, for example, opened in 1898, Philadelphia in 1899, and Chicago in 1900 and are still fine institutions today.

The first college of osteopathy had the legal right to confer the degree MD (Doctor of Medicine) but Still chose DO (Doctor of Osteopathy). This was argued over a number of years until 1909 when the American Osteopathic Association finally settled the question. By that time surgery and all other subjects necessary to the specialist as well as the general practitioner were present in the osteopathic schools. The MD and DO were equivalent.

Osteopaths throughout the United States had to fight hard through the courts to obtain legal licence to practise. Much opposition was raised by the MDs but despite many setbacks all states obtained legal backing. Similar difficulties occurred in Canada.

The standard set by the American Osteopathic Association in the early 1900s was high and, despite many earlier mistakes, the association strove to learn from their experiences. Several schools were suspended for not meeting standards, which were above those required by the medical profession at that time. There was a continual process of enlarging and enriching the curriculum. A regular four-year course was established for all recognized colleges by September 1916, a year before Still died.

Comparative educational requirements in 1923–24 between medical practice, osteopathy and chiropractic showed osteopathy ahead of medicine and chiropractic a poor third.

Osteopathy was the only one to cover information about food and diet in relation to health.

As the range of skills and educational requirements increased Still nevertheless insisted that students should not do just what they saw someone else do. 'Don't be an imitator,' he said. 'Know your anatomy and your physiology, what structures are involved and what nerves control their function and you need not worry.'

He was concerned that some thought bones should be adjusted until they 'popped'. He was adamant that 'popping' was not important, since bones do not always 'pop' when going back into their proper place, nor does it mean they are properly adjusted when they do 'pop'. 'The "pop",' he said 'is fraught with such significance to the patient who considers the attempts at adjustment have proven effectual. The osteopath should not encourage this idea in his patient as showing something accomplished.'

Although Still used certain methods of adjustment he knew other ways were just as good. In his own words

I want to make it plain that there are many ways of adjusting bones. The choice of methods is to be decided by each operator and depends on his own skill and judgment. Every operator should use his own judgment and choose his own method of adjusting all bones of the body. It is not a matter of imitation and doing just as some successful operator does, but the bringing of the bone from the abnormal to the normal.

Hippocrates said 'nature is the first physician' which is exactly what osteopathy has always claimed. A physician never cures but relieves. The only curative agencies are the inherent self-reparative forces and substances found in every person.

In conclusion Andrew Taylor Still stands out for me as a great man of many talents who combined his practical skills with his spiritual sense; who with great courage, despite opposition, began the development of a continuing science to cure disease; who recognized that there was more than one way to treat disease and encouraged individuality in approach, only to be guided by that inner sense of intuition that is God within.

PRESENT–DAY OSTEOPATHIC EDUCATION

In America there are now fifteen accredited colleges of osteopathic medicine including several within universities. The regular four-year course is preceded by a minimum three years of pre-professional training in which the majority gain a bachelor's degree in either the sciences or humanities. In addition a new medical college admission test is required. Following graduation and an intern year further postgraduate training is offered for all medical specialties including osteopathic manipulative therapy (OMT). Continuing medical education credits are compulsory to enable all graduates to keep up their skills and absorb new knowledge. There is a growing number of women and ethnic graduates and special encouragement for establishing osteopathic hospitals in less favoured areas. For any information on osteopathic education contact the Department of Education of the American Osteopathic Association.

OSTEOPATHY IN GREAT BRITAIN

Osteopathy in Great Britain did not develop with the same strong legal footing as found in America, and because of this the practice of osteopathy is not strictly the same system. In America all osteopaths are equivalent to medical doctors, and the principles and practice of osteopathy is spread throughout all medical disciplines including osteopathic manipulative therapy. It is the manipulative element direct to the somatic body tissues (body framework) that has gained predominance in Britain. The wider concepts and use of osteopathy within medicine have not penetrated the medical establishment to any great degree as yet. However, there are moves to establish the science more strongly in the eyes of the law.

We can recognize two main links leading from the first school in Kirksville. One was the arrival of American-trained osteopaths in Britain who formed the British Osteopathic Society in 1911, and the other a breakaway group of these same osteopaths led by John Martin Littlejohn. Littlejohn was one of the first teachers at Kirksville and became the second Dean there, later to establish the Chicago School of Osteopathy before coming to Britain. For various reasons of opinion and personality these two groups failed to combine as a united force of osteopathy but grew into two distinct teaching colleges namely: the British School of Osteopathy (1917) under the auspices of Dr John Markin Littlejohn; and the London College of Osteopathy (1946), now known as the London College of Osteopathic Medicine.

The earliest American-trained osteopath was J. Dunham who arrived in 1902 and practised in Belfast. His son, T. Dunham, also trained in America and continued to practise until his death in 1984. I had the privilege of knowing him for nineteen years and being first introduced to osteopathy by him when I was a medical student at Queen's University. He encouraged me and taught me several aspects of osteopathy.

The next to come, in 1907, were L. Willard Walker and Franz Joseph Horn. The first organization attempt was the formation of the British Osteopathic Association on 1 July, 1911 following a meeting at the Midland Hotel, Manchester, under the auspices of Dr Franklyn Hudson of Edinburgh. This Association was confined exclusively to graduates of the American Osteopathic schools who were practising in Great Britain and included Dr John Martin Littlejohn.

The breakaway group under the guidance of Dr Littlejohn founded the British School of Osteopathy in 1917. He became President of the British Osteopathic Association in 1925 and at this stage it appeared likely both links would merge. However, differences over educational policy prevented this. It is not possible because of lack of records to assess fully the important differences, but a major issue was the fact that the British Osteopathic Association wanted to wait until legal recognition of osteopathy paved the way for a teaching college of the highest standards on the lines of the American colleges, whereas Littlejohn felt the best school then possible was better than none. This is one of the main reasons why osteopathy did not receive acceptance by the British Medical authorities to include treatment within the National Health Service when it was formed in 1948. Unfortunately at the same time numerous practitioners with incomplete osteopathic training from schools in America not recognized as up to the standard of the schools of the American Osteopathic Association made their appearance in Britain conducting classes whose quality or value was difficult to assess. In 1925 several responsible practitioners not eligible for membership of the British Osteopathic Association formed the Incorporated Association of Osteopaths. Their main concern was the growing number of people with little knowledge or training in osteopathy taking responsibility for treating patients. The Society aimed at protecting their interests against this growing band of people, a development not dissimilar to experience in the United States.

Meanwhile, the British Osteopathic Association had established a registered charity clinic at Vincent Square, London, in 1927 opened by George Bernard Shaw. Its rapid success led to a move in 1931 to larger premises at 24–25 Dorset Square, London NW1 with a back entrance into Boston Place, and named Andrew Still House. A college management committee was formed in 1935 when the possibility of opening a college and hospital with nurses training centre on the lines of the American counterpart was mooted. An appeal for finance was launched in 1937 but this was abandoned due to lack of support. However, in 1946 the British Osteopathic Association established the London College of Osteopathy exclusively for teaching medical graduates the principles and practice of osteopathy. Courses ran successively until 1975 when the College ceased for three years during which the major part of Andrew Still House facing Dorset Square was sold. The College and Association regrouped in the back section of the building facing Boston Place. Courses began again in 1978 and the college was renamed the London College of Osteopathic Medicine to reflect its link with doctors of the American and Canadian Osteopathic Associations. Although small, with only between four and nine graduates a year, the college is thriving and planning future expansion. Postgraduate and education of a wider public, particularly the medical profession, are continuing aims.

Since 1982 a third school of osteopathy has reached a high enough standard to give graduate eligibility to the Register of

Osteopaths: the European School of Osteopathy. The school was founded in 1951 as the École Française d'Ostéopathie in Paris, later to move to London in 1965 and then to its present site in Maidstone, Kent in 1971. It provides, like the British School of Osteopathy, a four-year full-time course.

The promotion of legislation to regulate osteopathy and protect both qualified practitioners and the public was championed by Dr Wilfred Streeter. The chief proposal of a bill presented to Parliament was to enable the public to distinguish between the qualified osteopath and the large number of inadequately trained people who called themselves 'osteopaths'. It was intended to provide the same protection that the Medical Act of 1858 gave to registered medical practitioners. Due to various factors the bill did not succeed. The various osteopathic groups were not properly prepared, and opposition from the established medical associations, including the British Medical Association, was too powerful and well co-ordinated.

The House of Lords Select Committee report following the unsuccessful bill suggested that those practising osteopathy had a choice open to them if they were dissatisfied with their present status: either to qualify for admission to the medical register; or constitute a voluntary register of osteopaths and develop effective training institutions in this country with appropriate qualifications for persons to be admitted to that register in the future.

As a direct result of these events the General Council and Register of Osteopaths was born on the 22 July 1936. One of its primary tasks was to supervise and raise osteopathic educational standards, and it first turned its attention to the British School of Osteopathy which has continued to develop to the present high standard today.

The origin and development of osteopathy has been full of colourful characters, setbacks and successes with the main and continuing aim of providing a sound and efficient science to serve humankind.

OSTEOPATHY IN AUSTRALIA AND NEW ZEALAND

Osteopathy began in New Zealand and Australia in the early

39

part of this century with the arrival of both American and British doctors of osteopathy.

In Australia the federal and state governments, and both private and public health agencies, recognize osteopathic treatment as a separate and essential part of health care. The emphasis is on general practice rather than specialization. Nearly all states of Australia have already or are in the process of enacting the registration of osteopaths, who are restricted to manipulative practice as is the case in Britain and therefore cannot prescribe drugs or perform surgery like their American counterparts. Two colleges are fully recognized in Sydney and Victoria (see addresses on p.102). There are several British and American-trained doctor osteopaths active in Australia in both private practice and hospital work.

The New Zealand register of osteopaths began in 1973 to be followed in 1978 by official recognition when the New Zealand Register of Osteopaths Incorporated Act was passed. It is hoped to pass a further 'Osteopathic Bill' through Parliament this year. It is gratifying to see the progress of osteopathy in both Australia and New Zealand, with a distinct openness between allopathic doctors and osteopaths which is beneficial to patients.

4 *Who Practises Osteopathy?*

The work of the osteopath is to adjust the body from the abnormal to the normal; then the abnormal condition gives place to the normal and health is the result of the normal condition.
ANDREW TAYLOR STILL

In choosing an osteopath there are several useful, sound ways of establishing his or her competence and personal suitability. Recommendations by a friend or acquaintance is an obvious and widely used means of deciding on a particular osteopath, or perhaps your general practitioner or specialist may recommend one to you as many doctors are aware of the benefits of osteopathic treatment; only a few are non-commital.

In Britain two directories give names of professionally trained osteopaths. The General Council and Register of Osteopaths maintain a published list of all 'registered' osteopaths while the British Osteopathic Association provides a directory of all doctor graduates of the London College of Osteopathic Medicine. Both lists are available in libraries, or alternatively by post. Similarly, in America the name of a licensed osteopathic doctor can be obtained from the American Osteopathic Association while the respective osteopathic associations in Canada, Australia and New Zealand have a list of suitably registered practitioners. These same organizations can also advise on those individual osteopaths practising in several countries worldwide.

The yellow pages directories carry an entry under osteopaths that you may wish to consult or, alternatively, the local Citizens Advice Bureau may be able to help. Increasingly your own doctor will know of an osteopath whom he or she can recommend.

QUALIFICATIONS

In order to check the qualifications of an osteopath it is helpful to know what the letters DO mean – Diploma in Osteopathy if a British qualification or Doctor of Osteopathy if American-trained. There are very few American-trained osteopaths spread throughout the world and of these the majority are found in Britain and Australia. They usually have the name of their college in brackets after the DO (for example Kirksville). In the United States both the osteopathic and the traditional medical schools follow the same curriculum. The osteopathic doctor (DO) is the same as the medical doctor (MD). In addition to the standard medical and surgical therapies the osteopathic doctor has training in the philosophy and practice of osteopathy including osteopathic manipulative therapy throughout his or her medical course. FAAO indicates a Fellow of the American Academy of Osteopathy.

Britain tried but failed to open a similar school in the '30s, but Australia has two colleges in Victoria and Sydney with DO courses accredited by their respective tertiary education state boards. They are not yet recognized as of an equivalent educational standard to the American osteopathic colleges because their graduates do not prescribe drugs or perform surgery. By Australian state law osteopaths are restricted to manipulative practice. However, in Britain qualified doctors obtain training in osteopathy as postgraduates at the London College of Osteopathic Medicine where successful graduates are awarded the MLCOM. Apart from this a sound and professional full-time four-year course is available under the guidance of the General Council and Register of Osteopaths (the development of this Register is explained in Chapter 3).

An MRO is a Member of the Register of Osteopaths and is entitled to use the term 'registered osteopath'. Not all osteopaths who are eligible to join do so but those who are members have a sound professional training.

There are three British training colleges at present which meet the high professional standards of the General Council and Register of Osteopaths: the British School of Osteopathy, the London College of Osteopathic Medicine, and the European School of Osteopathy (addresses can be found on p.101). The letters MRO will always be preceded by DO or MLCOM (see below). Similar letters such as MSO and MCO only indicate membership of the Society of Osteopaths and College of Osteopaths respectively. These are just professional organizations and do not in themselves indicate a professional qualification or additional expertise.

The letters MLCOM (Member of the London College of Osteopathic Medicine) are awarded to registered medical practitioners who have completed a thirteen-month training in osteopathy some eight years or more after medical graduation. Some graduates, by recommendation, become fellows of the college and are entitled to use FLCOM.

The letters MBNOA signify graduates of the British College of Naturopathy and Osteopathy who receive a separate diploma in these subjects. The emphasis leans towards naturopathy (using 'natural' treatments with food, diet and exercise in contrast to 'unnatural' manmade medicines), and the osteopathic content of the course is still not considered sufficient to be accepted by the General Council and Register of Osteopaths. The College is at present trying to improve the educational content with the aim of joining the Register, and I have no doubt this will occur in the near future. This can only strengthen the osteopathic base in Britain.

Several other smaller training establishments have appeared in the last ten to twenty years providing courses run at weekends over four to six years with examinations that lead to a diploma in osteopathy. Although many of these graduates are no doubt competent they are not eligible to join the Register of Osteopaths. They keep their own independent registers and have their own osteopathic societies. These training schools, nevertheless, have the option to develop their courses up to the standard required by the General Council and Register of Osteopaths. Since the law in Britain does not prevent anyone from calling himself/herself an osteopath however minimal their knowledge, care should be taken in finding a competent practitioner.

The above-mentioned qualifications cover all those who have received a satisfactory training in osteopathy. Don't be confused by other letters used by some who claim to be osteopaths. Physiotherapists, for example, are different from osteopaths. Certain manipulative techniques are part of a physiotherapist's training and some choose to develop their manipulative skills, many being excellent in what they offer, but they do not generally cover the wide range of skills of an osteopath.

A group of doctors are members of the British Association of Manipulative Medicine (BAMM) founded in 1973, and all doctors interested in manipulation can apply for membership. It is a charitable company whose principal activity is the promotion of education and research in the science and art of manipulative medicine, and comprises both associate and full members. Around 40 per cent of full members have trained at the London College of Osteopathic Medicine and obtained the MLCOM. The remainder have taken a series of weekend courses over two years at which time, although no examination is taken, they become eligible for full membership. These are shown in capital letters in the BAMM membership list, available in libraries. These doctors, mainly general practitioners, use simple manipulative skills in the surgery although some will develop a full-time manipulative practice.

The British Association of Manipulative Medicine is affiliated to the International Federation of Manual Medicine (FIMM) an organization of European nations which promotes the art of manipulative and allied techniques for the relief and/or cure of disease. FIMM is formed entirely of registered medical practitioners and in common with most medical manipulative training some osteopathic concepts and treatment methods are incorporated within their teaching. Perhaps your own general practice has a doctor so trained who will be able to help or alternatively refer you to a doctor/osteopath or lay osteopath whom they can trust.

Some laymen such as bonesetters or football trainers develop certain manipulative skills, and some do have a great gift for dealing with dislocated joints and displaced ligaments. You will be fortunate if you meet one of them, but sadly there will be others who learn one or two techniques and set themselves up as osteopaths, only to give the profession a bad name. It is a reality of life that there are 'cowboys' in all professions. Indeed, in the early days of osteopathy, Still had to contend with people who, after a few hours talking about osteopathy, went out and declared themselves osteopaths.

MEETING YOUR OSTEOPATH

After having obtained a recommendation or found a name in a suitable directory or yellow pages, when you ring for an appointment you will have the opportunity to make your choice. Is the receptionist clear and helpful over the phone? Does she give you a feeling of confidence? Are your questions answered in a firm and polite manner? Of course it is virtually impossible to tell you over the phone if your problems will definitely respond to treatment. Consultation and assessment will be needed to be sure of your suitability for osteopathic treatment and to explain the likely benefits and outcome.

Having made an appointment arrange to arrive on time or even a little early if you don't know the premises. Be clear about nearby facilities for parking or access to public transport. Remember to ask the receptionist for clear instructions on how to get there.

On arriving note how you feel about the welcome. Is it warm and inviting or just brisk and cold? Do you feel the osteopath has a professional and efficient manner and is one you can trust? After your initial consultation you will be in a position to know whether you have made a good choice. If the answer is yes, put your trust in him or her and give the treatment a fair chance. Follow instructions and don't hesitate to ask why you should or should not do something. It is your own health and wellbeing that are in question and taking an active part in treatment will speed up your recovery. Knowing more about how your body works can only be beneficial in using your body to its best advantage, and in avoiding ways that might damage your health. Be prepared to make some changes in your daily habits and activities.

YOUR GENERAL PRACTITIONER AND YOUR OSTEOPATH

Many people are concerned about seeking their general practitioner's approval for osteopathic treatment. This concern, even fear, of disapproval by the general practitioner has been common in the past with many patients going to an osteopath without their general practitioner's knowledge. A lot has changed in the last ten years, and it is now considered normal and desirable for referral to an osteopath to be with the knowledge and even active assistance of a patient's general practitioner. As an adult, in the final analysis, you must make the decision whether or not to inform your general practitioner. In Britain the primary entry to medical facilities is through your general practitioner and it is helpful to inform him or her for reasons of safety, efficiency and good manners. You may not be fully aware of the implications of some medical problems you might have, and your doctor may want to write to the osteopath of your choice. Some doctors will also advise you of a suitable osteopath. They may also be able to talk about and make clear your reasons for seeking help. Do not be put off by the feeling that your own doctor is too busy to listen. Be direct and say what you think. The more knowledge you have of what is wrong with you the better you can decide how best to put it right. Seek your doctor's advice, but make the final decision yourself.

My own personal approach is to obtain the name and address of a patient's doctor and ask whether or not their doctor knows of the visit. I will usually write direct to the general practitioner concerned or ask patients to speak directly with their own general practitioner. However I also respect the few individuals who do not wish their doctor to have knowledge of their visit; and I do not deny treatment because of this unless I need to know some important fact of medical history that might influence whether or not treatment is appropriate. I would then insist on contacting a patient's doctor before treatment. Fortunately this is rare. Some feel afraid of their doctor's possible disapproval, others feel that their doctor would not be interested, while others say their doctor only gives them drugs like valium or painkillers 'which don't get to the root of the problem' and therefore feel it is 'a waste of time' to let their doctor know. I can understand their concerns but I also know, from the doctor's position, that he or she is trained primarily towards treatment with medicines and feels most comfortable using this approach. However, many doctors are coming to realize that medicines are not always as useful as was hoped, particularly when given over a long period, and they are only too aware of their disadvantages. We are partly limited by the medical system we have learnt and practised and change needs to take place from within each system to value other approaches. Medicine and osteopathy have already begun this process.

OSTEOPATHY AND THE NATIONAL HEALTH SERVICE

The British National Health Service (NHS), being under the direct control of the Department of Health and Social Services (DHSS) together with the General Medical Council (GMC) which licenses the doctors who work in the NHS has, up to the present, not recognized the inclusion of osteopathy as an available treatment. Only a minority of doctors will use osteopathic or other manipulative techniques in their own surgery and offer it as a treatment within the NHS. Generally osteopathy is a private treatment and must be paid for. The various schools of osteopathy already mentioned do run clinics where treatment is given by a student under supervision. A donation is usually required but anyone unable to pay is not turned away. Many private osteopaths will also make fee adjustments for genuine inability to pay. There is no standard fee for treatment and the fee can vary. Whether you feel a particular fee is expensive or not will depend on many factors, but if osteopathic treatment can relieve you then it is money well spent and proves to be so time and time again.

INSURANCE SCHEMES FOR FEES

In Britain those who belong to provident associations such as BUPA, PPP, WPA and other more recent insurance schemes like Allied Medical and Commercial Union for example, can claim for osteopathic treatment provided treatment is by a medically qualified osteopath. There are certain guidelines for medical doctors, so you should always make a point of asking whether the doctor of your choice is eligible for a claim on your private insurance. At the time of writing BUPA has become more restrictive on allowing claims from doctor osteopaths.

Those who belong to the Civil Service Medical Aid obtain consideration for claims for benefit in respect of osteopathy 'if treatment by a *named* osteopath has been recommended by a general practitioner or a consultant, or if the osteopath himself is a registered medical practitioner'. There may possibly be other exceptions so always check with your osteopath or insurance scheme.

In America all osteopathic medical treatment including osteopathic manipulative therapy is eligible for claims from a wide range of private medical schemes, Medicare and Medicaid.

In Australia where the majority of states have registration of osteopaths via state registration boards fees are covered by private health insurance, workers' compensation and third party. In New Zealand private insurance together with the Accident Compensation Corporation will cover fees for treatment by an approved osteopath.

5 Examination and Treatment — What to Expect

An intelligent person will soon learn that a soft hand and a gentle move is the way to obtain the desired result.
ANDREW TAYLOR STILL

Once you have chosen your osteopath what can you expect when going for treatment? The most important factor is an osteopath who is professional, confident and caring, and able to help you relax. If you prefer to have a female osteopath your choice is not difficult. A large proportion of osteopathic graduates are women, so check in the directories.

I have touched on the reception you may receive on ringing up to make an appointment and on the welcome you find on entering the osteopath's premises (see p. 45). These will range from a room in the practitioner's home to a large or small clinic encompassing several different therapies. I feel you must always expect a warm welcome to help put you at ease when you are likely to be in pain and feeling miserable, even angry with yourself for being ill.

The sense of clarity of appointments and explanations by the staff, adequate and clean premises properly heated, and a businesslike approach are all things to be expected. Osteopaths are professional people. Gowns should be available if needed, though treatment is usually undertaken wearing underclothes because a thorough examination is necessary before the commencement of treatment. The state of undress will depend on the area of the body being treated, and in practically every patient the whole spine must be examined.

Your perceived pain in one area of the spine or limbs may actually originate in a different area of the spine or skull, so examination of other areas is required. Visual observation of the body is second only to touch in making a diagnosis before starting treatment.

Treatment is not simply in one direction from osteopath to patient. An interaction is taking place. A relationship between therapist and patient is present and a certain trust builds up. You have to expect to be touched, to be in close proximity, and to be moved into certain positions both for examination and treatment. This involves co-operation on your part and consideration and explanation by your osteopath. Do speak up if a position or movement is uncomfortable. Slight alteration might make all the difference between comfort and discomfort. True osteopathic treatment aims at minimal disruption for greatest effect. It is not a painful treatment.

If you change osteopaths do not expect to have exactly the same treatment. As Still said, each osteopath's approach, although having the same intent to restore normal function followed by nature's cure, is not necessarily the same.

There is a variety of ways of manipulating and moving the joints and muscles; it is the results which matter. During training each osteopath learns a wide range of techniques and then, using his/her own skill and judgement, applies those that suit him or her best as an operator. Right-handed and left-handed people use different approaches. A small or large person will find certain manipulative methods more comfortable to use and therefore more effective in his or her hands. Anatomical variations in patients require variety in technique.

Some use mechanical devices for positioning or providing rhythmical movements of joints – special types of couch or traction tables, as useful adjuncts to direct use of the hands. The osteopath always has your comfort in mind in the process of achieving normal function of the joints and tissues, although certain techniques can be more uncomfortable than others. In the following explanation of treatment it is impracticable as well as unhelpful to describe all the methods of examination or the many specific treatment positions.

HISTORY

First, be prepared to give the history of your problem, how it began, what makes it better or worse, and the character of your pain and disability. The length and depth of history will depend on the extent of importance laid by each individual osteopath on this aspect of the treatment as compared, for example, to the visual and physical examination. Expect to talk about your past medical problems, your family situation, personal stresses and upsets, work conditions or other environmental factors, exercise, diet and nutrition, attitudes to life and general lifestyle. These can all, either singly or in combination, influence the particular problems pain or disability you are experiencing. Some changes will undoubtedly have to be made in your attitudes and lifestyle to help you become better, with the aim of preventing any recurrence.

EXAMINATION

One of the essential distinguishing features of osteopathy is its great reliance on touch – the use of the hands as organs of diagnosis and treatment. A tremendous amount of information is gained by palpation with the hands and fingers without which the osteopath could not function. Examination will usually be carried out in three main ways, namely: standing; sitting; lying.

Standing

When standing, the osteopath will first assess general body posture, including how you walk. Do you walk with a limp or have flat feet? Is there any obvious difficulty in standing upright? Is there a tilt of the pelvis, shoulders or head which might show that a particular part of the spine needs more careful evaluation? Is there a short leg present? Is there an increased lumbar curve or rotation of the spine that indicates deviation?

Spine. You will be asked to go through the movements of the spine, forward movement (flexion), backward movement (extension), rotation, and side bending. More specific testing of the fine movements of each spinal segment (vertebra) will come later when sitting or lying. Our spines are comprised of a series of box-like structures called vertebrae, which through a series of interlocking joints produce our spinal column or back bone. The vertebrae are so shaped to contain and protect our spinal cord, from which a series of spinal nerves emerge through holes between each vertebra. It is at this point that inflammation, swelling from a collection of fluid or overgrowth of bone tissue, can result in the 'trapped nerve', a term you will commonly hear in diagnosis. The 'trapped nerve' is not always physically irritated, but is the result of reflex activity elsewhere in the nervous system producing pain felt at a more distant area of the body from the spine.

The osteopath will take note of any swellings or deformities of the body, any scars indicating operations, tension in the muscles, and these observations will add to the assessment of the cause of your problem. The osteopath assesses your spine as a whole functioning unit from head to tail bone.

Sitting

Sitting gives further information. For example, if the hip bones are level on sitting and tilted when standing it strongly suggests an anatomical short leg, a common cause of pain in the pelvis and lumbar spine. Sitting allows further specific testing for joint movement or restriction, particularly in the neck and upper spine. Rib movement is noted with breathing, and skin and muscle palpated for tissue changes which, added to other information, help localize the source of trouble.

Lying

While on your back the osteopath will check leg length and examine the joints at the bottom of your spine, the hips, knees and ankles as necessary. He or she will check reflexes and muscle strength, sensation and movement to cover a basic examination of the nervous system. Blood pressure is usually taken. Lying on your back also allows for further examination of your neck. The osteopath will then ask you to lie on your side to examine the extent of movement between the vertebrae in your back. By bending your knees and placing one hand behind your knees to provide a lever for guidance the other hand is placed on your back to feel for movement and tissue changes along the spine. Lying prone on your stomach provides a further opportunity to test each of the joints. The osteopath will check each joint for its position and movement, and muscles and skin for tension or tightness. You might be asked to kneel on your hands and knees as another position that can help him or her in making a diagnosis.

The osteopath will gently pass fingers over the skin to feel for texture, dryness, dampness and consistency. He or she will press more firmly to assess the tone (elasticity) and suppleness of the muscles. Areas of floppiness, bogginess, thickening or increased tension will be noted and are often tender to touch. You will often be asked to indicate tender points from pressure with the fingers.

The osteopath needs to know the difference between the range of normal and abnormal in respect of joint positions, movement and end feel of all joints. Fine movements of the joints will be tested. He or she knows what healthy skin and muscle look and feel like, and what happens when something is wrong.

THE NEXT STEP

The osteopath will by now have gathered together an historical pattern of your problem, its origin, development and present state; hereditary factors, emotional interactions; stress factors; lifestyle. He or she will have looked at your overall pattern of body movement, posture, muscle bulk and shape of your spine. Specific testing movements and procedures will demonstrate abnormal position and movement of the joints and muscles etc. that show where the problem is. Medical conditions not suitable for osteopathic treatment will have become more clear, and whether to obtain further specialized opinion will hopefully have been established. Any X-rays or other tests required will have been considered and arranged.

PLAN OF ACTION

A plan of treatment is now ready to be put into action. Your initial consultation may only be for assessment and a further appointment for treatment will need to be made. Often, however, a new patient will receive treatment during the initial visit. Don't expect a single magic treatment. I have met several patients who have expected a quick manipulative 'click' and all will be well. It rarely happens like that.

A full history, examination and assessment with explanation should be expected at the first visit. The initial plan of action may need to be altered with further sessions because treatment may involve other aspects of a problem which did not surface at the first consultation. This may be because of some new historical fact which comes to light, perhaps an underlying emotional problem or an admission of a lifestyle which, if not changed, will perpetuate the problem despite treatment. It may also be because certain body changes will direct attention to an area of the spine not formerly thought to be significant in terms of the overall problem. Pain which is very persistent or recurs soon after osteopathic treatment may indicate some further underlying factor that needs investigation, and steps will be taken to elucidate this.

Three plans of treatment form the basis of osteopathic techniques: soft tissue work, articulation, and more specific thrusting manipulation.

Soft Tissue Work

Soft tissue work is the name given to a range of techniques used on the soft tissues of the body. These comprise the skin; fascia (a fibrous-like membrane that envelopes muscles, arteries, veins and nerves acting as a support to these structures and as a buffer between them); muscles; musculotendinous junctions (that part of the muscle attached to bone); and ligaments. Using various stretching, rolling, kneading movements with the hands and fingers circulation is stimulated, lymphatics drained, muscles and ligaments relaxed. Significant improvement can take place with this alone. Gentle pressure is used at first; then, depending on the state of the tissues and your own sensitivity, more firm pressure is applied. Patients remark how satisfying a firm pressure on the muscles can be. The feeling is a pleasurable 'pain' or sensation.

Articulation

Articulation describes a range of techniques designed to articulate the joints, that is to move each joint or series of joints through their range of movement. This is achieved by manual or sometimes mechanical means and involves repeated rhythmical movement. It can be very relaxing and extremely effective in restoring normal function of the joints. The repeated movement stretches attached ligaments and muscles and encourages the joint surfaces to move in their correct pattern. The underlying problem is largely related to abnormal patterns of movement of joints and their associated structures, with blockage of the correct movement, and articulation goes a long way to relieving this.

Specific Manipulation

A commonly used method is direct thrusting manipulation of joints of the spine and the limbs. This manipulation for the technically minded involves a high velocity low amplitude movement directed precisely at adjacent joint surfaces to regain the correct joint position and movement. You may be asked for respiratory co-operation – to take a breath in or let a breath out to help a particular manipulation.

This is perhaps the technique most associated with manipulation, and one in which several misconceptions occur about what takes place. It is only one of several techniques used and common to all techniques the art is a subtle one. It depends on accurate positioning, correct angle of thrust and precise timing to achieve movement at a point of relaxation by the patient. It requires confidence on the part of the osteopath, choice of correct technique for the condition assessed, and trust on the part of the patient. It can be momentarily uncomfortable but only very rarely painful.

The technique is highly effective. Although many times a 'pop' or 'click' is heard which may be perceived by some as satisfying, reassuring or perhaps disconcerting, this noise is *not* essential to release the block. What *is* essential is obtaining normal joint position and movement with freedom from pain.

A commonly used alternative to the high velocity thrust is that of muscle energy technique. It involves resistance by the patient's muscles against those of the osteopath after being placed in the same positions used for the thrusting techniques described above. It is comfortable and very effective. It is now as widespread in its use as the direct thrust technique. As well as these more direct methods, indirect techniques – such as functional and counterstrain technique – are used to guide through positioning the body joints and muscles towards freedom of movement and freedom from pain.

THE CRANIAL CONCEPT

Additionally your osteopath might use some cranial techniques. The pattern or examination and treatment in cranial work requires the same high skill in touch and visual diagnosis. The cranial osteopath will observe how you hold your head, the shape and position of your jaw, nose, eyes and mouth looking for asymmetry. Gentle touching of the skull including the likely placing of fingers in your mouth to move the jaw will be necessary. The same principles of diagnosis and checking for abnormal or blocked movement is used on the skull as it is in the spine. This is followed by releasing those blocks to obtain normal function.

Diagnosis and treatment require a delicate and gentle touch. Movements are so gentle that a common reaction is one of 'feeling hardly anything is being done', yet remarkable effects are achieved. Hands and fingers are placed on your head to palpate the skull movements and rhythm. Small corrective movements are made by tapping, stretching and holding to balance the movements and rhythm. They are not painful.

Cranial work is sometimes used to obtain relaxation before general treatment although it has far wider applications, and is a powerful and effective treatment when used in trained hands.

OTHER IMPORTANT ASPECTS OF TREATMENT

As well as the three main treatment plans of soft tissue work, articulation and direct or indirect manipulation with the additional use of cranial techniques, several further areas of action will need to be considered. These will include: nutritional suggestions, exercises, both in the short and long term; posture advice, guidance on work positions both in the home and outside the home; methods of relaxing; encouragement in changing lifestyle to show more positive ways to feel and be healthy; support in emotional crises that have inevitably been reflected in ill health; guidance to ways of improving environment. Some or all of these may be suggested. Your osteopath will be likely to know other practitioners from whom you may gain appropriate help and guidance in addition to or instead of osteopathic treatment. You may be asked to consult or return to your general practitioner.

6 *Pattern of Treatment*

Always treat the person as your reasoning faculties tell you treatment should be. Don't be an imitator.
ANDREW TAYLOR STILL

The first thing to remember is that there is no 'typical' pattern of treatment.

The main aim is to restore normal body function by means of various manual techniques. The range of osteopathic techniques is extensive. Any one osteopath will learn and use a selection of these adapting their use to his or her own size, weight, ability and inclination. Different patients need different techniques. An osteopath will use those techniques that he or she feels will most benefit the patient. People from all groups including women during pregnancy and people with mental or physical handicap, can benefit from treatment through childhood to old age

Do tell your osteopath what you feel about any technique used, especially if experiencing some difficulty with it. I know from personal experience that this feedback is helpful. One patient of mine finds the 'crossed arm technique' for the upper back too uncomfortable. I use a different method. Remember it is a relationship so don't hesitate to express your feelings.

The number of treatment sessions required will vary and the obvious first concern as to the financial cost has to be discussed. Further treatment will obviously involve more cost. However, the need for ongoing treatment when necessary must be appreciated by each individual patient. Osteopathic treatment has to be paid for and costs are not hidden as in the 'free' NHS.

MAIN AREAS OF TREATMENT

From my experience I would suggest that we can usually look at four main areas of osteopathic treatment patterns that together show what influences the success of treatment:

(1) the complaint;
(2) the patient;
(3) the osteopath;
(4) other factors.

The Complaint

The severity and extent of a complaint will determine the amount of treatment required hopefully to effect a cure. Often an osteopath can say 'Yes, your condition can be relieved but I cannot easily say how soon.' In practice it may take four to eight sessions or more. A good analogy is learning to drive and the number of driving lessons needed — some people will only require six lessons, while others will need twice that or more. Longstanding problems, say of sciatica in the leg or neck pains, take more treatment over a longer period of time than acute conditions such as a 'crick in the neck' or a strained low back joint following a specific fall. Usually the earlier treatment is obtained, the fewer sessions will be required. The longer a problem in the joints and muscles is present, the more restricted movement becomes because of stiffness and tightness. Repeated treatment is then needed to free these tight tissues and restore movement.

The number of sessions must be balanced against the period of time treatment continues. To say you will require six to twelve sessions might sound a lot but spread over a year it sounds more realistic and acceptable. It is common to have treatment initially four to seven days apart for the first few sessions, occasionally more frequently. After that, time between treatments is gradually increased until no further treatment is required. Many people need regular checks or 'maintenance' sessions anything from a month to a year apart.

The Patient

Any fear of treatment or over-anxiety causes muscles to tighten and makes treatment technically more difficult. A good osteopath will help you with this. Overweight or over-developed muscles add their own problems in examination and treatment. Sometimes, as with all healing professions, a patient becomes a little over-dependent on osteopathic treatment. If this can be recognized some discussion may take place to understand what further benefit treatment can offer to improve the condition, or a second opinion may bring a fresh light to the problem. Recurrence of illhealth, and therefore more treatment, is often due to factors such as inherent weakness from an old injury or disability, continuing bad posture, the wrong environment, or personal/relationship problems.

These comments are not meant in judgement but rather as a realistic attempt to put treatment into perspective. Osteopaths offer guidance, support and expertise but the final result, as in all healing processes, is also dependent upon each individual person and co-operation with life's natural forces.

The Osteopath

The extent of knowledge, experience, skill in diagnosis and technical ability of your osteopath obviously has a bearing on determining the treatment. Professional zeal or pride in his/her work should not stand in the way of the wish to achieve a perfectly functioning spine, and consultation with a colleague is always an option and used when necessary by any good osteopath.

Other Factors

Sadly, I sometimes sense a patient is going to be ill for a long time, and until such a person learns that change must also come from within, treatment directed from outside is unlikely to lead to a cure on its own. Illness or disease often has a purpose, which may not become clear until later. It can force us to stop for a while, it can provoke a change in our attitudes to life and to other people, it can create the necessity to change jobs, to move house; all of these produce different challenges, losses and benefits. After a period of adjusting the change can work out better than we might have considered possible. There is always a positive side to any disaster. Look for it and work towards it. Seek help and support in the process. Further factors such as social disruption, lack of money, pressure from relatives or other outside pressures may determine the extent of treatment.

AIM OF TREATMENT

The aim of treatment is to work with the structure of the body to obtain normal function. I have observed four main patterns of response but even these can only give a broad picture and must not be seen as the only patterns that may occur in any one individual.

Patterns of Response

Immediate response with relief of pain and symptoms over the next few days with lasting effect. This response is not so common but is more likely when visiting a familiar osteopath with a recurrence of an old problem or for a specific acute episode of spinal pain with early and accurate treatment. A few respond with dramatic and immediate improvement followed by rapid deterioration which may then only slowly respond to treatment or not at all. This is rare but can indicate a wrong diagnosis, and further investigation is required.

Progressive step-by-step response to effective cure. This is the most common response pattern that I see and is related to the majority of musculoskeletal (muscles, tendons, fascia, joints, bony structures) problems that are seen in osteopathic practice. I use the words 'effective cure' because this includes not only those with total cures who don't need further treatment but also those who respond well yet need regular continuing (maintenance) treatments every one to three months to keep them pain free.

Delayed response. Some people show a delayed response with no real improvement for at least three to four treatments after which time step-by-step changes occur.

No response. There are those who, for whatever reason, do not achieve any obvious improvement after several sessions following assessment and expected change. Fortunately this is a very small group.

Other Factors in Treatment

While remembering that an interactive process is taking place with the osteopath, there are other factors to consider which involve both the patient and the osteopath. The motivation to get well at both a conscious and unconscious level is relevant. Is there a motive for staying unwell? To avoid work; to avoid travelling; to punish oneself for guilt feelings; perhaps for some other personal reason known only to yourself? It can be upsetting to think like this but unexpressed fears are common to us all and are nothing to be ashamed about.

This sharing of the burden of a problem has a positive effect in treatment. To know that a physical cause for your symptoms has been found and that something can be done brings relief. When you are aware that you respond better to a gentle technique or a more firm technique, do tell your osteopath.

Treatment brings various beneficial effects apart from relief of pain. These can be variously described as a feeling of wellbeing, euphoria, a sense of freedom in the body, an increased energy level, a readiness to get on with life. Relaxation of muscles can also bring emotional release from feelings of depression, hurt, anger, resentment that have been stored up in the body for whatever reason. It is possible sometimes to feel quite drained for several hours after treatment, perhaps wanting to cry, to just be on one's own. These, if they occur, are quite normal feelings and soon pass. For these reasons it is best to have a quiet evening on the day of treatment and avoid strong mental or physical stimulus.

The osteopath is intent on giving you the right 'dose' of treatment, in the right place and at the right time. A relaxation response will depend on his/her technique. In theory, symptoms will disappear when the cause has been found and removed, and symptoms in themselves are therefore not crucially important from the treatment point of view. Naturally, most people will be most interested in just obtaining relief from their symptoms so that they can continue their lives without pain.

However, your osteopath, as well as helping to relieve your symptoms, is also aiming to remove the underlying cause to prevent the problem recurring. This will usually need more treatment. Stop for a minute and think about your symptoms. Have they any more meaning than that of being just a nuisance? Does your pain suggest you are overloading yourself in some way at home or at work? Remember what happens when you overload the electricity wiring – a fuse blows! Does your illness have any link with anxiety towards your spouse or other members of your family? Are you being affected by some of your own attitudes and prejudices that now demand a change? These are challenging questions that many people won't want to hear or do anything about. Nevertheless I believe they often need to be asked in order to achieve wellbeing. Isn't that what you want?

Try not to be like the patient who came to the doctor and said 'Doctor, I have not come to be told I'm burning the candle at both ends, I've come for more wax!'

REACTIONS TO TREATMENT

Several specific reactions may follow osteopathic treatment, mostly mild but sometimes unpleasant. The majority of treatments do not have reactions. During treatment on the muscles the skin commonly becomes flushed and those with very sensitive skins may get some bruising which soon disappears. Mild headache may follow neck treatment, and relief of pain in one part of the spine may result in some minor discomfort elsewhere which is very rarely permanent and not incapacitating. Be prepared 'to get worse before you get better'. Any reaction, when it occurs, can last for several hours before clearing. Everyone will react a little differently. But remember that most people improve with treatment.

RECURRENCE OF SYMPTOMS

Pain and other symptoms that come back again are frustrating, annoying and often restrict lifestyle. They can be distressing yet challenging to your osteopath. A careful reassessment between both patient and osteopath is needed.

Stopping treatment too soon with only relief of symptoms without the proper healing of joints and tissues is a common cause of recurrence. Increasing activity too early by going back to heavy work or repeating awkward body positions is a major reason. Perhaps there is a need for support in the form of a strapping or rest, and seating or work height may need to be altered. Overdependence on treatment by a patient, either consciously or unconsciously, may invoke recurring pain to obtain more treatment. An osteopath will always be happy to check your spine at intervals.

Recurrence may be inevitable due to old injury and persistent weakening of muscles or ligaments. This results in a constant stimulus of the nervous system leading to pain. Regular treatment becomes necessary at intervals to break this pattern and give relief.

A missed diagnostic factor by the osteopath may be responsible or it may be a new problem with symptoms that appear the same as the last. Further assessment is needed and perhaps a second opinion if the problem persists. A common reason for return of a problem is failure for whatever reason to remove or alter deeper underlying causes. These are usually related to stress mainly of an emotional nature. This points to the necessity, as I have already mentioned, of looking beyond just the symptoms to what they may mean in any one individual's life. Mental, emotional, physical and spiritual aspects may be important. For some people osteopathic treatment acts as a tremendous support with relief of body aches and pains that occur during stressful life events such as bereavement following death of a close relative or friend, divorce, job loss or relationship difficulty. These of course can be ongoing situations for varying lengths of time and determine the amount of treatment given.

REGULAR (OR MAINTENANCE) TREATMENT

Maintenance treatment can be likened to Andrew Taylor Still's simile of the osteopath as the master mechanic, your body the engine and the need for regular servicing. Many chronic problems need regular maintenance treatment over various periods of time, most commonly monthly to three monthly. Periodic treatment also acts as a preventive to keep healthy in our stressful, technological, instant-gratification age of living. Opportunity is also provided to discuss further development of healthy living patterns, alteration of habits, encouragement to exercise etc. We all need a little push now and again to keep ourselves going. I thoroughly recommend this positive use of regular checks.

STOPPING TREATMENT

While considering what I've just said, how and when does one stop treatment? Financial reasons are often put forward, but a genuine inability to pay needs to be discussed with your osteopath. A personality clash may mean stopping treatment with one osteopath and looking elsewhere. Stop when you feel you are well and don't need another appointment, but keep in mind some of the reasons already given as to why problems return and whether any apply to you. Please don't cancel without some explanation if possible and don't make an appointment and then not turn up. It is rude when unnecessary. A cancellation fee may be charged.

Treatment may need to be stopped because of some medical complication that needs medical treatment, for example a severe rise in blood pressure. A further specific example concerns a lady I was treating who came for a third treatment session having fallen the day before. She was highly agitated, in a lot of pain and I sent her for X-ray which confirmed that she had a crush fracture of one of her vertebrae for which it was necessary to refer her to her own doctor. Finally, your osteopath may simply feel that no further benefit is likely with further treatment.

WHEN NOT TO USE OSTEOPATHY

There are several medical conditions where direct treatment with local manipulation must not be used. This is either because it is not safe to use or because no benefit is likely. They are mostly obvious and a good osteopath will be on the lookout for these problems in order to send you to your own doctor. The main conditions are:

active infections;

fractures;

bone disease;

cancer;

gross structural deformities;

severe general medical conditions such as gross high blood pressure or heart attack;

vascular disease, for example, thrombosis;

neurological conditions with nerve damage;

spinal cord damage;

severe prolapse of an intervertebral disc.

If you are concerned about osteopathic treatment for a medical condition talk to your doctor or ask your osteopath to contact him or her.

Although I have mentioned fractures, prolapsed discs or heart attacks as unsuitable for osteopathic manipulation there are certain circumstances when it *is* useful. This is more commonly used in the United States and Canada where osteopathic doctors are trained in osteopathic principles as well as medicine. For example, when treating heart attacks in hospital recovery has been shown to be quicker by using osteopathic treatment to the ribs and spine which helps blood circulation, breathing and speeds up elimination of waste products from the damaged heart muscle.

Osteopathic assessment and treatment is also useful in the rehabilitation of a patient after a fracture when the bone has healed, usually after four to six weeks. Earlier treatment can be given to the spine and adjacent joints while the fractured joint is supported in plaster. This is because the fall or blow causing the fracture will transmit strain to other joints and reflex spasm to the spine. Osteopathy is also indicated when pain persists after 'disc' surgery. This is because, although the surgery has dealt with the local problem, other areas of the spine will have reacted with tension and restriction which will often respond well to osteopathy. This is another example of the usefulness to recovery that a combination of traditional medicine and osteopathy can bring. Unfortunately at the present time this integration is less well understood in Britain in contrast to the United States.

7 How Does Osteopathy Work?

The rule of the artery is supreme. Remove the cause which stops or clogs the blood flow or blocks the nerve which controls the blood flow and the blood itself will work the cure.
ANDREW TAYLOR STILL

Nature has been thoughtful enough to place in man all that the word 'remedy' means.
ANDREW TAYLOR STILL

An osteopath must find the true corners as set by the Divine Surveyor.
ANDREW TAYLOR STILL

How *does* osteopathy work? It seems a simple question. But the answer is extremely complex and evolving all the time with each succeeding scientific discovery and understanding of how the body and mind function in health and disease. We are in a period of great expansion and rapid progress in many fields of scientific and technological endeavour.

IN THE PAST

During the original development of osteopathy the mechanical aspects of spinal pain were of prime importance. The clinical effects on the body were recognized by an osteopath using fingers to touch skin and muscle and test joint movement. The various symptoms of pain and disability were found to be linked to areas of warm and moist skin, thickened ligaments, tense muscles and restricted joints in the back. Each area of body abnormality was given the name 'osteopathic lesion'. The first theories spoke of both the circulation and nervous system as probable factors in how treatment worked. Andrew Taylor Still was insistent on finding the specific focus in the skeleton that was causing the pain — 'find it, fix it and leave it alone' was his dictum.

The emerging ideas and understanding of the osteopathic lesion were soon confirmed by observations of other scientists worldwide. With further growth it became clear the role of the osteopathic profession was of central importance in medical science in relation to health. To increase communication with other doctors and scientists the diagnostic term 'osteopathic lesion' was renamed 'somatic dysfunction'. The words soma/somatic are medical terms which collectively describe several body tissues — skin, muscle, ligament, fascia and tendon.

The joint problem of 'somatic dysfunction' is a major factor causing the pain of an illness or strain, but it must be seen to occur simultaneously with other 'causes' such as the environment, our relationships, stress etc., a theme recurring throughout this book. It is because of these links that treating a specific joint problem directly with osteopathic manipulation sets in motion a chain of events that effects a cure.

IN THE PRESENT

The discovery in America, Europe and Russia that nerves produce and carry substances around the body is very exciting. These substances are made up of proteins and, it would appear, act to keep our tissues (skin, muscle etc.) healthy. These functions of the nerves are known as 'trophic' functions and are independent of the more usual nerve activity of moving muscles. It would appear that osteopathic treatment stimulates this movement of fluid.

There is an increasing realization that the natural world functions as a complete whole, each part having an effect on every other part — a sort of knock-on effect. Therefore we can understand that nations and people are not isolated from events going on elsewhere in the world. Similarly, our bodies act as a whole unit affected by the environment in which we live and the feelings we have within us. These concepts of linkage from one part of the world to another and from one body part to another have a special relevance to osteopathy. This is because of two main body structures: the blood circulation throughout the body; and the numerous nerve connections in the brain and the spinal cord within the backbone, and the nerves that reach to all parts of the body. The pattern of nerves that spread throughout the brain looks like the pattern made by a tree in winter, silhouetted against the sky with hundreds of little branches.

Continuing research is beginning to show the central role that the nervous system plays in controlling our bodies and our experiences of both physical and mental pain. A continuous level of nerve activity is needed to keep us healthy, yet overactivity or lack of activity in the nerves results in symptoms of distress and pain. Similarly, increased or decreased circulation has widespread effects. As we continue to build the jigsaw together we can show how one part of the body affects another part, often at a distance. Pain in the arm, for example, is often caused from problems in the neck. Pain inside the knee can be caused by arthritis in the hip joint. A person with one leg shorter than the other will have a curve in the spine and may have back pain, headaches and neck pain.

Scientific evidence shows that the links between body parts can be complex and the pattern is organized by the spinal cord. The range of symptoms felt from disease or injury is controlled by the section or segment of the spinal cord that supplies the part of the body affected. Because this same section of the spinal cord has nerve connections to other parts of the body it is common to feel a variety of symptoms. A chain of events continues in the body independently from the original body part affected. Thus long after a strain, injury or infection we can continue to have symptoms because they are organized by the nervous system. A dramatic example occurs when a person loses a leg. They can still feel pain in the leg even though it is obviously not there — phantom limb pain. Understanding this has a profound relevance to osteopathic treatment methods.

Therefore it would appear that increased activity of certain nerve pathways has a damaging effect on those organs or tissues which they supply. Thus your osteopath, in listening to your complaint of pain and disability, will direct his or her attention to your body to discover which section of the nervous system is overactive. By the various osteopathic treatment techniques this overactivity of the nervous system will be reduced as the body adjusts towards its own normal level. Symptoms will therefore be removed, the nerves will act normally, any reduced blood flow will be increased, muscles relaxed and activity in the body cells balanced.

The osteopathic profession owes a great debt to the hard work, sincerity and vision of the physiologist Irvin M. Korr. He realized that 'physiological processes and their disturbances in the individual human could be fully understood only in the context, not only of human life but in the specific context of that person's total life and his or her total physical and sociocultural environment, past and present'.

This understanding of the relationship between the body processes of blood flow, heart rate, muscle contraction, joint movement etc., and the various events in a person's life, produced a great boost to his research. Who hasn't noticed the flushed face and increased heart beat on falling in love, or the tightness of the body when anxious or afraid? He became involved in studies of many areas that lay outside the traditional laboratory approach. He was an early pioneer of the now more accepted theories of dependence of one body system on another and the effects on the body of both internal and external factors — in other words the growth of whole person or holistic medicine. Before continuing further I shall briefly outline some facts about the nervous system.

THE NERVOUS SYSTEM

We divide our nervous system into three main groups depending on their function — motor, sensory and autonomic.

Motor

The motor system, as its name implies, comprises those nerves which activate our muscles to carry out movements like walking, sitting, shaking hands etc. The pathways of most nerves in the body and the specific body tissues or organs they supply are well known. The nerves exert their effect by the release of certain chemicals at nerve endings resulting in the particular movement or activity required. Thus when you turn the pages of this book your brain activates the motor nerves that send a message to your hand and arm muscles to produce the necessary movement.

Sensory

The sensory nerve system gives us information about touch — soft or rough, hot or cold feelings; smell — pleasant or unpleasant; a range of taste from sweet to sour; our sight through our eyes; and the sense of where our joints are as we move them about. These combine to give a wide range of information for living. The particular development of touch through the use of the hands is an osteopath's most important skill.

Autonomic

The autonomic nerve system functions automatically in the body through a complicated pattern of nerve messages that help to keep our body in balance and harmony. There are two parts to the system: the sympathetic and parasympathetic. The *sympathetic* controls our sweat glands — most of us are familiar with the excess sweating that occurs in hot weather and helps to cool our system. The sympathetic also controls the contraction or tightening of the smooth muscle which lines our gut, blood vessels and heart muscle, helping our heart to contract and pump blood round the body. The *parasympathetic* in contrast relaxes these same smooth muscles and, using the same example, allows the heart to relax between each contraction (you can feel that beat or contraction at the pulse on each wrist). The parasympathetic also regulates male and female hormones. A further example of the two systems at work is the pupil in the eye. The sympathetic makes the pupil smaller when exposed to light, while the opposite effect of enlargement of the pupil that occurs in the dark is a function of the parasympathetic. The pupil is rather like the aperture in a camera which opens and shuts to control the amount of light reaching the lens.

The sympathetic system is also believed to have much wider effects on the body that are not yet fully clarified. It could perhaps turn out to be a common link to many normal and abnormal physiological body functions.

Interaction between the autonomic nervous system and the muscles, joints and body organs has only slowly been accepted in medical circles. Although the existence of these reflex pathways was known over thirty years ago, it is only the recent actual demonstration of observed nerve pathways that is providing the 'scientific proof' to allow a widespread acknowledgement of these interactions that show how the body responds in disease and how manipulation affects these disease processes.

How does osteopathic manipulation affect the body to bring about change? With our present understanding three main areas stand out:

(1) circulation of blood and lymph fluids which carry away body waste;
(2) mechanical changes in joints and muscles;
(3) activity of the nervous system.

All these areas interlink and we cannot isolate one part of the human anatomy from another.

EFFECTS ON CIRCULATION OF BODY FLUIDS

Our bodies are formed of a higher percentage of liquid than solid content. Free fluid flow is a basic requirement of a healthy body. Blood is the main fluid, flowing through a wide network of arteries and veins from the pumping pressure of our heart. Then there is lymph which flows through its own system of tubes carrying waste products from the body tissues to empty into the venous system on its way back to the heart. The cerebrospinal fluid bathes our brain and spinal cord to supply nutrition.

Our blood continually flows round the body in a circulation under pressure from the heart. It leaves the heart through the arteries that carry oxygen to feed the muscles and body organs, and returns to it via the veins and lymph channels. As the blood passes through the lungs it picks up oxygen from the air we breathe which is then transported around the body. It may come as a surprise that William Harvey who discovered that the blood circulated around the body was totally disbelieved and thought a quack by fellow doctors and scientists. This was a very similar experience to Andrew Taylor Still when he first developed the practice of osteopathy.

The veins hold about 75 per cent of the amount of blood

circulating and are rather like a reservoir from which the heart pumps blood. The sympathetic nervous system helps the muscles lining the blood vessels stay toned up to keep the circulation moving.

The functions of the blood are essentially those of supplying oxygen and other materials for energy, growth and repair and removing waste products from activity of the cells throughout the body tissues. It also helps temperature control.

Because the flow of blood is essential to healthy body tissues and organs such as heart, liver and kidneys any reduction or obstruction to normal flow will cause effects to all those parts of the body dependent on the flow. On the distal or far side of the obstruction pressure increases, enlarging the blood vessels (such as varicose veins), while on the proximal or near side blood vessels will collapse giving symptoms due to lack of oxygen and nutrition or inability to remove waste products (for example, angina, or pain in the heart due to lack of blood to muscle).

Problems experienced as pain or other symptoms can have their main basis as mechanical, chemical, through nerve activity or fluid obstruction. Sometimes what appears to be mechanical has a deeper cause in the circulation, and the osteopath's ability to check through the various links in the chain and treat the source of obstruction will gain better and more long-lasting relief.

One law of fluid flow states that 'the pressure on a confined fluid is transmitted equally and undiminished in all directions'. Because our blood circulation is confined, if there is an obstruction its effects spread throughout our body system. This is in contrast to a river which can release extra pressure by overflowing its banks when an obstruction occurs. This is one reason why your osteopath will check through various parts of your body to release the primary cause.

Fluid flow can be affected by several factors: the consistency or thickness of the blood; the shape of the blood vessels (tubes); friction or rubbing of fluid against the vessel walls; the ability of the muscles lining the blood vessels to relax and contract; mechanical problems; increased pressure or stress due to everyday social and economic aspects of life.

In treatment, rhythmical stretching and pumping

movements will encourage circulation, and increase the oxygen supply and the ability of the blood to take away waste products. Tensions are relaxed. Gentle force is best used so as not to aggravate symptoms and therefore allow the body to release its own energy for healing. You will be encouraged to exercise within your limits, to avoid unchanging positions that slow blood flow, or excesses that might cause your problem to recur. Understanding the processes that occur and preventing their disruption is the best cure. The osteopath will assist you but you must also help yourself.

EFFECTS ON MECHANICAL CHANGES IN JOINTS AND MUSCLES

Joints are formed between two adjacent bones, the ends of which are lined by smooth cartilage and surrounded by a supporting capsule containing synovial fluid which bathes the joint and acts as a lubricant. Joints are strengthened by strong bands called ligaments and moved by muscles attached to the bone by tendons.

Joints and muscles provide a mechanical system for movement and leverage. When we function normally we don't give a second thought to our joints, but when they are painful or restricted we don't stop moaning. This can come from many causes that include local problems such as strain or injury, as well as more distant ones as, for example, obstruction to blood flow or disease of internal organs. Direct release of blocked joints with treatment will relieve symptoms, but if some cause in a distant part of the body is not also treated the joint problem is likely to recur. An osteopath will make a thorough search for linking causes throughout your body.

The limited joint movement that follows a strain, injury or some other cause is dependent on the relaxation or contraction of the muscles that move a joint. Osteopathic treatment can be given direct to the joint and/or to the muscles around the joint. The continuation of symptoms appears to be more dependent on the nerve activity following a joint strain than the strain itself. Nerve activity and manipulation are discussed further in the next section.

CHANGES IN THE NERVOUS SYSTEM THROUGH OSTEOPATHY

The nervous system has been recognized for some time as a major factor in explaining how manipulation works. Its precise mechanisms are still obscure, despite continuing research work. Briefly, the following are the main areas of thinking.

Referred Pain

This is pain originating from one part of the body and felt somewhere else in the body, often at a distance. The phenomenon occurs because the two parts of the body affected are supplied by the same nerve in the spinal cord. A good example is that of angina pain from the heart muscle which is referred to the chest wall, the left arm, neck and jaw. All these distant areas have the same spinal nerve supply as the heart muscle. We usually describe the pain distribution in terms of a dermatome (area of skin) or myotome (area of muscle). A body map of the common types of referred pain has been produced (Figure 7.1), and further additions are continually being discovered. This helps an osteopath in making a diagnosis.

Several scientific experiments have been carried out that show these links. The patterns show a close similarity to the pain and symptoms produced by actual disease of body organs such as kidney, stomach, bowel. A good example is when an irritant solution is injected into the back at the level of the first lumbar vertebra. A person will experience all the characteristic pain distribution of a stone in the kidney (renal colic). Some of the volunteers in this experiment who had experienced real renal colic said that they could not distinguish it from the pain produced by the experimental injection.

The Facilitated Segment

When a particular segment or part of the spinal cord (the main nerve that lies within the vertebrae in the back) becomes overactive on receiving nerve messages from injured joints, muscles etc., it is known as a 'facilitated segment'. It is very sensitive to any nerve impulse which reaches it and acts rather like an accelerator in a car; it increases (or decreases) or

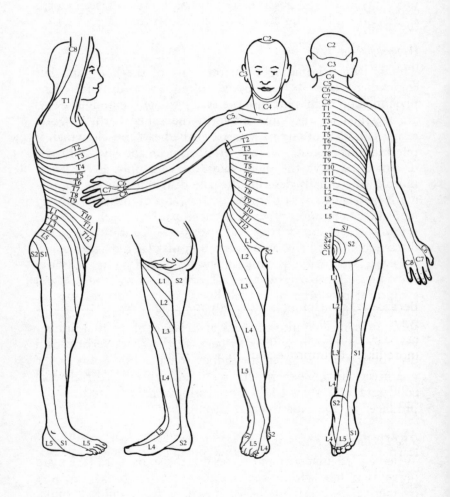

Figure 7.1 BODY MAP OF SKIN ZONES (DERMATOMES)
THAT AID DIAGNOSIS

'facilitates' nerve activity. As this activity is continued so will the corresponding pain and disability continue. The functions of all those body structures receiving a nerve link from this facilitated segment are potentially liable to be influenced by change in nerve activity and therefore in the range of symptoms experienced. In other words pain may be felt at a distance from the original injury — referred pain again.

What affects the facilitated segment. Two types of influence affect this concentrated area of nerve activity making it worse and giving more symptoms:

(1) *Internal factors* including the facilitated segment itself; influences carried down from the brain centres controlling both emotional and mental aspects – when you get angry the pain often gets worse; the particular state of health of an individual before the problem started, for example, if weakened from chronic infection, lack of food or stress of some sort. Healing is usually slower or blocked unless these areas are also looked at.

(2) *External factors* such as further injury, life disasters, bereavement, environment about us, our socio-economic state including unemployment, and emotional and practical support or lack of it from relatives and friends.

Because of these influences the osteopath will suggest additional ways of helping to improve the condition through diet, exercise, relaxation etc. By treating several 'causes' a patient is more likely to improve and get well again.

These additional forms of help may include nutritional advice from a dietician, exercise classes from the local authority or sports centre – perhaps joining a club for a specific sport, relaxation through yoga, posture training through the Alexander technique (see pp.93-4), attending a back school to learn more about coping with longstanding back problems, counselling from marriage guidance or other counselling agency, pastoral care from your minister, and encouragement to learn some new skills.

Primary and secondary problems. Primary problems in the joint and muscles in the spine and limbs are those which have resulted from some direct injury or strain. These types of problems are those most commonly treated by osteopaths.

Secondary problems in the joints and muscles are so named because they are secondary to some internal disease in body organs. Usually there will be a few symptoms felt in the back, but a trained osteopath can detect changes in skin, muscle and joint movements etc. For example, an ulcer in the stomach produces changes in the spine between the shoulder blades. By treating these (somatic) changes in the spine the body is stimulated to heal itself and help cure the ulcer.

The use of osteopathy here can minimize the use of drugs which, although essential in acute ulcer pain, can be more quickly dispensed with. The osteopathic approach is particularly relevant when symptoms keep recurring. Direct treatment of the somatic component (skin, muscles, ligaments) in the spine then becomes necessary to achieve a cure, and the mutual benefit to a patient of this combined approach becomes obvious.

It must be emphasized that osteopathy (that is, treatment) for disease of internal organs is not necessarily a replacement for the use of drugs and other traditional treatment. Like all treatment methods there is a time and a place for the use of each one. The correct use of osteopathic manipulative techniques will depend on the severity and extent of any disease process. However, its value in combination with more traditional treatment has not been experienced in Britain to the same extent that it has in the United States.

Manipulation that is effective will result in re-establishing normal integrated nerve activity and thus eliminate the symptoms of pain and disability. This return of normal nerve response is gained by the direct adjustment of joints, muscles, ligaments and supporting fascial tissues. The important fact in treatment is that the somatic component of dysfunction in the body, whether directly caused from the joint or muscle itself (primary), or indirectly from a viscera (secondary), is easily reached by touch and palpation. The appropriate treatment of this component will, through action in the nervous system, benefit all the structures involved and lead to healing the body.

Several types of experiment help to confirm some of these nerve reflex patterns and their associated tissue changes, such as the one on renal colic mentioned above. A wide range of measurement devices are used. One particularly useful instrument is called a 'thermograph', which produces thermal photographic images of the body by measuring the infrared energy emitted by the skin. Various technical processes transfer this energy into electrical energy which, on final conversion to light, acts on a polaroid camera film to produce a permanent picture. Warm and cold areas are found in a normal picture pattern and these are found to change in disease. The photographs so produced can be used both for diagnostic purposes and for monitoring improvement or deterioration in disease.

EVERYBODY IS NOT THE SAME

It would be simple if everybody produced the same specific spinal dysfunction pattern for the same diagnosis of ulcer or high blood pressure, joint strain, pain patterns etc. However, patient has a unique pattern of dysfunction; so in ulcer disease, for example, all the vertebrae between the shoulder blades from two to eight must be checked. Although these local changes are occurring within the spine, a patient is often unaware of them because they do not produce local symptoms. The osteopathic approach, therefore, is one of checking the whole spine for areas of observable spinal dysfunction with the aim of optimum health response in any particular patient.

Take as an example a recent patient. He last had osteopathic treatment thirty years ago in London for low back pain. He noticed at that time that his indigestion cleared up. On this occasion he came for a general check of his spine because of a recurrence of his low back pain and hoped that his mild chronic indigestion would be relieved as before. He had demonstrable tenderness with skin sensitivity between the shoulder blades which reflected his stomach irritation, and as well as relieving his low back pain, his indigestion cleared up again with treatment.

The rationale behind the preventive use of osteopathy is early detection of areas of spinal dysfunction that are often without symptoms. This dysfunction of the tissues can be reversed with treatment and prevent the likely build-up of nerve activity, blood circulation obstruction or joint obstruction which, if prolonged, will produce symptoms. An example is a person born with one leg shorter than the other, usually between one and two inches (2.4–5 cm). This results in a slight tilt downwards to the short side and in order to maintain the upright posture the spine will make some adjustments that produce abnormal tensions on the tissues.

This leads to gradual onset of low back pain which can begin as late as mid-life. Releasing the tense muscles and ligaments by osteopathic manipulation and inserting a small raise in the shoe can effectively banish the pain. The prolonged period of overactivity of the nerves is reduced by these means, and the spine and surrounding tissues regain their normal adaptive position without pain.

8 Prevention and Osteopathy?

We adjust the machinery and depend upon nature's chemical laboratory for all the elements necessary to repair, give ease and comfort while nature's corpuscles do all the work necessary.
ANDREW TAYLOR STILL

The prevention of disease, illness and deformity is surely a sound objective. However, it is a part of medicine which gains little acclaim in contrast to the glamour of lifesaving surgery or the application of hi-tech techniques. Prevention is variously seen as impracticable and expensive. It is seen to be neither cost-effective nor important enough for doctors to involve themselves in; it is mainly a sociopolitical problem. In truth it is probably part of all these, and yet there is a positive side depending on your viewpoint. Preventing disease *can* save money. The educational role of medicine is a worthwhile one. Positive political action can lead the way for changes in health, and if preventing disease results in each of us living a happier, more productive life then it is worth achieving.

OSTEOPATHY AND PREVENTION

What has all this to do with osteopathy? Every consultation with your osteopath involves, whether you realize it or not, a preventive message, both through discussion of lifestyle and in treatment. Examination of your spine and limb joints will include areas other than the painful parts. The aim is not only to remove the present problem but also encourage a healthier and more balanced body able to resist further insult or injury. Skin or muscle tension, tenderness and limited movement will often be found in your back which, if left untreated, would result in pain and other symptoms. Our bodies are excellent at adapting to insult and disruption. Numerous minor stresses and strains

81

are absorbed and dispersed without significant symptoms. However, when these disruptive forces rise above a certain level symptoms will appear. The ability to adapt, and thus the point at which symptoms appear, will vary from individual to individual. Those blessed with a strong constitution will outshine us all, seemingly against odds which would affect most of us. In contrast others will inherit disease through our family line. The majority of us will be somewhere in between these two extremes. We must work with what we have and a regular annual or biannual check by an osteopath is certain to result in improved wellbeing and a better understanding of your health needs.

UNDERSTANDING OURSELVES

Are you satisfied with the health you have? What is health anyway? The World Health Organization defines health as physical, mental and emotional harmony. Health is said to be absence of disease, but what is disease? Most of us would agree that disease involves some physical or mental disruption, injury, insult, infection or degeneration of parts of the body that results in pain and disability. If disease persists this will usually restrict our activities in some way and may require a change of job, or even worse the loss of our job. We will then need courage, adaptability and determination together with support from family, friends and professionals. I believe understanding ourselves more fully is a major key to prevention, and we can minimize our likelihood of developing disease. It is not an easy task. Your osteopath is one important source to help identify aspects of your lifestyle that with change will help you achieve optimum health.

We seem to grow up, generation after generation, with a rather negative approach to the care of our body and minds. They only become important to us when something goes wrong. We are more likely to put effort in the form of time and money into looking after animals or other people than in looking after ourselves. When we feel ourselves as important as others, then we are more likely to aim for prevention of illness and disease. As we continue to gain a fuller understanding of how the body works we will be in a better position to prevent problems arising. Osteopathy has and is increasing this knowledge.

SCIENTIFIC TESTS

One useful approach is the development of various objective scientific tests by which we can:

(1) predict likely disease and then take steps to change that likelihood;
(2) detect early disease and then apply early treatment with a high chance of success.

Research Projects

An example of the first is that of research projects which explored low electrical resistance measurements of skin areas in large numbers of apparently healthy people. Many developed signs and symptoms of disease such as ulcer or chest pain (angina) months or years after showing prominent areas of low electrical skin resistance in those areas of the skin directly related (by the same spinal nerve segment) to the affected organs, that is, stomach in the case of ulcer, heart for angina in the above examples. For some of this large group, symptoms of disease appeared following severe stress in the form of emotional conflicts, infections, important examinations or job changes.

This links with the osteopath's recognition of an area of muscle or joint abnormality as found in the body on examination by observation and touch. These areas of tissue change correspond with the demonstrated skin areas of low electrical skin resistance. The measurement of skin resistance can be used as an early signal that indicates alteration in our normal physiological adaptation and therefore the likelihood of disease following. Osteopathic treatment will remove the abnormality (dysfunction) and the electrical skin resistance returns to normal.

Smear Tests

An example of the second type of test is in the detection of early cancer of the cervix by regular smear tests. Early treatment has been shown to lower the death rate significantly and like many forms of cancer, effective cure is achieved by early detection and treatment.

BENEFITS OF OSTEOPATHY IN PREVENTING DISEASE

Although many of the problems seen by an osteopath are not life and death ones, nevertheless the earlier problems are found the quicker treatment can be given and the more likely it is to be effective. In osteopathy the particular skill of touch can be used as a potent tool in prevention. Posture, tissue tensions and alteration in joint movement present to the osteopath a guide to both physical disturbance, and areas of reflex tension that may be related to internal disease. With regular check-ups an alert osteopath can minimize the development of serious disease by re-establishing structural imbalance. For example, problems in the feet and lower extremities, if not treated, may later lead to compensatory problems at the top of the back and neck with headaches, shoulder pains etc.

A good example of the art of osteopathy in prevention concerns a boy of eight who came to see an experienced osteopath with whom I was working at the time. The boy had been playing in the school playground when he was suddenly lifted by the head from behind by an older boy and then dropped. He developed a lack of concentration and loss of his usual energy. The general practitioner could not find anything obviously wrong, but fortunately the boy's mother brought the child to us. Examination revealed a positional slip of the skull on the first vertebra confirmed by X-ray. The manipulation treatment resulted in a complete cure with a normal happy and energetic boy able to concentrate at school and at play. Without treatment the boy would likely have remained depressed and tired, headaches would have developed and probably arthritis in later life.

In the words of Irvin Korr

Osteopathic manipulation is not just another form of therapy; it is a whole strategy, a whole approach in itself. It is not merely a treatment of 'lesions'; in effect it is the putting of influences into the whole man through the accessible tissues in the body, influences which deflect his life processes to more favourable paths, and which help put the man in better command of his situation, whatever it is, whatever it may become, whatever his illness and whatever its etiology.

Regular osteopathic examination and treatment throughout life acts as an aid in balancing the body tissues, keeping a full range of joint movement, encouraging blood circulation and drainage of waste products such as lactic acid from muscle activity, stimulating muscle tone and elasticity, and guarding against poor posture development. These examinations are particularly useful in the often overactive teenage years expressed through work and sport. The rough and tumble of everyday activities results in many stresses and strains to which the body may react with pain and disability. Osteopathic treatment encourages the correct use of the body, relaxes muscles and deals with the factors already mentioned above. Babies who have difficulty in feeding or severe crying bouts may do so because of pain from spinal irritation. Very gentle stretching of these tissues in the neck and base of the spine, in the absence of any more specific cause, may be all that is needed.

Women and Pregnancy
Women, during and after pregnancy, form another group where prevention is particularly relevant. Persistent backache in pregnancy is due to a number of causes and osteopathic treatment will help most of them. There is a need for all women to have their spine assessed around the time of the postnatal examination at six weeks after the birth. Any misalignment or imbalance can then be corrected and the start of chronic backache prevented. It is also an opportunity to discuss lifting and other activities that may damage the body.

Sport
Similarly for those who are active in sports of all kinds osteopathic assessment and treatment has value in dealing with many of the strains and injuries received. Other problems will

need a different specialist approach, such as that available from sports medicine clinics which are open to anyone, not only top professional sports people. Indeed your own club may have an osteopath member from whom advice can be obtained. Prevention of injury is crucial when taking part in sport. This means having the correct clothing and equipment, particularly footwear, proper training using the correct techniques, and obeying the rules of the game. One is responsible to others as well as oneself. Going back to a sport too soon following injury is a common cause of further problems. Advice for all these can be found from your osteopath, doctor, coach or trainer, fellow sports people and clothing and equipment manufacturers. Sport is fun and enjoyable. Make sure yours is.

Ageing

Growing older affects all of us. Osteopathy cannot prevent it but it *can* help to prevent aches and pains and make life more comfortable. Regular check-ups and treatment are the best forms of insurance for old age. They feel good too. Our bodies normally lose flexibility, strength and endurance as we age and we have to adapt to this change as best we can. Many of us know of relatives who have appeared to grow smaller. This is because the discs between the vertebrae in the back lose their water content and therefore dry out and become thinner, hence the loss of height. One way to minimize this effect is to stay gently active since movement of the joints acts as a pump to keep the fluid levels up in the discs. Osteopathy as a regular treatment helps this process. It has a similar effect on the joints as oil has on stiff and rusty hinges, freeing their movement.

Many other groups of people might be mentioned, from musicians and dancers to builders and office workers. The common denominator is our minds and bodies and how effectively we use what we have. Periodic osteopathic assessment and treatment is, therefore, appropriate for many different people from birth to old age. It enables creation of a fitness reserve in lungs, digestion, muscle tone and balance that provides a benefit in throwing off likely insults of disease and injury which befall us all.

9 Allied Techniques

*I want to make it plain that there are many ways of adusting bones . . . .
the choice of methods is a matter to be decided by each operator and depends
on his own skill and judgment.*
ANDREW TAYLOR STILL, 1892

Osteopathy is continuously evolving with new techniques
being developed to restore body function. Although described
here under allied techniques, the first two, functional technique
and spontaneous release by positioning, are now incorporated in
osteopathic techniques. Although originating with the
osteopathic framework in the United States, the former and to a
lesser extent the latter are used by therapists in other disciplines.
Traction, injections, exercise and posture training are universal
and not exclusive to osteopathy. I have rather chosen them as
representative of some of the commonest additional treatment
methods used by osteopaths. The Alexander technique, applied
kinesiology and the 'back school' are further developments of
interest.

FUNCTIONAL TECHNIQUE

Functional technique evolved through the observations of an
osteopath called Harold Hoover. He found that in joint
disorders the neutral anatomical position for the joints resulted
in asymmetrical muscle tension – he envisaged a position of
greatest harmony or balance which he named 'dynamic neutral'
in which the tensions around a joint would be equal.

   In this technique, therefore, the joint is moved in the
direction of least resistance and greatest comfort. This is the
position called dynamic neutral in which there is a progressive
lessening of the need for an abnormal position. The joint is
continuously moved in the most comfortable direction until the

dynamic position is the same as the joint's anatomical position. At this point the joint returns to normal function and pain is relieved.

This technique requires both a lot of skill by the osteopath in feeling the joint position and muscle tension, and co-operation and trust from a patient in the osteopath's movements.

SPONTANEOUS RELEASE

Spontaneous release by positioning or counterstrain technique evolved out of observations made by Lawrence H. Jones over many years of osteopathic practice. Spontaneous release (of joints) by positioning results in the relief of spinal or other joint pain by passively placing the joint into its most comfortable position. In more scientific terms this involves reducing or stopping the inappropriate proprioceptor nerve activity that is producing the pain.

Abnormal function and pain in joints results from an increased nerve and muscle response as the body reacts to some strain or trauma. Evidence of the injury typically persists long after the original strain has stopped. This neuromuscular response is activated through special nerve endings within the muscle fibres close to the joint. These are the nerves that give the brain information about the positions our joints are in at any one time. On examination of a strained joint the problem is found not in the overstretched muscles but in the muscles opposite those affected. For example, a strain to the biceps muscle in the front of the upper arm will result in a tender spot in the triceps muscle at the back of the upper arm. Similarly a low back strain will commonly result in a reaction by the abdominal muscles in which one or several tender spots may be found. These tender spots are not normally recognized until palpated and pressed by the osteopath.

Treatment is accomplished by obtaining the most comfortable position for the joint and the tender spot in the muscle. By holding this comfortable position for 90 seconds the nervous system is given the opportunity to stop reacting, and pain and dysfunction is removed. The joint is always returned slowly from the treatment position to the starting position to avoid triggering the nerve reflex again.

This technique needs constant feedback through talking between a patient and osteopath to enable the most comfortable joint position to be found. It is a gentle technique which must not be rushed. It is extremely effective and like functional technique is being used more often in place of the sharp thrusting techniques (high velocity; low amplitude) which are so much a part of osteopathy. Although a gentle technique, muscle reactions are not uncommon and twenty-four to forty-eight hours, discomfort can often be expected.

SPINAL TRACTION

Spinal traction is a very ancient technique, probably of Greek or Egyptian origin. It has a limited yet useful place in the treatment of back pain. Careful selection of those who might benefit is essential. A rotated pelvis will usually not respond and pain will be increased; an acutely inflamed spine caused by rheumatoid disease or ankylosing spondylitis, together with cancer in the spine must not have traction.

Spinal traction is particularly useful following manipulative treatment for neck and low back sprains and in aiding recovery from 'disc' surgery. Two forms are used – static and dynamic. Static or still traction can be performed by hand or machine. Hand traction is commonly used in the neck to stretch and ease tight neck muscles. Dynamic or moving traction is only machine produced and involves rhythmical stretching with varying tensions provided mechanically.

Traction is most commonly used in physiotherapy departments in hospital. Osteopaths are less likely to use traction, but individual preferences for offering this form of treatment will naturally vary. If your osteopath provides this treatment arrange not to be left alone on a traction machine without some audible alarm as a warning if discomfort increases in any way.

INJECTIONS

Injections for musculoskeletal pain and dysfunction will only be used by doctor osteopaths. Injections comprise three main types:

(1) injection of local anaesthetic into joints or tender trigger points in muscles as a diagnostic procedure;

(2) injections of local anaesthetic mixed with steroid (cortisone) to reduce inflammation in joints or adjacent soft tissues; this includes epidural injections into the epidural space surrounding the spinal cord at the base of the spine in the treatment of sciatica and 'disc' protrusion;

(3) injection into ligaments mainly in the pelvis and lower spine, often referred to as 'sugar' injections. This involves accurate placing of a special solution into the point where the ligament is attached to bone. It is effectively an irritant solution that tightens the ligament giving better stability to the joint mechanism and thus relieving pain. Before use it is essential that all joints, particularly the sacroiliac joint, are in correct position and moving freely.

Although other doctors use these injection techniques more commonly, doctor osteopaths will only use them if manual techniques fail, or a specific indication shows an injection to be the treatment of choice.

EXERCISE AND POSTURE TRAINING

Exercise

Many books have been written on exercise and posture training, and the reader is encouraged to look in the local bookshop or library. Here only some of the most important principles will be highlighted.

Exercise has many important benefits; it:

produces a feeling of wellbeing;
aids healthy skin and body tissues;
maintains muscle tone and flexibility, and thus posture;
stimulates blood flow to bring nutrition to our body cells;
hydrates our spinal 'discs' to maintain their integrity and
    slow down degeneration;

is essential in following any slimming programme;
helps us to learn discipline;
can be done alone or in groups when it provides for social
contact.

Exercise needs to be relevant to your age, state of health and aims in life. Obviously as you age body tissues are not so flexible, and sudden effort after a long period without exercise is progressively damaging to those over thirty-five to forty years. The older you become the more regular exercise needs to be.

Exercise must begin gradually and increase to a level that does not overstrain the heart and lungs. To monitor the heart take the pulse reading at the wrist. First check your resting pulse as to rate per minute (normal range 70–80 for the average person; athletes often have a lower rate). The pulse should be checked after exercise and return to normal within five minutes of stopping exercise. If not, you have overdone your exercise.

Several excellent exercise clinics are now open throughout the country and your osteopath will know of one near you. The various machine facilities provided for assessing lungs, heart, muscles and blood flow, although more directed to athletes initially, are open to anyone who wants to use them. These clinics provide a useful baseline before starting exercise. The BUPA and PPP clinics, among others, also offer health assessments. If in doubt, and particularly if middle-aged or above, see your doctor or osteopath before commencing exercise.

Purpose of exercise. Exercise is used for three main physical purposes:

(1) mobility;
(2) stamina;
(3) strength.

Certain sports emphasize these different aspects depending on your aims. For general fitness mobility is most important. If your job or hobby requires lifting, pushing or carrying, more strength and stamina is required. Physically demanding jobs need a physically fit person. All sport is exercise but all exercise is not sport. When you experience the benefits of exercise you will want to continue. Try different forms of exercise to find the one or several that suit best; here are some suggestions:

> walking, running, skipping, trampolining, circuit training, weight training, aerobics, cycling, rowing, dancing, horse-riding, tennis, badminton, golf, volley ball, skating, rugby, soccer, hockey, yoga, tai chi (a form of disciplined movement akin to dancing), acrobatics, swimming, judo.

Your osteopath will be happy to discuss with you various forms of exercise or direct you to those people who can help.

Posture

Good posture gives some of the benefits of exercise such as a feeling of wellbeing and keeps the tissues healthy. Bad posture can result in poor circulation and weak muscles, backache, headache etc. Posture awareness leads to a more balanced body. Knowing the best way to stand, walk, sit and rise from a chair, how to lift, the most advantageous work positions for different tasks, and how to relax are all part of good posture. For example, research has shown that the pressure on the spinal discs recorded on rising from a chair can be reduced by 50 per cent using pressures from the hands to aid rising. The most relaxed and least pressured position for the spine is lying down on your back with the feet raised on a cushion or stool with the knees at 90°. It is known as the semi-Fowler position. Use it for ten minutes every day or after strenuous activity when you feel stiff and sore.

Good posture acts, therefore, as a prevention of body discomfort and illness. Posture is dependent on an intact nervous system and a willingness to maintain adequate tone and strength in our muscles, which in turn requires exercise. Strengthening and balancing the muscles which hold our posture, especially the gluteal or buttocks muscles, is extremely effective for ligament sprain in the low back and pelvis.

There is no ideal posture; it varies with individual build and we will all have slight mechanical or postural irregularities which are our 'norm' and with which we function adequately.

The comfortable position is not always the best for good posture. Corrective training for posture can take a long time, months or even years.

Kneeling chairs. In any one day sitting is a major activity after time spent sleeping in bed. Designers continue to improve seating especially for the office where tilting seats combined with an angled work surface improve the comfort of staff. One particular form of tilting chair is the kneeling chair, the original being the Balans range of chairs from Scandinavia, suitable for both children and adults. They encourage correct back posture, prevent abdominal organs being compressed and allow freer rib cage movement for breathing. They are not so suitable for those with knee problems that produce pain on kneeling, and like any form of chair should not be used for long periods. These and other chairs with tilting seats are available from both office and home furnishing suppliers, as well as from more specialist shops selling 'health' products.

ALEXANDER TECHNIQUE

One of the best posture training methods is the Alexander technique which encourages through body positioning and movement the most relaxed and advantageous body posture and balance by making you more consciously aware of tensions in your body. It forms part of the training of many actors, actresses and dancers enabling them to maintain more relaxed control of their bodies while performing in what is very demanding work.

The technique is well established in Britain and Israel, less so in Europe and North America. It originated at the turn of the century when Frederick M. Alexander, an Australian actor, sought to correct his recurrent hoarse throats. He learnt that far from being a simple voice problem the whole muscle pattern of his body was involved together with his mental attitude.

Learning the technique involves one-to-one teaching by directly experiencing body position and movement with encouragement to continue practice through everyday living. It is a gradual process and an excellent preventive of body aches and pains. Emotional and mental wellbeing improves in parallel with physical improvement. The technique can be thoroughly recommended. The address is given in the Appendix, p.102.

APPLIED KINESIOLOGY

There are several forms of kinesiology, which is the study of the mechanics of body movement.

Applied kinesiology is the study of muscle activation that leads to excess activation (tightness and spasm) or reduced activation (weakness). Those using this form of knowledge use specific muscle testing to find out which ones are weak or tight. Then using muscle balancing techniques muscles are returned to their normal shape, posture is improved and health with it.

Because the body is one coherent whole and has many links from one part to another through the nervous system (see above), this technique consists of more than muscles being treated. The muscles all relate to some specific joint or organ system such as heart or stomach, so variable symptoms can be helped throughout the body. It is particularly useful following osteopathic treatment especially when problems keep recurring.

Some of you may have heard of touch for health, which is a method of treatment using applied kinesiology on muscles and is something everyone can learn and use within families and with friends. Just like the Alexander technique, touch for health helps you become more aware of your body, and prevent small body disturbances getting out of hand and becoming serious illness. Touch for health can also be used in testing for food allergy or intolerance by showing what foods to avoid.

The address is given in the Appendix, p.102. Several therapists including osteopaths and chiropractors have incorporated these muscle-testing methods into their own work.

THE BACK SCHOOL

Back schools have developed over the last ten years and are found both in Europe and the United States. The main function of the back school is to teach people how to manage their back pain better and to avoid recurrence. The methods used will vary from clinic to clinic but usually comprise a limited number of sessions, usually six. Participants are taught about: back movements and posture; what can be done to minimize or avoid back pain, especially in the work environment; exercises for their problems and methods of relaxation.

The British School of Osteopathy has set up a back school here and several hospitals throughout the country have similar clinics.

10   *The Future of Osteopathy?*

Restating the quote at the beginning of this book: Will you dare to be different in living your life? Will you do what is right for you and not follow what everyone else is doing? It is not easy being different because people find challenge and change threatening. However, we can be different in small ways that enlarge our responsibilities for not only our health but how we live our lives. Small ways can become large ways and with them confidence in ourselves, courage to learn new skills, an awareness of the inner strength we all have and a commitment to live life fully sharing what we have with others.

We can't all be like Andrew Taylor Still and found an original philosophy of treatment, or like Einstein discover new laws of physical matter, but we can in our own ways discover more about ourselves. By aiming for our own optimum health we are providing the essential basis for living and working. Those with mental or physical disabilities, those in wheelchairs, or bed bound can all discover more about themselves.

There are many practical ways we can begin or continue to seek our optimum health. Look at our posture. Are we slumping in a chair? Are we holding our shoulders tight? Do we lift weights that are too heavy? What about the foods we eat? There is some truth in the statement 'We are what we eat.' Are we following the latest understanding of a balance of food intake that requires less fat and sugar, sufficient roughage like bran and wheat, plenty of vegetables and fruit and less red meat? That means less alcohol too. Cigarettes, although well publicized as a health hazard, are still consumed in large quantities. For those who smoke: ask a friend who has stopped smoking if he or she feels more healthy. The answer will surely be yes.

The self-regulating mechanisms that maintain our internal balance or homeostasis are finely tuned to keep our temperature, blood pressure, breathing etc. at their best level as we go about our lives. Just think for a moment of the wide range of environments throughout the world and the various ways human beings have adapted over thousands of years. We have a very adaptable body with its own self-healing abilities. Osteopathy aims to harness this natural ability to maintain optimum health. As I have previously explained, it achieves this through a wide range of manual and allied techniques to influence blood flow, nutrition, nerve reflexes, joint movement and muscle balance, always mindful of the emotional and physical state of each individual receiving treatment.

Osteopathic medicine is practised in its widest sense in the United States where the full range of allopathic medical procedures, treatments and surgery are integrated with osteopathic principles and practice that include osteopathic manipulative therapy. The important concepts of body unity, self-regulation and the interrelationships between structure and function are three main principles used with every patient. The examination of the easily reached somatic (body framework) tissues through touch gives much information about a patient's problems while manipulative technique applied to the muscles and joints brings about freedom from pain and return of normal body function.

Outside the United States it is this latter aspect of osteopathy, the osteopathic manipulative therapy, that is used and has come to be seen as the whole of osteopathy. The majority of osteopaths worldwide, mainly found in Britain, Australia and New Zealand, are not doctors (registered or licensed physicians). Doctors in these countries who have trained in osteopathy come closer to the American model, though they lack the hospital status and university backing of the American colleges and hospitals of osteopathic medicine.

Osteopathy is still growing in the United States where the American Osteopathic Association has an active continuing advancement programme to encourage osteopathy's unique concepts, education and research. In particular those states with small numbers of osteopathic doctors or hospitals receive special assistance. The American Osteopathic Association is also, upon request, resolved to offer help or guidance to any country to provide practice rights for osteopathic physicians. They are also ready to help promote and develop osteopathic medical schools that intend to demonstrate a similar educational level to accredited American colleges of osteopathic medicine. A representative of the American Osteopathic Association has inspected the osteopathic training establishments in Australia, for example, in pursuit of this policy.

In Britain continuing negotiations aim towards a bill to obtain parliamentary recognition and registration of osteopathy. It *is* spreading its message of healing. The future is open for further advancement of this unique philosophy of healing, a whole-person therapy that originated through the mind of Andrew Taylor Still over 100 years ago.

Appendix: Useful Addresses

GREAT BRITAIN

London College of Osteopathic Medicine
8–10 Boston Place, London NW1 6QH. Telephone 01 262 5250.
Professional association: British Osteopathic Association (BOA)

British School of Osteopathy
1–4 Suffolk Street, London SW1Y 4HG. Telephone 01 930 9254
Professional association: The General Council and Register of Osteopaths Ltd

European School of Osteopathy
104 Tonbridge Road, Maidstone, Kent ME16 8SL. Telephone 0622 671558
Professional association: Society of Osteopaths

All graduates from the above three colleges are trained to a high standard and are eligible to join the Osteopathic Register under the auspices of the General Council and Register of Osteopaths at 1–4 Suffolk Street, London SW1Y 4HG

British College of Naturopathy and Osteopathy
6 Netherhall Gardens, London NW3 5RR. Telephone 01 435 8728
Professional association: British Naturopathic and Osteopathic Association (BNOA)

The Cranial Osteopathic Association
478 Baker Street, Enfield, Middlesex EN1 3QS. Telephone 01 367 5561

UNITED STATES OF AMERICA

American Osteopathic Association
212 East Ohio Street, Chicago, IL 60611. Telephone (312) 280 5800
(Includes information about colleges of osteopathic medicine and licensed physicians)

American Academy of Osteopathy
12 West Locust Street, PO Box 750, Newark, OH 43055.
Telephone (614) 349 8701

The Cranial Academy
1140 West Eighth Street, Meridian, ID 83642. Telephone (208) 888 1201

CANADA

Canadian Osteopathic Association
575 Waterloo Street, London, Ontario, Canada N6B 2RZ.
Telephone (519) 439 5521

AUSTRALASIA

Australian Osteopathic Association
71 Collins Street, Melbourne 3000, Victoria, Australia

International Colleges of Osteopathy
148 Barker Street, Randwick 2031, Sydney, Victoria, Australia

Phillip Institute of Technology
Plenty Road, Bundoora, Victoria, Australia
(Five-year bachelor of science degree DO course)

New Zealand Register of Osteopaths
PO Box 33-768, Takapuna, Auckland 9, New Zealand

ALSO MENTIONED IN THE TEXT

Society of Teachers of the Alexander Technique
3b Albert Court, Kensington Gore, London SW7. Telephone 01 584 3834
The Society will provide a directory of all recognized teachers in the United
Kingdom.

The Association for Systemic Kinesiology (including Touch for Health)
39 Browns Road, Surbiton, Surrey KT5 8ST. Telephone 01 399 3215

British Wheel of Yoga
80 Leckhampton Road, Cheltenham, Gloucestershire

Iyengar Yoga Institute
223a Randolph Avenue, London W9. Telephone 01 624 3080

OTHER NON–OSTEOPATHIC ORGANIZATIONS USING MANIPULATION

British Association of Manipulative Medicine (BAMM)
62 Wimpole Street, London W1M 7DE

North American Association of Manipulative Medicine
5021 Seminary Road, Suite 125, Alexandria, VA 22311 Canada
Telephone (703) 931 0233

Federation Internationale de Medecine Manuelle
c/o Dr H. Baumgartner, Klinik Wilhelm Schulthess, Neumunsterallee 10, CH-8032, Zurich, Switzerland.

Bibliography

J. C. Boileau Grant, *An Atlas of Anatomy*. Baillière Tindall & Cox, 5th Edition, London, 1962.

E. R. Booth, *History of Osteopathy and Twentieth Century Medical Practice*. The Caxton Press, London, Memorial Edition 1924 incorporating the 1905 Edition

Dennis Brookes, *Cranial Osteopathy*, Thorsons, Wellingborough, 1981.

H. H. Fryette, *Principles of Osteopathic Technique*. Academy of Applied Osteopathy, Carmel, 1954.

Laurie Hartmann, *Handbook of Osteopathic Techniques*. Heinemann Medical, London, 1985.

Lawrence H. Jones, *Strain and Counterstrain*. American Academy of Osteopathy, 1981.

I. M. Korr, *The Collected Papers of Irvin M. Korr*. American Academy of Osteopathy, 1979.

G. Lowry, *From Mons to 1933* Simpkin Marshall Ltd, London, 1933.

Andrew Taylor Still, *Autobiography*. Published by the author Kirksville MO, 1908.

Andrew Taylor Still, *Osteopathy Research and Practice*. Published by the author Kirksville MO, 1910.

Andrew Taylor Still, *Philosophy of Osteopathy*. Published by the author Kirksville MO, 1899

Year Book, American Academy of Osteopathy, 1973.

Index

Spine, 51-2, 69
Spontaneous release, 88-9
Sporting injuries, 18, 85-6
Still, Dr Andrew Taylor, ix, xi,
    29-36, 44, 50, 64, 67, 72, 98
Stomach, 25
Streeter, Dr. Wilfred, 39
Stress *see* Lifestyle
Surgery, 12, 23-4
Sutherland, William, 7-8
Symptoms, 62
    recurrence of, 63-4

Tendonitis of the shoulder, 21
Tennis elbow, 21
Thermograph, 79
Tinnitus, 27
Tissue change, 83
Touch, 2, 7, 50, 51
    for health, 94
Training in osteopathy, 34, 36-
    7, 43-4

Trapped nerve, 15, 52
Treatment, 4, 18
    description of, 49-57
    individuality of, 58
    pattern of, 58-65
    termination of, 65
    with drugs, 22, 24
Trust, 50

Ulcers, 78

Vertigo, 26

Walker, L. Willard, 37
Whiplash injury, 20
Whole person approach, 1-7,
    27-8, 33, 50-1, 70
    see also Lifestyle

X-rays, 3, 9, 12, 15, 53

Is Acupuncture for you?

Professor J. R. Worsley

As the number of qualified practitioners of traditional Chinese acupuncture increases, and as public awareness of acupuncture as an effective therapy increases, so does the demand for reliable information.

Professor J. R. Worsley – founder of The College of Traditional Chinese Acupuncture (U.K.) and The Traditional Acupuncture Institute (U.S.A.) – draws here on his thirty years of experience as teacher and practitioner to answer the questions most commonly asked about acupuncture by those who are wondering whether to have treatment as well as those who have already begun to have it.

Element Books Ltd

LONGMEAD, SHAFTESBURY, DORSET

ISBN 0 906540 67 4

The Healer's Hand Book

A step-by-step guide to developing your latent healing abilities

Georgina Regan and Debbie Shapiro

Most of us know someone who is capable of calming us down; who is soothing to be with; perhaps someone who is known to have 'healing hands'. But what many of us don't realise is that potentially we all have these abilities.

This book is based on the work of Georgina Regan, an internationally known healer who has been developing her techniques and understanding of the healing process for over fifteen years. In it she shows that channelling energy for healing is a completely natural ability that we are *all* capable of, and are all able to learn.

Including relaxation and meditation techniques, a step-by-step guide to energy channelling, and a fully illustrated practice section, *The Healer's Hand Book* contains all you need to enter the fascinating and fulfilling world of hands-on healing.

Element Books Ltd

LONGMEAD, SHAFTESBURY, DORSET

ISBN I 85230 022 I

The Visual Handbook

John Selby

We receive over 70% of our sensory experiences through our eyes. Most of our physical movements, our emotional responses, our mental performance, and even our deeper spiritual insights, are intimately linked with the successful functioning of our visual system. But how much of this link do we understand and how much are we aware of the process? And can we improve it?

In *The Visual Handbook,* John Selby offers a comprehensive view of how the eyes function, how they sometimes misfunction, and how we can act to regain optimum visual health and vitality.

Whether you have 20:20 vision, myopia or glaucoma, this book shows that you can still improve your eyesight and learn to see more clearly.

Element Books Ltd

LONGMEAD, SHAFTESBURY, DORSET

ISBN I 85230 018 3

If you would like to know more about these titles or other titles on the Element List, and would like to receive regular copies of our catalogue. Please write to:

ELEMENT BOOKS
LONGMEAD, SHAFTESBURY
DORSET SP7 8PL

Telephone
Shaftesbury (0747) 51339